Trauma and Resilience Among Displaced Populations

Gail Theisen-Womersley

Trauma and Resilience Among Displaced Populations

A Sociocultural Exploration

Springer

Gail Theisen-Womersley
Institut de Psychologie et Education
University of Neuchâtel
Neuchâtel, Switzerland

The open access publication of this book has been published with the support of the Swiss National Science Foundation.

ISBN 978-3-030-67711-4   ISBN 978-3-030-67712-1 (eBook)
https://doi.org/10.1007/978-3-030-67712-1

This Springer imprint is published by the registered company Springer Nature Switzerland AG
The registered company address is: Gewerbestrasse 11, 6330 Cham, Switzerland

The original version of the book was revised: Open-access funder information has been updated. The correction to this book is available at https://doi.org/10.1007/978-3-030-67712-1_13.

Contents

1 **Introduction** ... 1
Mental Health of Refugee Populations ... 2
The Problem with PTSD ... 3
Calls for a More Contextualised Understanding of Trauma ... 7
Adapting Clinical Practice ... 8
Addressing the Gap in the Literature—Implications for Research ... 9
The Context of the Research ... 11
Why Read This Book ... 11
Theoretical Framework ... 12
Conceptualising Experiences of Trauma and Migration from a Collective, Sociocultural Perspective ... 15
Applications for Professionals ... 17
Conclusion ... 21
References ... 21

2 **Trauma and Migration** ... 29
Pre-migration ... 30
Torture ... 31
Migration ... 33
Requesting Asylum ... 34
Prolonged Detention ... 36
Court Proceedings ... 37
Being Denied Asylum ... 38
Post-migration ... 38
Reception in the Host Country ... 39
Multiple Losses and Social Isolation ... 40
Continual Exposure to Trauma ... 41
Unemployment ... 41
Race-Related Trauma ... 42
Language Proficiency ... 43

Gender 44
Daily Stressors 44
Considering the Interrelation of Factors 45
Case Study One: Trauma Among Displaced Victims of Torture in Athens, Greece 48
Case Presentation 48
First Feedback Loop: Breakdown of Interpersonal Relations 51
Second Feedback Loop: Delayed Asylum Procedure 51
Third Feedback Loop: Living Conditions 52
Fourth Feedback Loop: Hospitalisation and Interpersonal Encounters in Medical Consultations 52
Case Study Two: Self-immolation Among an Asylum Seeker in Switzerland 53
The Self-immolation of Armin 53
Analysis 55
Concluding Remarks 57
References 59

3 Prevalence of PTSD Among Displaced Populations—Three Case Studies 67
Case Study One: Durban, South Africa 68
Method 69
Results 69
Case Study Two: Yezidis in Iraq 70
Method 72
Results: Topline Findings 72
WHO-5 73
Harvard Trauma Questionnaire 73
Case Study Three: Marawi, Philippines 76
Method 76
Results 77
Conclusion 78
References 80

4 Beyond PTSD 83
Models of Trauma: Conflicting Theoretical Traditions 84
What Is “Trauma”? 87
Conflicting Concepts of Trauma 90
The Problem of Pathologization 92
Criticism of the Use of PTSD as a Diagnosis Among Refugee Communities 94
The Instrumentalisation of the Diagnosis Among Asylum Seekers 97
Conclusion 100
Case Study 101
Representations of Trauma Among Refugee Victims of Torture in Athens 102

Representations of Trauma Among Medical Professionals Across Europe ... 103
References ... 105

5 **Culturally Informed Manifestations of Trauma** ... 113
Defining Culture from a Sociocultural Perspective ... 114
Culturally-Informed Narratives of Trauma: Perspectives of Diverse Theoretical Traditions ... 115
The Impact of Trauma ... 118
The Interplay of Factors ... 120
Culturally-Informed Responses to Trauma: Attributing Meaning to the Experience ... 122
Pathways to Healing ... 125
Case Study 1: Mass Fainting Spells Among the Murle Tribe of South Sudan ... 130
Introduction to the Context ... 130
A Case of "Mass Hysteria"? ... 131
Reflections ... 132
Case Study 2: Psychotherapy with a Guinean Refugee Victim of Torture in Athens ... 133
Conclusion: Introducing a Collective, Sociocultural Approach to Understanding Trauma and Recovery ... 135
References ... 139

6 **Collective Trauma, Collective Healing** ... 147
Loss of "Home" as Container ... 149
Collective Responses to Trauma ... 150
Collective, Culturally-Based Interventions ... 151
Case Study One: The Displaced Yezidi Community of Northern Iraq ... 152
The Impact of Events ... 154
Manifestations of Trauma ... 155
Collective Trauma ... 155
Culturally Informed Idioms of Distress ... 156
Perceptions of Mental Health Services ... 157
Case Study Two: Displaced Populations Affected by ISIS in Marawi, Philippines ... 157
Origins and Layers of Trauma ... 158
Intergenerational Transmission ... 159
Effect on Adults and Children ... 159
Self-awareness of Trauma ... 159
Thematic Analysis of Qualitative Data ... 159
Subjective Experiences of the Marawi Siege ... 161
Individual Trauma Narratives—Specific Focus ... 162
Psychological Avoidance ... 164
Multiple Levels of Loss ... 164

Community Response 165
Impact on Children 166
Religious Values and Beliefs 167
Uncertainty About the Future 168
Post-Traumatic Growth and Resilience 168
Conclusion 169
References 170

7 Collective Resilience and Imagination 175
Collective Resilience Among Displaced Populations 175
Imagination, Trauma and Migration 177
Imagination from a Sociocultural Perspective 180
Case Study: Resilience and Imagination Among Victims of Torture in Athens, Greece 182
The Case of Jules 183
Discussion 188
Conclusion 190
References 191

8 Collective Aspirations 195
Case Study: Collective Aspirations of Refugees in Europe 198
Analysis 199
The Case of Mr B 199
Discussion 204
Conclusion 206
References 206

9 Working with Shame and Trauma 209
Migration and Post-traumatic Shame 210
Cultural Manifestations of Shame and Implications for Clinicians 211
Case Study One: Research Among Displaced Victims of Torture in Athens, Greece 212
Applied Approach to Dealing with Shame: The Case of Sylvain 215
The Shame of Dependence 215
Implications for Transformation 216
The Shame of Social Discrimination 216
Implications for Transformation 217
The Shame of Being Unemployed 217
Implications for Transformation 218
Case Study Two: Female Survivors of Sexual Violence in Cape Town, South Africa 219
Analysis 221
Conclusion 228
References 229

10 Working with Cultural Mediators 233
Case Study: Cultural Mediation Among Victims of Torture in Athens 237
Cultural Mediators as Negotiating Different Interpretations of Trauma 239
Translation: Accuracy Versus Interpretation 239
A Game of Alliances Between Refugees and Health Professionals 241
Working with Health Professionals Perceived as "Culturally Inexperienced" 243
Conclusion 244
References 245

11 Working with PTSD in the Asylum Procedure 249
PTSD Among Refugee Populations 250
The Importance of Correctly Identifying Trauma in the Refugee Determination Process 251
PTSD and the Question of Legal Causality 252
The Refugee Determination Procedure as a System of Activity 254
Case Study 256
Asylum Seeker Perspectives 257
Discrepancies in Narratives of Trauma 258
Asymmetries in Trauma Narratives, Asymmetries of Power: The Case of Dilraj 259
Adapting the Trauma Narrative: The Case of Jules 260
Health Professionals' Perspectives 262
Conflicting Narratives Across the Activity System 265
Discussion: An Overview of the Various Critiques of PTSD Within the Asylum Process 266
Deconstructing the "Traumatized Refugee" Narrative 267
Implications for Health Professionals Working with Asylum Seekers 268
Conclusion 269
References 271

12 Conclusion 277
Towards a Sociocultural Definition of Trauma 282
Implications for Mental Health Clinicians 285
The Role of Narrative Activity 285
The Collective Cultural Frame 286
Temporality 287
The Permeable Self 291
Universality of Experience 291
Implications for Mental Health and Psychosocial (MHPSS) Interventions in Humanitarian Settings 293
A Community-Based Response 294

A Culturally Relevant Response 295
A Longitudinal, Contextually Situated Response 296
A Depathologizing Response 296
A Resiliency-Based, Forward-Looking Response 297
References 300

Correction to: Trauma and Resilience Among Displaced Populations C1

Chapter 1
Introduction

We are now witnessing the highest levels of displacement on record. According to the United Nations High Commission for Refugees (UNHCR), there are 70.8 million forcibly displaced people worldwide. This includes over 41 million internally displaced people, 25 million refugees and 3.5 million asylum seekers. This is a challenge of historic proportions. Evolving responses having now become one of the defining challenges of the early twenty-first century (Farhat et al., 2018; *Médécins Sans Frontières*, 2016; UNHCR, 2015). Not least among the difficulties are public health challenges of the multiple traumas faced by displaced populations. The loss of loved ones or caregivers and/or livelihood, the destruction of property, insecure living conditions, war, torture, imprisonment, terrorist attacks, abuse, and sexualised violence are among the traumatic experiences that characterizes experiences of displacement. Furthermore, trauma does not stop at the border. A plethora of literature attests to the traumatic impact of post-migration factors with which many refugees[1] are faced upon arrival in host countries (Bhugra & Gupta, 2011; Greene et al., 2017; Greene et al., 2019; Heeren et al., 2014; Schick et al., 2018; Schouler-Ocak et al., 2016; Sijbrandij et al., 2017; Silove et al., 2017; Ventevogel et al., 2019; Wenzel & Drožđek, 2018). In the post-migration context, stress and trauma may be related to harsh living conditions, the erosion of mutual social support mechanisms, limited access to basic needs and services and lack of opportunities for maintaining livelihoods and education (Greene et al., 2019; Weissbecker et al., 2018). Furthermore, displaced populations may be facing these stressors in situations where the capacity for self-help and mutual support has been negatively impacted by forced migration, the separation from families and communities, collective violence and mistrust (Sijbrandij et al., 2017).

The severe impact of exposure to potentially traumatic events on the mental health of this population are pervasive and profound. Trauma constitutes an urgent threat to human, social, cultural, and community development (d'Halluin, 2009; *Médécins*

[1] Throughout the book, the term "refugee" as defined by the Geneva Convention of 1951 is used to include both refugees legally recognised in a host country as well as asylum-seekers.

G. Theisen-Womersley, *Trauma and Resilience Among Displaced Populations*,
https://doi.org/10.1007/978-3-030-67712-1_1

Sans Frontières, 2016; Ventevogel et al., 2019; Wilson & Drožđek, 2004). It is transmitted intergenerationally. The unprecedented number of displaced populations around the world are not only carrying the emotional scars of the traumatic events to which they've been exposed, and to which they continue to be exposed. Many are suffering from the effects of intergenerationally transmitted trauma—and may risk continuing to transmit these effects in a way which perpetuates ongoing cycles of violence and conflict.

The impact of trauma has become an object of increased attention since the turn of the century, both in the scientific domain but also within public discourse regarding the influx of migrants into Europe and North America (d'Halluin, 2009). In the realms of journalism, social media and public discourse more generally speaking, the idea of trauma is revoked repeatedly to testify to the significant level of mental health difficulties (Summerfield, 2000b). Attention to trauma has also increased in the humanitarian field over the last decade in particular. Programmes focusing on mental health and psychosocial support now routine elements of a humanitarian response to refugee crises (Weissbecker et al., 2018). It has even been suggested that all forced migrants experience some degree of post-traumatic symptomatology (Copping et al., 2010). Furthermore, the psychological consequences of exposure to trauma and/or ongoing environmental stress in host contexts may impede process of adaptation and acculturation (Steel et al., 2016). The vastness of the phenomena of trauma and migration has therefore led it to become an urgent area of inquiry—with research into the ksey determinants of refugee trauma and potential opportunities to improve mental health now a pressing concern (Hall & Olff, 2016; Tessitore & Margherita, 2017).

Mental Health of Refugee Populations

The literature overwhelmingly attests to significantly high prevalence rates of post-traumatic stress disorder (PTSD), anxiety and depression among refugee populations when compared to the general population of host communities (Abbott, 2016; de Arellano & Danielson, 2008; Kirmayer et al., 2010; Lambert & Alhassoon, 2015; Schweitzer et al., 2006; Steel et al., 2009; Sturm et al., 2010; Van Ommeren et al., 2001; Weine et al., 2001). In a recent study of over one million people in Sweden, Hollander and colleagues (2016) found that refugees granted asylum were, on average, 66% more likely to develop schizophrenia or another non-affective psychotic disorder than non-refugee migrants from the same regions of origin. This finding confirms a previous meta-review of the literature by Porter and Haslam (2005) who found evidence that refugees from the former Yugoslavia suffered significantly more mental health impairment then non-refugees from the same region across multiple studies.

Exposure to torture has emerged as a particular triggering factor of PTSD symptomatology (Haenel, 2015; Hodges-Wu & Zajicek-Farber, 2017; Mollica et al., 1998; Silove et al., 2017; Song et al., 2017). This is no surprise, given the multiplicity of challenges to which refugee Victims of Torture (VOTs) are exposed. The dual trauma inherent in being both a VOT as well a refugee is related to a myriad of losses, human rights violations and other dimensions of suffering linked not only to torture experienced pre-migration, but to different forms of violence experienced during and after migration as well. Indeed, refugee VOTs "often present a complex constellation of symptoms further complicated by cultural variables and post-migration factors including immigration legal issues, economic challenges, diminished social networks, shifting power dynamics, bereavement, and other prolonged stressors" (Hodges-Wu & Zajicek-Farber, 2017).

Torture itself represents an extraordinary exception in the psychopathology field. The particularity of torture as pathogenic is linked to the fact that the act itself is taught, organized, elaborated, and perpetrated by humans against other humans (Sironi, 1999; Viñar, 2005a). It disrupts our connection to all that make us human (Viñar, 2005a). As such, the psychopathologic disorder of the survivor cannot be reduced to the intrapsychic plane. It is not an individual act, but a social one. It does not only have individual consequences, but social, legal, and political ones for those who survive. It damages different spheres of an individual including body, personality, hope, aspirations for life, identity, integrity, belief systems, the sense of being grounded and attached to a family and society, autonomy, community relationships, and a sense of safety. These far-reaching effects may interact and manifest in complex and diverse ways, mediated by culture, gender and other aspects of the context of the torture survivor, the context of torture and the context of the recovery environment (Esala et al., 2018; Patel et al., 2014).

The Problem with PTSD

Despite the high prevalence rate of PTSD noted among refugee populations, the authors of the above-mentioned meta-reviews examining epidemiological data have all highlighted the substantial variability of prevalence rates across symptoms—with a variability range as wide as 0–99% noted by Steel for example (2009). This discrepancy remains unexplained (Bogic et al., 2012). Larger and more rigorous surveys were found to report lower prevalence rates than did smaller studies, but significant variability persisted across the board (Fazel et al., 2005; Silove et al., 2017). Furthermore, a re-analysis of the data of the meta-review by Steel and colleagues (2009) conducted by the World Health Organization in 2013 yielded rates of only 15.4% for PTSD (Nickerson et al., 2018). A number of factors, such as the level of exposure to potentially traumatic events before, during and after migration, as well as resettlement conditions in the host country are thought to influence the prevalence rates—which appear to be dose-dependent (determined by the level of exposure to trauma) and occurring in a curvilinear pattern across the resettlement period (Copping et al., 2010; Schick et al., 2016; Turrini et al., 2017).

A growing body of research demonstrates the substantial and negative impact post-migration factors may have on mental health (Li et al., 2016). This includes socioeconomic difficulties, as well as stressors relating to the asylum seeking process. For example, a recent study conducted by *Médecins Sans Frontières* among asylum seekers in Italy (2016) found that significant differences in prevalence rates were related to gender, the state of vulnerability, nationality, the waiting time before being seen by a specialist, and exposure to traumatic events before, during and after migration. This is a particularly relevant consideration for the mental health of refugees in light of the multiple and arguably ongoing environmental stressors and potentially traumatic experiences with which they are faced. In a multi-agency guide on the mental health of refugee populations released in 2015, UN agencies and other international humanitarian organizations have highlighted the fact that—for most refugees and migrants—potentially traumatic events from the past are not the only, or even most important, source of psychological distress but that the majority of emotional suffering is directly related to current stresses and worries and uncertainty about the future (Eleftherakos et al., 2018; Médecins Sans Frontières, 2016; IASC, 2015; MHPSS, 2015).

So where and what exactly is the trauma? Cross-sectional epidemiological studies do not allow for a clear distinction to be made between symptoms of trauma related to current contextual stressors within the environment (for example, facing refugee populations in host communities) and a diagnosable mental disorder—based on a psychiatric formulation of mental health located at the level of the individual (Silove et al., 2017). The medicalisation of trauma on an individual level, linked to fixed 'traumatic' events in the past, risks rendering us blind to other ongoing aspects of interpersonal, political and social violence on a more global scale, including significant post migration factors which may be deemed equally traumatic by refugees (Maier & Straub, 2011; Silove et al., 1998; Silove et al., 2000; Weissbecker et al., 2018). It also neglects the broader socio-political context within which it occurs (Marsella, 2010; Summerfield, 2001; Young, 1995). Narrowing refugees to stories of trauma, it is argued, stabilizes their experiences too firmly within personal histories of victimisation and injury. It focuses attention on therapeutic outcomes rather than a political response to the structural issues that led to trauma (Pratt et al., 2015). Among refugees, this criticism could also extend to scant attention being paid to their current social, political and economic realities and lived daily experiences in host countries (Silove et al., 2000; Watters, 2001). As recently noted by Wenzel and Drožđek (2018), the emphasis on vulnerability tends to minimize refugee resiliency and agency, and may not adequately representing the heterogeneity found across refugee populations.

Furthermore, what about the influence of culture? There have been significant concerns raised in the literature over the relevance and cross-cultural validity of PTSD as a diagnostic construct being used among displaced populations (Bracken, 2001, 2002; Fisher, 2014; Hinton & Lewis-Fernández, 2011; Janoff-Bulman, 1985; L. Kirmayer et al., 2010; Marsella, 2010; Staeuble, 2004; Summerfield, 2001; Tummala-Narra, 2007; Wasco, 2003; Young, 1995). Notably, the diagnosis has been criticized for ignoring significant variability among symptoms evident in different cultural settings across the world (Hinton & Lewis-Fernández, 2011). One example of this variability which continues to attract considerable debate is the prevalence of psychosomatic symptoms found among some cultures and not others (Eagle, 2014). Not only do our reactions to trauma differ according to cultural norms, but the very appraisal of what is or what is not traumatic may similarly be informed by socio-cultural context. Various cognitive and psychodynamic theories purport that the individual's processing of traumatic events (i.e. their cognitive appraisal or making sense of the event) is informed by internalized representational constructs, both influenced by and reflected through language and culture (Brewin et al., 1996; Drožđek & Wilson, 2007; Sturm et al., 2007; Sturm et al., 2010). The way in which trauma is experienced is thus thought to be significantly determined by larger cultural systems and historic contexts (Carlson, 2005; Kirmayer et al., 2010; Marsella, 2010; Marsella et al., 1996; Mattar, 2011; Cecile Rousseau et al., 1997; Tummala-Narra, 2007; Wilson & Drožđek, 2004).

A singular construct of PTSD is simply inadequate to grasp the complexity inherent in how different human beings in different cultures respond to terrifying events (Marlowe, 2010; Steel, 2001; Summerfield, 2001). Scholars such as Momartin et al. (2003), Tummala-Nara (2007) and Afana et al. (2010) highlight how little attention has been given to the impact of traumatic experiences on migrants from diverse religious and cultural backgrounds. They argue that displaced populations in particular are exposed to a multiplicity of challenges including losses, human rights violations and other dimensions of suffering. However, the "benign universe" model inherent to the construct of PTSD, is inherently based on white middle-class populations where traumatic events are considered to be infrequent and outside of the range of normal human experience. The relevance of a PTSD diagnosis is therefore questionable among certain cultures continually exposed to traumatic stressors (Afana et al., 2010; Marsella, 2010) where traumatic events may actually validate instead of violate one's assumptive worldviews (Tang, 2007).

Briefly put, one could deconstruct the very notion of "PTSD" by breaking it up into its various linguistic constituents (Post, Traumatic, Stress and Disorder) in order to examine some of the major criticisms which have been levelled against it. The first word, 'Post,' refers to a discrete event of the past, thus denying the mental health impact of any ongoing factors of mental distress based on current economic, political and social hardships faced by displaced populations. The second word, 'Traumatic,' is problematic insofar as whether an event is perceived to be 'traumatic' or not is in part influenced by the individual's subjective perception of the event, in turn significantly informed by socio-cultural and historical context. The third word, 'Stress' implies a specific reaction to the event based on a pre-determined range of psychological symptoms, thereby neglecting the wide range of possible reactions an individual may have to a traumatic event. The fourth word, 'Disorder,' necessarily pathologises this reaction, placing it at the level of the individual and squarely within the framework of Western medical discourse. Such reductionist medical discourse arguably stabilizes experiences too firmly within personal histories of victimisation and injury (Pratt et al., 2015). Therefore, rather than portraying refugees as homogenous and pathologised "passive victims" suffering from mental health problems, critics have argued that attention should also be given to the resistance of displaced individuals and the ways in which they interpret and respond to experiences. This includes challenging the external forces bearing upon them and allowing space for the articulation of experiences in their own terms (Harvey, 2007; Tummala-Narra, 2007; Watters, 2001).

Apart from putting into question the validity of a PTSD diagnosis among displaced populations, the significant discrepancy among prevalence rates provides us with an important reminder that not all refugees are traumatized—a seemingly logical yet oft-neglected fact. The myriad of mental health experiences of displaced populations are indeed far more complex than can fit into overly simplistic discourses of trauma. Marlowe (2010) is among the many authors who have highlighted the importance of considering alternative discourses around forced migration "for developing more sophisticated understandings of how people have responded to trauma beyond the "event-worthy" underpinnings of forced migration" (p. 1). She implores a move beyond the "refugee" label, noting that "the story of a person's experience(s) of trauma associated with forced migration and how it has negatively influenced his/her life can overshadow other co-existing stories which can emphasize something very different about what a person values and readily identifies with." (p. 1). Loizos (2002) similarly problematizes the term "refugee" as often dependent on sometimes arbitrary political decisions. He criticises accompanying discourses around the label fuelling common myths such as the idea that a refugee is usually or necessarily traumatized by the experience of forced migration; that a refugee is a helpless and dependant person; that a refugee is socially isolated; that a refugee will have difficulty in adjusting to life in a new country because of 'cultural differences; and that a refugee needs 'across the board support. Indeed, it has similarly been noted that the process of migration may in fact reinforce internal and group psychological resources (Sturm et al., 2010). As noted by Papadopoulos (2002a), "refugees are defined not as a group of people exhibiting any specific psychological condition but merely as people who have lost their homes" (p. 9).

As neatly summarized by Ventevogel and colleagues (2019),

- Firstly, PTSD is not the only mental health problem in humanitarian setting
- Secondly, in many cultural settings, people do not have words or concepts for 'trauma-related' mental disorders, or, if they have, these are remarkably different from the prevailing psychiatric definition of PTSD
- Thirdly, there has been sharp conceptual criticism of posttraumatic stress disorder as a 'psychological construct' that obscures the driving socio-political causes of emotional distress and transforms human suffering into a mental disorder in need of treatment
- Lastly, the emphasis on past traumatic events in the development of current emotional distress may ignore the pathogenic role of everyday stressors and the multiple hassles to survive in situations of hardship

Calls for a More Contextualised Understanding of Trauma

Rather than portraying displaced individuals as "passive victims" suffering from mental health problems, critics have argued that attention should be given to the resistance of refugees and the ways in which they interpret and respond to experiences. This includes challenging the external forces bearing upon them and allowing space for the articulation of experiences in their own terms, including discourses of resilience and post-traumatic growth (Harvey, 2007; Tummala-Narra, 2007; Watters, 2001). The notion of "Adversity Activated Development" has similarly been conceptualised by Papadopoulos (2002a, 2002b, 2007) to refer to the phenomenon whereby individuals may not only be resilient in the face of exposure to potentially traumatic circumstances, but that such adversity may conversely lead them to develop as individuals with new psychological resources. A psychiatric diagnosis such as PTSD has the potential to deny these realities, to pathologise individuals and homogenously to identify all members of minority groups as passive victims. By placing human suffering within such an exclusively medicalised and trauma-focused paradigm, a thin description of the individual is created where other important socio-historical considerations are easily lost or hidden (Marlowe, 2010). It's an approach which neglects "a concern not to impose order on the world but instead to allow the emergence of other voices and visions, even if this involves increasing complexity and ambivalence" (Bracken et al., 1997).

Individual responses to trauma are thus increasingly understood as unfolding within the context of systems of relationships which form the environment, as defined by Bronfenbrenner's (1986) Ecological Systems Theory. As Harvey (2007) notes, this ecological perspective is needed to guide inquiries into the understanding of trauma resilience. This is because it incorporates a "resource perspective" which assumes that human communities, like other living environments, evolve adaptively and are deeply embedded in complex and dynamic social contexts in which resources are exchanged. Individuals within this system are capable of negotiating and influencing, as well as being influenced by, this system. Equally, symptom severity is not static but fluid and changing according to a continuum of pathological reactions (Drožđek, 2015b).

In recent years, there has indeed been a burgeoning of theoretical models for understanding trauma that situates individual refugee's trauma sequelae and recovery within inter-personal, political, and social context. Maercker and colleagues (Maercker & Hecker, 2016; Maercker & Horn, 2013) have recently elaborated and extended a social-interpersonal framework model of PTSD incorporating a host of influential factors external to the individual. Harvey's (2007) "ecological" model, Drožđek's (Drožđek, 2015b) model, Marsella's (2010) interactive model, and De Jong's (2007) ecological-cultural-historical model of "traumascape," similarly explore how culture influences the clinical parameters of the diagnostic criteria for PTSD by incorporating a systemic understanding of local representations and experiences of trauma. In the context of trauma among displaced populations in particular, Miller and Rasmussen's (2017) ecological model highlights how "mental health among refugees and asylum seekers stems not only from prior war exposure, but also from a host of ongoing stressors in their social ecology, or displacement-related stressors" (p. 1). Such multisystem, ecosocial frameworks consider trauma among displaced populations as

> the endpoint of an imbalance in the multiplicity of countervailing environmental factors that impact on refugees rather than an expression of innate or intrapsychic problems at an individual level. In that sense, the distinction between normative and pathological responses is somewhat blurred and fluid, the vicissitudes of the ecological context determining the direction and extent to which individuals shift on a continuum of stress (Silove et al., 2017, p. 133).

Such perspectives take into account the fact that symptom severity is fluid, ever changing due to a myriad of interacting intrapsychic and external factors. This requires that we pay attention to the "various, context-dependent, long-term, and complex social, political, and economic measures" affecting the mental health of refugee populations (Wenzel & Drožđek, 2018).

Adapting Clinical Practice

As recently noted by Goguikian Ratcliff and Rossi, (2015),

> if illness is individual, then we understand that health is collective: the status, place and experience of the human face of health and disease, the modes of social responses and institutions are reconfiguring themselves in a logic of supply and demand, strongly influenced by contemporary social and cultural transformations (p. 8).[2]

It is crucial that experiences of trauma are understood as being situated within a specific sociocultural and historical context. Indeed, the past several years of mental health interventions for refugee populations in particular has moved from being exclusively focused on PTSD (and accompanying specialist interventions) towards a more inclusive and communal approach which recognises cultural variance in mental health as well as the need to develop resilience within already existing health, social and community systems (Weissbecker et al., 2018)—despite ongoing divisions in the field regarding these two approaches (Silove et al., 2017).

Yet, despite this growing tend towards community based interventions aimed at privileging local cultural knowledge and practices, existing cultural and contextual information is rarely utilized effectively to inform the design of programs aimed at addressing the mental health of refugee populations (Greene et al., 2017). A significant void in our knowledge still exists regarding the relation of culture to trauma and the relevance of a PTSD diagnosis to refugee populations (Drožđek & Wilson, 2007; Mattar, 2011; Summerfield, 2000a). One striking example of this gap in our knowledge can be found in an interesting review of tools used to measure trauma among refugees conducted by Hollifield et al. (2002). They found that of the 125 different

---

[2]Loose translation from French.

instruments used among refugee populations, only 12 were explicitly developed in a refugee sample. This skewed focus on existing tools and concepts created for a western population is problematic as it neglects the cultural and linguistic heritage which influences which experiences are interpreted as 'traumatic,' the manifestations and expressions of post-traumatic symptomatology, the interpretation of symptoms, narratives of distress as well as healing models (Drožđek, 2007; Janoff-Bulman, 1985; Kirmayer et al., 2010; Kleinman & Good, 2004; Luno et al., 2013; Marsella, 2010; Steel et al., 2009).

Inflexible clinical practice drawing on Western diagnostic categories may not take into account the sociocultural context in which trauma unfolds for refugee populations—an understanding which could be essential in the interpretation and definition of a psychotherapy (*Médecins Sans Frontières*, 2016). From a public health perspective, the need for culturally relevant tools to accurately detect and predict traumatic responses among migrants is clearly of no small concern. Clinicians and academics working with refugee populations have similarly highlighted the continued lack of systematic knowledge regarding concepts of illness among traumatized patients, leading health professionals to ignore or misunderstand their needs (Faregh et al., 2019; Greene et al., 2017; Maier, 2006; Maier et al., 2010; Maier & Straub, 2011; Wenzel & Drožđek, 2018).

Addressing the Gap in the Literature—Implications for Research

As noted by Li and colleagues (2016) in a recent meta-review, the majority of research investigating the effect of post-migration stressors on mental health in refugees has focused on identifying which factors most strongly predict psychopathology in a rather static manner. Rather, there is a need to explore *how* the interaction of these factors affect mental health as it develops over time and within specific sociocultural and historic contexts. A plethora of key authors in the field have highlighted substantial gaps in the literature by calling for more longitudinal studies to add to our understanding of trauma from a more culturally, socially and politically relevant perspective. This includes a focus on life trajectories, dynamic processes and current material realities for refugees in host communities which goes beyond the individual to consider the interrelation of mind and society in human development (Eagle, 2014; Harvey, 2007; Nickerson et al., 2011; Goguikian Ratcliff & Rossi, 2015; Summerfield, 1996, 2001; Wilson & Drožđek, 2004). In addition, there are calls to enrich understandings of "historical trauma" (Gone, 2013) or collective, cultural, and identity-related trauma, with an emphasis on the social location of human subjects and a recognition that trauma responses may carry a sense of group burden and collective suffering beyond symptomatic individuals (Eagle, 2014).

This call for more research has been echoed not only in the world of academia but by many international humanitarian organisations engaged in the implementation of mental health and psychosocial interventions with refugees across Europe and who are looking for more culturally relevant tools (which consider more local idioms of distress, for example) to better address the mental health needs of this population (Einhorn et al., 2018; Faregh et al., 2019; *Médécins Sans Frontières*, 2016; Hecker et al., 2015; Inter-Agency Standing Committee (IASC) 2015; Tol et al., 2014; UNHCR, 2015; Ventevogel et al., 2019). Learning about the impact of dislocation, trauma and loss, of political persecution and human malevolence, and social systems involving abuse, neglect, and ethnic and cultural rejection is crucial in terms of guiding policy makers and clinicians to assist, and as advocates to address, the social and historical perspectives of trauma and their mental health consequences (Wilson & Drožđek, 2004). This is particularly pertinent given the migrant crisis currently being faced by Europe. What is needed is an increased understanding of the influence of context on psychological functioning and the empowering possibilities of ecologically informed interventions and public health strategies which do not unduly not unduly medicalize socio-political problems or psychologize human rights violations (Harvey, 2007; Wenzel & Drožđek, 2018). We have known for some time that culture matters when trauma is concerned; however, we need to fine-tune our knowledge of how culture matters in the definition of what is experienced as traumatic as well as the processes through which traumatic events are experienced and either accommodated or not:

> Intercultural trauma treatment is a new field, one whose time has come. It reminds us yet again of the basic values of human encounters, beyond all sophisticated treatment techniques and devices, and it offers us ways for expanding the borders of our profession … (Drožđek & Wilson, 2007)

Some key implications for researchers highlighted by experts in the field in a briefing paper on trauma and mental in forcibly displaced populations by the International Society for Traumatic Stress Studies (Nickerson et al., 2018) include:

- Implement community participatory designs to be conducted in collaboration with service providers, clinicians and policymakers where possible
- Investigate the full breadth of psychological disorders and symptoms in refugees, focusing on cultural conceptions of distress
- Implement longitudinal methods to identify mechanisms underlying refugee mental health and determine the temporal causal relationship between refugee experiences, mental health and other outcomes

They recommend that research should be undertaken in collaboration with refugee communities to increase understanding and treatment of psychological disorders amongst refugees and asylum-seekers, and that professional organizations can play an important role in facilitating, promoting and disseminating research on refugee mental health. In their reflections on research into the mental health of refugee torture survivors in particular, published in *Lancet Psychiatry,* Liddell and colleagues (2017) similarly state,

> a new research approach that considers the interactive effects of past trauma, contextual stress, and psychological symptoms on torture survivors could enhance the ecological validity of

research. We propose that multimodal research that merges robust clinical and experimental research within appropriate ecological frameworks is needed to advance the field [...] to fully understand the effects of torture, clinical science must go beyond the traditional boundaries of psychiatric research to account for the influence of sociocultural contextual factors "(p. 1).

It is now time to move on to broader and more operationally relevant research and for researchers to engage with contemporary notions of resilience and social ecology (Weissbecker et al., 2018).

The Context of the Research

This books aims to weave together both theory and practice. It is based both on my research as an academic, as well as my lived experience as a clinician working with displaced populations around the world: in police stations and clinics for rape survivors in South Africa, in refugee camps across central Africa, in prisons in the Ukraine, in clinics for torture survivors in Greece, and in shelters for Yezidi survivors of genocide in Iraq. I believe that both the theoretical knowledge and practical experience are needed for the exploration of refugee trauma I attempt to undertake in this book.

Why Read This Book

Globally, we are facing unprecedented levels of displacement. More than ever, we need to understand experiences of trauma—and of resilience—among displaced populations. More than ever, we need to understand the role of culture in these experiences. In order to address some of the needs for more research on trauma among refugee populations, this book aims to draw on a socio-cultural framework which focuses on the intersubjective, mediational space between the individual and culture-society-interaction (O'Connor, 2015) in order to try account for the experience of humans in time and in particular social and cultural environments. Such an approach presupposes human beings inhabit shared forms of life. Meaning is continually negotiated within the social sphere and "cultural products, like language and other symbolic systems, mediate thought and place their stamp on our representations of reality" (Bruner, 1991). As such, this theoretical framework thus highlights the heterogeneous, fluid and dynamic nature of individual subjectivities and the multitude of socio-culturally determined discourses which may be drawn upon to make sense of life experiences (Gee, 2014; Squire, 2008). As stated by Brunner, such an epistemological underpinning "brings profoundly into question not only the universality of knowledge from one domain to another, but the universal translatability of knowledge from one culture to another. For in this dispensation, knowledge is never 'point-of-viewless.'" (p. 2). As such, the book aims to consider the possibilities of building collective politics through the examination of case studies of trauma within social and political context (Pratt et al., 2015).

Chapters two to five offer the theoretical framework in which to understand experiences of trauma among forcibly displaced populations. Here I review the literature on pre-, peri- and post migration factors affecting trauma, examine prevalence rates of PTSD, and argue that we need to move beyond the diagnosis towards a more culturally relevant conceptualisation of trauma. Chapter's six to eight conceptualise experiences of trauma among displaced populations—as well as their resilience, imagination, and aspirations for the future—from a collective, sociocultural perspective. Chapter's nine to eleven address some applications for professionals: working with shame and trauma, working with cultural mediators, and working with PTSD in the asylum procedure. Final reflections are offered in the concluding chapter twelve.

Theoretical Framework

Chapter Two: Trauma and Migration
In a multi-agency guide on the mental health of refugee populations released in 2015, UN agencies and other international humanitarian organisations have highlighted that potentially traumatic events from the past are not the only, or even most important, source of psychological distress but that the majority of emotional suffering is directly related to current stress factors. A plethora of key literature from the field attests to the detrimental impact on mental health of the migration journey (including prolonged detention, stays in often unsafe refugee camps, exposure to trafficking rings) as well as the asylum-seeking process. Post-migration factors, such as unemployment, an insecure residency status and fear of repatriation, insufficient proficiency in a host language, social discrimination, and difficulties with integration have similarly been shown to be correlated with mental challenges among displaced populations. The psychological impact of these factors and other "daily stresses" are a relevant consideration in light of the additional critical life events with which displaced populations are faced. This chapter will explore the myriad of interrelating pre- and post-migration factors affecting the mental health of displaced populations.

Case study: Two case studies will be presented based on multiple interviews conducted with a victim of torture arriving in Greece and suffering from psychotic episodes exacerbated by his current living conditions, and of an asylum seeker from Switzerland after he set himself alight in a town square and survived—in his own words in order to protest asylum conditions. The cases will serve to illustrate the substantial psychological impact of current material realities of displaced populations, as they adapt to their new environment in transit and destination countries. An interpersonal-social model will be presented which examines various post-migration "feedback loops" influencing post-traumatic symptomatology.

Chapter Three: Prevalence of PTSD Among Displaced Populations

The literature attests to substantially higher prevalence rates of mental health challenges among displaced populations compared to the general norm, documenting statistically significant higher levels of post-traumatic stress, anxiety, and depression. In terms of PTSD prevalence specifically, a landmark meta-review conducted by Steel and colleagues in 2009 (2009) revealed an average prevalence rate of PTSD across all surveys of 30.6%. Prevalence rates of PTSD reported in other long-term refugee populations screened using the Harvard Trauma Questionaire (HTQ), include 45,5% among earthquake survivors in Wenchuan China (Kun et al., 2009), 37.2% among Cambodian refugees living on the Thai–Cambodian border camps (Cardozo et al., 2004), 29,3% among populations living in conflict-ridden southern Lebanon (Farhood et al., 2006), and 11.8% among displaced Guatemalans living in Chiapas, Mexico (Sabin et al., 2003).

Case study: This chapter will present prevalence rates of PTSD noted among displaced populations in Iraq, the Philippines, and South Africa, screened using the HTQ. These results are taken from three independent studies I conducted:

- A study in South Africa I conducted with *Médecins Sans Frontières* among refugees and asylum seekers from other African countries who fled to displaced camps after a flare-up of xenophobic violence occurred in Durban, revealing a prevalence rate of PTSD of 85%.
- A study in Iraq with the Free Yezidi Foundation, I conducted among displaced Yezidi communities in the context of an internal evaluation of the Free Yezidi Foundation's mental health intervention, revealing a prevalence rate of PTSD of 82%
- A study in the Philippines with the Global Initiative for Stress and Trauma Treatment (Gist-T), I conducted with colleagues among displaced communities affected by the recent conflict in Marawi in the context of a mental health needs assessment, revealing a prevalence rate of PTSD of 78%.

Chapter Four: Beyond PTSD

Despite the high prevalence of PTSD noted among displaced populations, there have been significant concerns raised in the literature over the cross-cultural validity of PTSD itself as a diagnostic construct. This is particularly problematic for humanitarian interventions. Critics argue that the medicalisation of trauma on an individual level, linked to specific "traumatic" events in the past, risks rendering us blind to other ongoing aspects of interpersonal, political and social violence on a more global scale. This includes significant post migration factors that may be deemed equally traumatic by displaced populations. Futhermore, treatment models developed in Western cultural contexts have been criticized for ignoring significant variability among explanatory models of distress evident in different cultural settings. There is a lack of standardized measurement tools for posttraumatic stress responses among culturally diverse populations. This speaks to the significant void in our knowledge regarding the relation of culture to trauma, and the way in which a diagnosis of PTSD is used and interpreted among displaced populations. This chapter will highlight the politicised history of the diagnosis, and discuss the implications for its use among displaced populations in humanitarian contexts.

Case study: The chapter will present a critical comparison of representations of trauma (and PTSD in particular) among refugees and health professionals. I compare the way in which trauma is understood and described by refugees (in interviews with victims of torture in Athens) to how it is understood and described by health professionals (in 43 interviews I conducted among psychiatrists and psychologists from thirteen different countries across the E.U., all of whom work with refugee populations). A specific focus will be on the ways in which a diagnosis of PTSD is contested, appropriated, and used strategically for different purposes.

Chapter Five: Culturally Informed Manifestations of Trauma
The burgeoning field of cultural psychiatry highlights how cultural variations in ways of life and social contexts shape the embodied experience of trauma. It demonstrates how particular symptoms or behavioral expressions of distress vary with cultural knowledge, beliefs, and interpretations and that individuals interpret and respond to their own symptoms with culturally varied coping strategies that may influence the experience of trauma. In other words, experience of trauma is an intersubjective, temporal, dynamic process shaped by culture, among other factors. This approach goes beyond a reductionist focus on "cultural differences," wherein "culture" is perceived as a reified, crystallised concept and viewed as a potential barrier to be overcome in a process of psychiatric classification. Instead, it focuses on ever-changing cultural and social systems which determine the various forms of an individual subjective experience of illness, an experience inevitably in constant flux.

Culture is considered in this chapter as both as a set of practices physically executed in a tangible and observable sense by the group, as well as integral to belief systems lying internally within individual members. Each level mutually reinforces the other. Furthermore, culture is not static but continually adapts to ever-changing environments: created, maintained and sustained among groups through dominant narratives or discourses. This chapter will provide a definition of culture from a dynamic ecological and sociocultural perspective. It will further explore the impact of cultural systems on the various ways in which the cultural environment informs the manifestation of trauma.

Case study: Examples of culturally informed manifestations of trauma will be explored by drawing on clinical examples from my work in the field—notably the case of 8 women from the Murle tribe affected by conflict in South Sudan who experienced an episode of mass fainting spells, as well as the case in Greece of a refugee victim of torture from Guinea confronted with a different cultural belief system of trauma between herself and her psychologist in Athens. These cases will notably explore belief systems around trauma, the meaning given to the traumatic event, culturally determined idioms of distress and symptom manifestations, as well as implications for health seeking behaviour and explanatory models of healing.

Conceptualising Experiences of Trauma and Migration from a Collective, Sociocultural Perspective

Chapter Six: Collective Trauma, Collective Healing
It is not only individuals who face traumatic events but entire communities. Over the past few decades, a plethora of research has highlighted the importance of the sociocultural environment for the way in which individuals, and indeed entire communities, experience trauma and recovery. The trauma associated with forced displacement has a psychosocial impact not only on the individual, but also their family, community and the larger society. At the family level, this includes the dynamics of single parent families, lack of trust among members, and changes in significant relationships and child-rearing practice. Communities tend to be more dependent, passive, silent, without leadership, mistrustful and suspicious. Additional adverse effects noted in the literature include the breakdown of traditional structures, institutions and familiar ways of life, and deterioration in social norms, ethics and loss of social capital (Somasundaram, 2014).

Saul's (2013) landmark definition of collective trauma highlights its larger social impact, occurring at multiple levels, with "shared injuries to a population's social, cultural, and physical ecologies" (p. 1). In another seminal work on collective trauma, Erikson (Erikson, 1976) defines it as "a blow to the basic tissues of social life that damages the bonds attaching people together and impairs the prevailing sense of communality" (p. 154). Considering the development of collective trauma as a process, this chapter will highlight elements of the temporality of collective trauma, as well as the continual interaction of factors influencing trauma in a given social and historical context. Particular focus will be on the socio-political context and power dynamics at play in influencing the mental health of entire populations. Implications for mental health interventions will be explored.

Case Study: To explore the collective impact of trauma on entire displaced communities, this chapter will draw on two case studies from my work in Iraq and the Philippines first introduced in chapter three: the forcibly displaced Yezidi community of Kurdistan Northern Iraq, (200 women whom I interviewed in the context of a project evaluation), and displaced communities affected by the recent conflict in Marawi, Philippines (factors of collective trauma and recovery explored by myself and colleagues among 80 participants in the context of a mental health needs assessment). The analysis aims to explore how individuals may be traumatized at multiple levels including collective/social, personal/physical, and role identity levels. Results will highlight the substantial impact of the political, legal, and sociocultural environment on both the prevalence of collective trauma, as well as processes of collective healing.

Chapter Seven: Collective Resilience and Imagination
Continuing with the theme of the impact of the sociocultural context on the collective mental health of entire populations, this chapter will explore resilience and imagination as experienced by displaced populations from a collective perspective. As

proposed by Ungar (2004, 2008, 2011, 2013), "resilience is both the capacity of individuals to navigate their way into psychological, social, cultural, and physical resources that sustain their well-being and their individual and collective capacity to negotiate for these resources to be provided and experienced in culturally meaningful ways" (Ungar 2008, p. 225). The burgeoning literature on resilience among displaced populations has begun to highlight the interaction of protective mechanisms with exterior risk factors. The more recent explicit focus is thus on the socio-ecological environment. Within this paradigm, resilience is not a fixed, individual trait. It is dynamic and variable. It reflects both the individual and the world around them. It's considered essentially as a social and environmental attribute (Lusk & Baray, 2017a), and the capacity of a person's "informal and formal social networks to facilitate positive development under stress" (Ungar, 2013, p.1). It is a collective endeavour. The chapter will argue that building resilience and imagining plans for the future are not solely individual projects, but communal processes involving reclaiming collective action, trust, and efficacy. Implications for community interventions will be explored.

The chapter further explores imagination among displaced communities. The paradoxes are multiple: (i) Migration is inherently imaginative, in the sense that the actualisation of migration begins with individuals imagining their destination (ii) however, trauma related to forced migration experiences in particular may impede imagination. To further add to the complexity: it may be imagination itself which acts as an essential component to resilience, and healing from trauma. The chapter explores the mobility choices of displaced populations and individual migration trajectories to provide insight into how the emotionality of subjective experiences, as well as the sociocultural context, are fundamentally involved in people's resilience, their plans to migrate, and the development of their ever-changing imagination of a better future elsewhere. How do displaced individuals the resilience to overcome trauma? How do they navigate the "brave new world" in which they find themselves? What helps them to find the strength to imagine and negotiate a new and better life?

Case study: In order to explore trauma, resilience, and imagination among displaced populations, I present the results of 12 months of research among refugees in a centre for victims of torture in Athens. This research includes 125 in-depth, qualitative interviews with victims of torture, health professionals, cultural mediators/interpreters, and leaders from refugee communities. The case study illustrates the substantial psychological impact of current material realities of refugee victims of torture as they adapt to their new environment and imagine a better future. Using a socio-ecological framework (Sleijpen et al., 2017), and drawing on the concept of imagination from the perspective of sociocultural psychology, the chapter explores the strategies used by this population in order to discuss additional insights of an interpersonal and communal perspective for the growing field of research on resilience after trauma.

Chapter Eight: Collective Aspirations
Not only are the aspirations of individuals constantly transforming as a result of sociopolitical developments; they are significantly shaped or contested by shared or collective aspirations of entire communities. This starts with collective aspirations

of communities in the country of origin. It also extends to the constantly developing shared aspirations of displaced communities in host contexts. The theoretical background of sociocultural psychology allows for an exploration of these nuances—of the ever-changing and dynamic development of aspirations over time, and within sociocultural context. It evokes a methodology incorporating an exploration "not only of the subjective perspective, but also the dynamics by which the social and cultural environment guide and enable the person's development" (Zittoun, 2017). Of particular interest in this chapter is the way in which aspirations are influenced by the encompassing fabric of the cultural collective, related both to the country of origin as well as humanitarian contexts of protracted displacement and a liminal permanent temporariness so often facing displaced populations.

Case study: Greece represents a unique context in which to explore the aspirations of asylum seekers entering Europe: perceived both as a country of transit as well as a final destination. Currently, many asylum seekers find themselves "stuck" in limbo in this context, unable to proceed with their asylum claim or continue their journey to the destination countries of Western Europe to which they continue to aspire. In order to explore the aspirations and experiences of integration of refugee communities within this context, I draw on the case of my fieldwork in Greece, introduced in chapter seven. To analyse the data, I emphasize the importance of non-linear temporality in the context of individual's changing subjective current realities—as they weave together images of the past, present and future. This includes tracking the developing aspirations of individuals as they configure, reconfigure, and make meaning of the new realities in a receiving country. The results are illustrated using qualitative case studies of individual trajectories, and highlight aspirations as a powerful motivating force for migration.

Applications for Professionals

Chapter Nine: Working with Shame and Trauma

Despite the psychically toxic nature of shame, it has historically been under-researched and under-theorised. However, a recent burgeoning of literature has brought an increasing awareness of shame as a pathogenic force. Research in trauma over the past decade has seen the development of the concept of "posttraumatic shame," with key authors stressing the importance of shame as a social emotion that impacts the severity and course of PTSD symptoms. Indeed, the experience of shame has even been revealed to potentially hold the same properties as traumatic events. Shame can trigger intrusions, flashbacks, strong emotional avoidance, hyper arousal, fragmented states of mind and dissociation. Shame and trauma are inextricably linked.

Unlike guilt (typically related to a particular action or behaviour), shame taints the entire landscape of the individual. It colours the very sense of self. It therefore could be considered to be a more complex intra-psychic process than guilt because it involves processes concerning attributes about the core dimensions of the self, identity, ego processes, and personality. Inasmuch as it lies within the interactional space between self and other, at the divide between the intimate and the public, the individual and society—it tries to hide itself by its very nature. As such, it often remains unnoticed. Its powerful yet seemingly invisible impact may be hidden behind a myriad of emotional cloaks—anger, dissociation, blame, and resentment. This is even more so in the context of clinicians working with displaced populations. In this context, a plethora of differently nuanced cultural cloaks may further obfuscate this noxious affect. Furthermore, shame-related cultural codes of behaviour might prevent migrants from directly reporting earlier traumatic experiences, from trusting the professional or from even attending appointments. As noted by Wilson and colleagues (2006), "the powerful emotions of posttraumatic shame are associated with a broad range of avoidance behaviours: isolation, detachment, withdrawal, hiding, nonappearance, self- imposed exile, cancellation of appointments, surrender of responsibilities, emotional constriction, psychic numbing, emotional flatness, and non-confrontation with others" (p. 138). These signs are easily misread.

Ethically, clinically, humanly, professionals working with traumatized populations cannot ignore shame. This is particularly true of work within multicultural contexts, where relations are so typically marked by power differentials in terms of race, class, nationality and socio-economic status. It is here, in this intersectionality of identities, that shame is located. In this chapter, aspects of migration and post-traumatic shame, and implications for professionals, will be discussed. New approaches to recognising and working with shame are needed for clinicians (both researchers and academics), which consider the interactive effects of shame and trauma within sociocultural contexts among such vulnerable populations.

Case study: As both a researcher and clinical psychologist working with displaced populations, I explore the myriad dimensions of shame within humanitarian contexts. This is based on personal reflections of my relationship with research participants as well as the burgeoning literature on this topic. Two case studies of shame will be presented, one a refugee victim of torture seeking asylum in Greece, the other a female survivor of sexual violence in Cape Town, South Africa. The analysis will track the ubiquitous manifestations of shame between researcher and researched to reveal how shame was unavoidably generated, exacerbated and maintained within the relationship. Implications for interventions are discussed.

Chapter Ten: Working with Cultural Mediators

As the number of refugee mental health programs increases, so has the use of cultural mediators. Without them, clinical services for displaced populations could not be provided. Here, the term "cultural mediator" is purposefully used instead of "interpreter," in order to reflect the dynamic and complex nature of their work. This work often extends far beyond that of simple translation. These professionals are often the mediators between the world of the health professional and that of displaced communities.

In this chapter, I will draw on Wang's (2012, 2016) notion that it is the complex "subjectivity" of the mediator that differentiates them from interpreters: they need to be focused on both the content and form of the discussion, as well as to pay attention to interpersonal relationships (Wang, 2016). This comes with challenges surrounding the need to be precise, emotionally detached, firm, to know how to behave in relation to a specific culture, and being neutral and impartial. This is particularly true in the context of mental health—a field which the literature highlights as being the most demanding for cultural mediators compared to their work with other professionals. This is a particularly pertinent consideration given the current influx of asylum seekers into Europe, many of whom have lived through horrors beyond description, indeed beyond words in any language.

Within this context, the role of cultural mediators is an essential one. These professionals have been shown in the literature to have to negotiate multiple positions including that of a cultural broker, community organizer and even a directly implicated co-therapist. Indeed, as stated by Summerfield (2005), the challenges they face are "not…of translation between languages but of translation between worlds" (Nicolas et al., 2015). They are active co-therapists. They are advocates of mental health. They are experts assisting health professionals to explore the culturally informed psychic worlds of displaced and traumatized individuals.

In this chapter, I will discuss issues affecting cultural mediators working with displaced populations. This includes an exploration of how the different representations and understandings of trauma are managed, contested, and negotiated in the complex relationship between patient, health professional and cultural mediator. Implications for health professionals and cultural mediators will be discussed.

Case study: The case study is based on my fieldwork in Greece—as seen in earlier chapters. The analysis will focus on cultural mediation within the intersubjective spaces between health professionals, cultural mediators, and refugees in consultation. Interviews with the cultural mediators highlight the variety of complex roles they play when translating between health professionals and refugee beneficiaries, particularly in the context of mental health. This involved assuming the role of the co-therapist, where many felt actively engaged in the therapeutic process and indeed often closer to the refugee beneficiaries on an emotional level than the health professionals themselves. In other cases, alliances lay more with the health professionals. For example, some saw their role as advocates of mental health when faced with refugee communities who don't appear to understand the role of the psychologist: their own role therein being to convince refugee populations of the value of a more westernized understanding of mental health. However, another challenge emerging in the interviews was the complexity involved in working with health professionals whom the cultural mediators deemed to be culturally incompetent.

Chapter Eleven: Working with PTSD in the Asylum Procedure

Asylum and trauma is an urgent area of inquiry—in particular given the unprecedented transnational migration occurring in Europe within the past few years. In terms of Article 1, Chapter 1 of the Geneva Convention of 1951, a refugee is defined as someone with a "well-founded fear of being persecuted for reasons of race, religion, nationality, membership of a particular social group or political opinion." The word "fear" here is of particular interest as it implies that a refugee is defined to some extent by his or her psychological response to events, not only by the events themselves. Furthermore, the burden of proof falls on the asylum seeker. When persecuted individuals seeking asylum cannot give evidence of marks on their body, they have the alternate possibility of proving the violence to which they have been exposed through what is sometimes designated as the "wounds of the soul," notably a diagnosis of post-traumatic stress disorder (PTSD). However, the literature highlights the risk of PTSD becoming a "pre-requisite" for validating the experiences of asylum seekers, reifying and reducing these experiences by placing them within an exclusively psychiatric paradigm in order to render their narrative accounts believable in asylum procedures. Such a politically loaded use of PTSD indeed leads to situations whereby victims of torture and other atrocities fear not being believed unless they can "check off the tick list of symptoms" required to be diagnosed with PTSD.

Among the factors that require sensitive consideration are risk of cultural and linguistic misunderstandings and the effect of posttraumatic stress disorder and depressive symptoms on the capacity to provide a coherent narrative. Trauma may be simply unspeakable. Such a consideration is particularly pertinent when seen in light of the literature, which demonstrates that the asylum process risks being a traumatic event in and of itself. Here, a culturally sensitive recognition of trauma may assist judges and other decision makers in recognizing and being more attentive to the difficulties asylum seekers may have in verbalising and constructing their case as a result of a compromised mental state which "may impede the applicant's ability to testify in a manner that appears direct, specific, and emotionally appropriate" (Linton, 2015, p. 1085). This recognition of impairment is critical to assist the comprehensive assessment of refugee claims—as it limits the risk of erroneous decision-making based on testimonies distorted by psychological trauma.

There is a need to explore tensions surrounding the controversial use of PTSD as evidence in court. There is equally a need to deepen the way in which the impact of trauma among displaced populations is understood. Nowhere is this more pertinent than in the asylum procedure. Here, questions of legitimacy are central. In this chapter, I argue that understanding trauma in the context of the asylum process should necessarily recognise the social-cultural context in which it occurs, in relation to the activity of which it is a part and within a broader systems of relations in which it has meaning. To do so, I explore the asylum process as a system of activity. I argue that such a systemic analysis allows for a broad contextualisation of practices around PTSD, revealing and exposing tensions and contradictions in how various actors involved in the asylum seeking process understand trauma among refugee populations and the implications this may have on their request for asylum.

In this chapter, I therefore explore the role of PTSD as a diagnosis functioning across an interconnected network of actors in the activity system of the asylum tribunal (including lawyers, health professionals, and asylum seekers themselves)—according to the various roles and activities of each actor concerned. By drawing on the case study of victims of torture claiming asylum in Greece, the numerous and changing functions of the diagnosis will be highlighted—including the way in which such functions may change over time even within the activity of each actor.

Case study: The case study is based on my fieldwork in Greece—as seen in earlier chapters. An analysis of the case study demonstrates how PTSD circulates among the different actors yet with specific meanings and functions within each activity system, and which change over time. It may be used by health professionals in certain activity systems to communicate among each other about the clinical symptoms experienced by the patient, and by the bureaucrats of the tribunal as evidence in court of the individual having survived a traumatic experience. The asylum seekers themselves experience the diagnosis in a myriad of different ways. Positioned as political subjects in the asylum procedure, as patients in the consulting room, as clients with their lawyers, as members of their community at home—PTSD appeared to have different meanings and functions across these activity systems. For the health professionals needing to address a variety of different actors outside of their clinical community, PTSD is helpful to explain (both to patients as well as to the bureaucrats of the asylum tribunal), to treat and, in some cases, to attest to the trauma experienced by the asylum seeker.

Conclusion

Chapter Twelve: Reflections on Working with Trauma in Humanitarian Contexts

In this chapter, I will conclude by summarizing the key themes raised throughout the book:

- There is significant evidence of alarmingly high rates of psychological disorders including posttraumatic stress disorder (PTSD) among displaced populations
- There is similarly evidence of significant resilience displayed by individuals faced with traumatic events
- Culture impacts on conceptualization, expression and treatment of psychological distress
- Not only do pre-migration factors influence trauma—the current political, social and economic environment has a significant impact on mental health
- Trauma may be experienced collectively, by entire communities.

References

Abbott, A. (2016). The troubled minds of migrants. *Nature, 538,* 158–161.

Afana, A.-H., Pedersen, D., Rønsbo, H., & Kirmayer, L. J. (2010). Endurance is to be shown at the first blow: Social representations and reactions to traumatic experiences in the Gaza Strip. *Traumatology: An International Journal, 16*(4), 73–84.

Bhugra, D., & Gupta, S. (2011). *Migration and mental health*. Cambridge: Cambridge University Press.

Bogic, M., Ajdukovic, D., Bremner, S., Franciskovic, T., Galeazzi, G. M., Kucukalic, A., et al. (2012). Factors associated with mental disorders in long-settled war refugees: Refugees from the former Yugoslavia in Germany, Italy and the UK. *The British Journal of Psychiatry, 200*(3), 216–223.

Bracken, P. (2001). Post-modernity and post-traumatic stress disorder. *Social Science and Medicine, 53*(6), 733–743.

Bracken, P. (2002). *Trauma: Culture, meaning and philosophy*. London, U.K.: Whurr Publishers.

Bracken, P., Giller, J. E., & Summerfield, D. (1997). Rethinking mental health work with survivors of wartime violence and refugees. *Journal of Refugee Studies, 10*(4), 431–442.

Brewin, C. R., Dalgleish, T., & Joseph, S. (1996). A dual representation theory of posttraumatic stress disorder. *Psychological Review, 103*(4), 670–686.

Bronfenbrenner, U. (1986). Ecology of the family as a context for human development: Research perspectives. *Developmental Psychology, 22*(6), 723–742.

Bruner, J. (1991). The narrative construction of reality. *Critical Inquiry, 18*(1), 1–21.

Cardozo, B. L., Talley, L., Burton, A., & Crawford, C. (2004). Karenni refugees living in Thai-Burmese border camps: Traumatic experiences, mental health outcomes, and social functioning. *Social Science & Medicine, 58*(12), 2637–2644.

Carlson, B. E. (2005). The most important things learned about violence and trauma in the past 20 years. *Journal of Interpersonal Violence, 20*(1), 119–126.

Copping, A., Shakespeare-Finch, J., & Paton, D. (2010). Towards a culturally appropriate mental health system: Sudanese-Australians' experiences with trauma. *Journal of Pacific Rim Psychology, 4*(01), 53–60.

d'Halluin, E. (2009). La santé mentale des demandeurs d'asile. *Hommes et migrations. Revue française de référence sur les dynamiques migratoires* (Vol. 1282, pp. 66–75).

de Arellano, M. A., & Danielson, C. K. (2008). Assessment of Trauma history and trauma-related problems in ethnic minority child populations: An INFORMED approach. *Cognitive and Behavioral Practice, 15*(1), 53–66.

De Jong, J. (2007). Traumascape: An ecological–cultural–historical model for extreme stress. In D. Bhugra & K. Bhu (Eds.), *Textbook of cultural psychiatry* (pp. 347–363). Cambridge: Cambridge University Press.

Drožđek, B. (2007). The rebirth of contextual thinking in psychotraumatology. In B. Drožđek, B., & J.P. Wilson (Eds.), *Voices of trauma: Treating psychological trauma across cultures* (pp. 1–26). New York, N.Y: Springer.

Drožđek, B., & Wilson, J. P. (2007). *Voices of trauma: Treating psychological trauma across cultures*. New York, N. Y.: Springer.

Eagle, G. (2014). From evolution to discourse: Key conceptual debates in the history and study of traumatic stress. *Psychology in Society, 47*, 1–20.

Einhorn, L., Rivière, M., Chappuis, M., Chevelle, M., & Laurence, S. (2018). Proposer une réponse en santé mentale et soutien psychosocial aux exilés en contexte de crise. L'expérience de Médecins du Monde en Calais (2015–2017). *Revue Européenne des Migrations Internationales, 34*(2), 187–203.

Eleftherakos, C., van den Boogaard, W., Barry, D., Severy, N., Kotsioni, I., & Roland-Gosselin, L. (2018). I prefer dying fast than dying slowly, how institutional abuse worsens the mental health of stranded Syrian, Afghan and Congolese migrants on Lesbos island following the implementation of EU-Turkey deal. *Conflict and Health, 12*(1), 38.

Erikson, K. T. (1976). Collective trauma: Loss of communality. In K. T. Erikson (Ed.), *Everything in its path* (pp. 186–245). New York: Simon and Schuster Inc.

Esala, J. J., Vukovich, M. M., Hanbury, A., Kashyap, S., & Joscelyne, A. (2018). Collaborative care for refugees and torture survivors: Key findings from the literature. *Traumatology, 24*(3), 168–185.

Faregh, N., Lencucha, R., Ventevogel, P., Dubale, B. W., & Kirmayer, L. J. (2019). Considering culture, context and community in mhGAP implementation and training: Challenges and recommendations from the field. *International Journal of Mental Health Systems, 13*(1), 1–13.
Farhat, J. B., Blanchet, K., Bjertrup, P. J., Veizis, A., Perrin, C., Coulborn, R. M., et al. (2018). Syrian refugees in Greece: Experience with violence, mental health status, and access to information during the journey and while in Greece. *BMC Medicine, 16*(1), 40.
Farhood, L., Dimassi, H., & Lehtinen, T. (2006). Exposure to war-related traumatic events, prevalence of PTSD, and general psychiatric morbidity in a civilian population from Southern Lebanon. *Journal of Transcultural Nursing, 17*(4), 333–340.
Fazel, M., Wheeler, J., & Danesh, J. (2005). Prevalence of serious mental disorder in 7000 refugees resettled in western countries: A systematic review. *The Lancet, 365*(9467), 1309–1314.
Fisher, M. P. (2014). PTSD in the U.S. military, and the politics of prevalence. *Social Science & Medicine, 115,* 1–9.
Gee, J. P. (2014). *An introduction to discourse analysis: Theory and method*. London: Routledge.
Goguikian Ratcliff, B. G., & Rossi, I. (2015). Santé mentale et sociétés plurielles. *Alterstice-Revue Internationale De La Recherche Interculturelle, 4*(2), 3–12.
Gone, J. P. (2013). Redressing First Nations historical trauma: Theorizing mechanisms for indigenous culture as mental health treatment. *Transcultural Psychiatry, 50*(5), 683–706.
Greene, M. C., Jordans, M. J., Kohrt, B. A., Ventevogel, P., Kirmayer, L. J., Hassan, G., et al. (2017). Addressing culture and context in humanitarian response: Preparing desk reviews to inform mental health and psychosocial support. *Conflict and Health, 11*(1), 21.
Greene, M. C., Rees, S., Likindikoki, S., Bonz, A. G., Joscelyne, A., Kaysen, D., et al. (2019). Developing an integrated intervention to address intimate partner violence and psychological distress in Congolese refugee women in Tanzania. *Conflict & Health, 13*(1), 1–16.
Haenel, F. (2015). Special problems in the assessment of psychological sequelae of torture and incarceration. In M. Schouler-Ocak (Ed.), *Trauma and migration* (pp. 95–107). Cham: Springer.
Hall, B. J., & Olff, M. (2016). Global mental health: Trauma and adversity among populations in transition. *European Journal of Psychotraumatology, 7,* 31140.
Harvey, M. R. (2007). Towards an ecological understanding of resilience in trauma survivors: Implications for theory, research, and practice. *Journal of Aggression, Maltreatment and Trauma, 14*(1–2), 9–32.
Hecker, T., Braitmayer, L., & van Duijl, M. (2015). Global mental health and trauma exposure: The current evidence for the relationship between traumatic experiences and spirit possession. *European Journal of Psychotraumatology, 6*(1), 29126.
Heeren, M., Wittmann, L., Ehlert, U., Schnyder, U., Maier, T., & Müller, J. (2014). Psychopathology and resident status–comparing asylum seekers, refugees, illegal migrants, labor migrants, and residents. *Comprehensive Psychiatry, 55*(4), 818–825.
Hinton, D. E., & Lewis-Fernández, R. (2011). The cross-cultural validity of posttraumatic stress disorder: Implications for DSM-5. *Depression and Anxiety, 28*(9), 783–801.
Hodges-Wu, J., & Zajicek-Farber, M. (2017). Addressing the needs of survivors of torture: A pilot test of the psychosocial well-being index. *Journal of Immigrant & Refugee Studies, 15*(1), 71–89.
Hollander, A.-C., Dal, H., Lewis, G., Magnusson, C., Kirkbride, J. B., & Dalman, C. (2016). Refugee migration and risk of schizophrenia and other non-affective psychoses: cohort study of 1.3 million people in Sweden. *BMJ, 352,* i1030.
Hollifield, M., Warner, T. D., Lian, N., Krakow, B., Jenkins, J. H., Kesler, J., et al. (2002). Measuring trauma and health status in refugees: A critical review. *JAMA, 288*(5), 611–621.
IASC. (2015). *Inter-agency standing committee (IASC) reference group for mental health and psychosocial support in emergency settings: Guidelines on mental health and psychosocial support in emergency settings*. Geneva: Inter-Agency Standing Committee.
Janoff-Bulman, R. (1985). The aftermath of victimization: Rebuilding shattered assumptions. *Trauma and Its Wake, 1,* 15–35.
Kirmayer, L. J., Kienzler, H., Afana, A. H., & Pedersen, D. (2010). Trauma and disasters in social and cultural context. *Principles of Social Psychiatry, 2,* 155–177.

Kleinman, A., & Good, B. (2004). Culture and depression. *New England Journal of Medicine, 351*, 951–952.
Kun, P., Chen, X., Han, S., Gong, X., Chen, M., Zhang, W., & Yao, L. (2009). Prevalence of post-traumatic stress disorder in Sichuan Province, China after the 2008 Wenchuan earthquake. *Public Health, 123*(11), 703–707.
Lambert, J. E., & Alhassoon, O. M. (2015). Trauma-focused therapy for refugees: Meta-analytic findings. *Journal of Counseling Psychology, 62*(1), 28.
Liddell, B. J., Nickerson, A., & Bryant, R. A. (2017). Clinical science and torture survivors' rights to rehabilitation. *The Lancet Psychiatry, 5*(2), 101–103.
Linton, R. (2015). A presumption of disclosure: Towards greater transparency in asylum proceedings. *Seattle UL Rev., 38*, 1069–1139.
Li, S. S., Liddell, B. J., & Nickerson, A. (2016). The relationship between post-migration stress and psychological disorders in refugees and asylum seekers. *Current Psychiatry Reports, 18*(9), 82.
Loizos, P. (2002). Misconceiving refugees. In R. Papadopoulos (Ed.), *Therapeutic care for refugees. No place like home* (pp. 41–56). Karnac
Luno, J. A., Beck, J. G., & Louwerse, M. (2013). Tell us your story: Investigating the linguistic features of trauma narrative. *The Cognitive Science Society, 35*, 2955–2960.
Lusk, M., & Baray, S. C. (2017). Mental health and the role of culture and resilience in refugees fleeing violence. *Environment and Social Psychology, 2*(1), 1–13.
Maercker, A., & Hecker, T. (2016). Broadening perspectives on trauma and recovery: A socio-interpersonal view of PTSD. *European Journal of Psychotraumatology, 7*, 29303.
Maercker, A., Brewin, C. R., Bryant, R. A., Cloitre, M., Reed, G. M., van Ommeren, M., et al. (2013). Proposals for mental disorders specifically associated with stress in the international classification of diseases-11. *The Lancet, 381*(9878), 1683–1685.
Maier, T. (2006). Procédure d'asile et rapports médicaux. *Bulletin des médecins suisses| Schweizerische Ärztezeitung| Bollettino dei medici svizzeri, 87*, 25.
Maier, T., & Straub, M. (2011). My head is like a bag full of rubbish: Concepts of illness and treatment expectations in traumatized migrants. *Qualitative Health Research, 21*(2), 233–248.
Maier, T., Schmidt, M., & Mueller, J. (2010). Mental health and healthcare utilization in adult asylum seekers. *Swiss Med Wkly, 140*, w13110.
Marlowe, J. M. (2010). Beyond the discourse of trauma: Shifting the focus on Sudanese refugees. *Journal of Refugee Studies, 23*(2), 183–198.
Marsella, A. J. (2010). Ethnocultural aspects of PTSD: An overview of concepts, issues, and treatments. *Traumatology, 16*(4), 17.
Marsella, A. J., Friedman, M. J., & Spain, E. H. (1996). *Ethnocultural aspects of posttraumatic stress disorder: Issues, research, and clinical applications*: American Psychological Association.
Mattar, S. (2011). Educating and training the next generations of traumatologists: Development of cultural competencies. *Psychological Trauma: Theory, Research, Practice, and Policy, 3*(3), 258–265.
Médecins Sans Frontières (M.S.F.). (2016). *Obstacle Course to Europe: A policy-made humanitarian crisis at EU borders*. Retrieved from https://www.msf.org/sites/msf.org/files/msf_obstacle_course_to_europe_0.pdf. On the February 12, 2020.
Miller, K., & Rasmussen, A. (2017). The mental health of civilians displaced by armed conflict: An ecological model of refugee distress. *Epidemiology and Psychiatric Sciences, 26*(2), 129–138.
Mollica, R., McInnes, K., Poole, C., & Tor, S. (1998). Dose-effect relationships of trauma to symptoms of depression and post-traumatic stress disorder among Cambodian survivors of mass violence. *The British Journal of Psychiatry, 173*(6), 482–488.
Momartin, S., Silove, D., Manicavasagar, V., & Steel, Z. (2003). Dimensions of trauma associated with posttraumatic stress disorder (PTSD) caseness, severity and functional impairment: A study of Bosnian refugees resettled in Australia. *Social Science and Medicine, 57*(5), 775.
Nickerson, A., Bryant, R. A., Brooks, R., Steel, Z., Silove, D., & Chen, J. (2011). The familial influence of loss and trauma on refugee mental health: A multilevel path analysis. *Journal of Traumatic Stress, 24*(1), 25–33.

Nickerson, A., Liddell, B., Asnaani, A., Carlsson, J., Fazel, M., Knaevelsrud, C., Morina, N., Neuner, F. Newnham, E., & Rasmussen, A. (2018) *Trauma and mental health in forcibly displaced populations: an International Society for Traumatic Stress Studies Briefing Paper*. ISTSS, Chicago. Retrieved from https://istss.org/getattachment/Education-Research/Briefing-Papers/Trauma-and-Mental-Health-in-Forcibly-Displaced-Pop/Displaced-Populations-Briefing-Paper_Final.pdf.aspx. On the February 12, 2020.

Nicolas, G., Wheatley, A., & Guillaume, C. (2015). Does one trauma fit all? Exploring the relevance of PTSD across cultures. *International Journal of Culture and Mental Health, 8*(1), 34–45.

O'Connor, K. (2015). Activity theory. In K. Tracy (Ed.), *International Encyclopedia of language and social interaction* (Vol. 1, pp. 27–34). Hoboken, NJ: John Wiley & Sons.

Papadopoulos, R. (2002a). Refugees, home and trauma. *Therapeutic care for refugees: no place like home, 9*.

Papadopoulos, R. (2002b). *Therapeutic care for refugees: No place like home*: Karnac Books.

Papadopoulos, R. (2007). Refugees, trauma and adversity-activated development. *European Journal of Psychotherapy and Counselling, 9*(3), 301–312.

Patel, N., Kellezi, B., & Williams, A. (2014). Psychological, social and welfare interventions for psychological health and well-being of torture survivors. *Cochrane Database of Systematic Reviews, 11,* Art. No.: CD009317.

Porter, M., & Haslam, N. (2005). Predisplacement and postdisplacement factors associated with mental health of refugees and internally displaced persons: A meta-analysis. *JAMA, 294*(5), 602–612.

Pratt, G., Johnston, C., & Banta, V. (2015). Filipino migrant stories and trauma in the transnational field. *Emotion, Space and Society, 24,* 83–92.

Rousseau, C., Drapeau, A., & Corin, E. (1997). The influence of culture and context on the pre- and post-migration experience of school-aged refugees from Central America and Southeast Asia in Canada. *Social Science & Medicine, 44*(8), 1115–1127.

Sabin, M., Cardozo, B. L., Nackerud, L., Kaiser, R., & Varese, L. (2003). Factors associated with poor mental health among Guatemalan refugees living in Mexico 20 years after civil conflict. *JAMA, 290*(5), 635–642.

Saul, J. (2013). *Collective trauma, collective healing: Promoting community resilience in the aftermath of disaster*. London: Routledge.

Schick, M., Zumwald, A., Knöpfli, B., Nickerson, A., Bryant, R. A., Schnyder, U., et al. (2016). Challenging future, challenging past: The relationship of social integration and psychological impairment in traumatised refugees. *European Journal of Psychotraumatology, 7*(1), 28057.

Schick, M., Morina, N., Mistridis, P., Schnyder, U., Bryant, R. A., & Nickerson, A. (2018). Changes in post-migration living difficulties predict treatment outcome in traumatized refugees. *Frontiers in Psychiatry, 9,* 476.

Schouler-Ocak, M., Wintrob, R., Moussaoui, D., Villasenor Bayardo, S. J., Zhao, X.-D., & Kastrup, M. C. (2016). Background paper on the needs of migrant, refugee and asylum seeker patients around the globe. *International Journal of Culture and Mental Health, 9*(3), 216–232.

Schweitzer, R., Melville, F., Steel, Z., & Lacherez, P. (2006). Trauma, post-migration living difficulties, and social support as predictors of psychological adjustment in resettled Sudanese refugees. *Australian and New Zealand Journal of Psychiatry, 2*(40), 179–187.

Sijbrandij, M., Acarturk, C., Bird, M., Bryant, R. A., Burchert, S., Carswell, K., et al. (2017). Strengthening mental health care systems for Syrian refugees in Europe and the Middle East: Integrating scalable psychological interventions in eight countries. *European Journal of Psychotraumatology, 8*(sup2), 1388102.

Silove, D., Steel, Z., McGorry, P., & Mohan, P. (1998). Trauma exposure, postmigration stressors, and symptoms of anxiety, depression and post-traumatic stress in Tamil asylum-seekers: Comparison with refugees and immigrants. *Acta Psychiatrica Scandinavica, 97*(3), 175–181.

Silove, D., Steel, Z., & Watters, C. (2000). Policies of deterrence and the mental health of asylum seekers. *JAMA, 284*(5), 604–611.

Silove, D., Ventevogel, P., & Rees, S. (2017). The contemporary refugee crisis: An overview of mental health challenges. *World Psychiatry, 16*(2), 130–139.
Sironi, F. (1999). *Bourreaux et victimes: psychologie de la torture*: Paris: Odile Jacob.
Sleijpen, M., Mooren, T., Kleber, R. J., & Boeije, H. R. (2017). Lives on hold: A qualitative study of young refugees' resilience strategies. *Childhood, 24*(3), 348–365.
Somasundaram, D. (2014). Addressing collective trauma: Conceptualisations and interventions. *Intervention, 12*(1), 43–60.
Song, S. J., Subica, A., Kaplan, C., Tol, W., & de Jong, J. (2017). Predicting the mental health and functioning of torture survivors. *The Journal of Nervous and Mental Disease, 206*(1), 33–39.
Squire, C. (2008). Experience-centred and culturally-oriented approaches to narrative. In M. Andrews, C. Squire, & M. Tamboukou (Eds.), *Doing narrative research* (pp. 42–63). London: Sage.
Staeuble, I. (2004). De-centering Western perspectives: Psychology and the disciplinary order in the first and third world. In A. C. Brock, J. Louw, & W. van Hoorn (Eds.), *Rediscovering the history of psychology: Essays inspired by the work of Kurt Danziger* (pp. 183–205). New York, NY: Kluwer.
Steel, Z. (2001). Beyond PTSD: Towards a more adequate understanding of the multiple effects of complex trauma. In C. Moser & D. Nyfeler (Eds.), *Traumatiserungen von Flüchtlingen und Asyl Schenden: Einflus des politischen, sozialen und medizinischen Kontextes* (pp. 66–84). Zurich: Seismo.
Steel, Z., Chey, T., Silove, D., Marnane, C., Bryant, R. A., & Ommeren, M. V. (2009). Association of torture and other potentially traumatic events with mental health outcomes among populations exposed to mass conflict and displacement: A systematic review and meta-analysis. *JAMA, 302*(5), 537–549.
Steel, J., Dunlavy, A., Harding, C., & Theorell, T. (2016). The psychological consequences of pre-emigration trauma and post-migration stress in refugees and immigrants from Africa. *Journal of Immigrant and Minority Health, 19*(3), 1–10.
Sturm, G., Baubet, T., & Moro, M. R. (2007). Mobilising social and symbolic resources in transcultural therapies with refugees and asylum seekers: The story of Mister Diallo. In B. Drožđek & J. Wilson (Eds.), *Voices of trauma: Treating psychological trauma across cultures* (pp. 211–231). New York: Springer.
Sturm, G., Baubet, T., & Moro, M. R. (2010). Culture, trauma, and subjectivity: The French ethnopsychoanalytic approach. *Traumatology, 16*(4), 27–38.
Summerfield, D. (1996). *L'impact de la Guerre et des Atrocités sur les Populations Civiles: Principes Fondamentaux pour les Interventions des ONG et une Analyse Critique des Projets sur le Traumatisme Psychosocial*. London: Overseas Development Institute.
Summerfield, D. (2000). Childhood, war, refugeedom and trauma: Three core questions for mental health professionals. *Transcultural Psychiatry, 37*(3), 417–433.
Summerfield, D. (2000b). Myths over the field of intervention. *Psychosocial*, 45. Retrieved from https://health.iom.int/sites/default/files/pdf/iom_notebook1.pdf#page=47. On the February 12, 2020.
Summerfield, D. (2001). The invention of post-traumatic stress disorder and the social usefulness of a psychiatric category. *British Medical Journal, 322*(7278), 95–98.
Tang, C.S.-K. (2007). Culturally relevant meanings and their implications on therapy for traumatic grief: Lessons learned from a Chinese female client and her fortune-teller. In B. Drožđek & J. P. Wilson (Eds.), *Voices of trauma: Treating psychological trauma across cultures* (pp. 127–150). New York: Springer.
Tessitore, F., & Margherita, G. (2017). A review of Asylum Seekers and Refugees in Italy: Where is the psychological research going? *Mediterranean Journal of Clinical Psychology, 5*(2).
Tol, W. A., Barbui, C., Bisson, J., Cohen, J., Hijazi, Z., Jones, L., et al. (2014). World Health Organization guidelines for management of acute stress, PTSD, and bereavement: Key challenges on the road ahead. *PLoS Med, 11*(12), e1001769.

Tummala-Narra, P. (2007). Conceptualizing trauma and resilience across diverse contexts. *Journal of Aggression, Maltreatment and Trauma, 14*(1–2), 33–53.
Turrini, G., Purgato, M., Ballette, F., Nosè, M., Ostuzzi, G., & Barbui, C. (2017). Common mental disorders in asylum seekers and refugees: Umbrella review of prevalence and intervention studies. *International Journal of Mental Health Systems, 11*(1), 51.
Ungar, M. (2004). A constructionist discourse on resilience: Multiple contexts, multiple realities among at-risk children and youth. *Youth and Society, 35*(3), 341–365.
Ungar, M. (2008). Resilience across cultures. *The British Journal of Social Work, 38*(2), 218–235.
Ungar, M. (2011). The social ecology of resilience: Addressing contextual and cultural ambiguity of a nascent construct. *American Journal of Orthopsychiatry, 81*(1), 1–17.
UNHCR. (2015). *The sea route to Europe: The mediterranean passage in the age of refugees.* Geneva: United Nations High Commissioner for Refugees.
Van Ommeren, M., de Jong, J. M., Sharma, B., Komproe, I., Thapa, S. B., & Cardeña, E. (2001). Psychiatric disorders among tortured bhutanese refugees in nepal. *Archives of General Psychiatry, 58*(5), 475–482. https://doi.org/10.1001/archpsyc.58.5.475.
Ventevogel, P., Ryan, G. K., Kahi, V., & Kane, J. C. (2019). Capturing the essential: Revising the mental health categories in UNHCR's refugee health information system. *Intervention, 17*(1), 13–22.
Viñar, M. N. (2005). La spécificité de la torture comme source de trauma. *Revue Française De Psychanalyse, 69*(4), 1205–1224.
Wang, S. (2012). Analyses sociologiques des pratiques de l'interprétariat-médiation en pédopsychiatrie: l'exemple des familles d'origine chinoise à Paris. *Enfances and Psy, 3,* 136–145.
Wang, S. (2016). Aidez-nous à comprendre vos Chinois! *Genèses, 4,* 141–156.
Wasco, S. M. (2003). Conceptualizing the harm done by rape applications of trauma theory to experiences of sexual assault. *Trauma, Violence, & Abuse, 4*(4), 309–322.
Watters, C. (2001). Emerging paradigms in the mental health care of refugees. *Social Science and Medicine, 52*(11), 1709–1718.
Weine, S., Kuc, G., Eldin, D., Razzano, L., & Pavkovic, I. (2001). PTSD among Bosnian refugees: A survey of providers' knowledge, attitudes and service patterns. *Community Mental Health Journal, 37*(3), 261–271.
Weissbecker, I., Hanna, F., El Shazly, M., Gao, J., & Ventevogel, P. (2018). Integrative mental health and psychosocial support interventions for refugees in humanitarian crisis settings. In T. Wenzel & B. Droždek (Eds.), *An uncertain safety: Integrative health care for the 21st century refugees* (pp. 117–153). New York: Springer.
Wenzel, T., & Droždek, B. (2018). *An uncertain safety: Integrative health care for the 21st century refugees.* New York: Springer.
Wilson, J. P., & Droždek, B. (2004). *Broken spirits: The treatment of traumatized asylum seekers, refugees and war and torture victims.* London: Routledge.
Wilson, J. P., Droždek, B., & Turkovic, S. (2006). Posttraumatic shame and guilt. *Trauma, Violence, and Abuse, 7*(2), 122–141.
Young, A. (1995). *The harmony of illusions.* Princeton: Princeton University Press.
Zittoun, T. (2017). Modalities of generalization through single case studies. *Integrative Psychological and Behavioral Science, 51*(2), 171–194.

Chapter 2
Trauma and Migration

Over the past two decades, there has been an increasing interest in the question of trauma among refugee populations. This body of research has largely focused on the immediate psychological aftermaths of armed conflicts in light of the well-described associations between these psychiatric disorders, displacement, and generalized forms of violence (Morina et al., 2018). In general, the literature attests to the greater mental health difficulties among refugees compared to general populations within host communities. High levels of post-traumatic stress, anxiety and depression have been documented, as well as other mental health issues such as psychosomatic disorders, grief related disorders and crises of existential meaning (Copping et al., 2010; de Arellano & Danielson, 2008; Kirmayer et al., 2010; Lambert & Alhassoon, 2015; Morina et al., 2018; Schweitzer et al., 2006; Steel et al., 2009; Sturm et al., 2010; Van Ommeren et al., 2001; Weine et al., 2001). Significant rates of medically unexplained pain and somatoform disorder have also been highlighted (Droždek et al., 2003; Van Ommeren et al., 2001).

This high prevalence of mental health problems is not surprising. Refugees are typically exposed to a multitude of traumas—not only in their countries of origin but all along their migration journey (Crepet et al., 2017). As summarized by Neace et al. (2020)

> refugees are also people who have survived the severe trauma not only of whatever caused them to flee their homelands in their first place – things like war, famine, genocide, natural disaster—but of all of the trauma associated with fleeing. Their contexts tend to be of the need-thwarting type, and most refugees do not leave their home by choice, causing a loss of autonomy (p. 13).

Yet, increasingly, studies focusing on pre-migration traumas exclusively have been criticized for a skewed focus on isolated traumatic events experienced pre-migration. The argument is that this focus neglects the repeated and prolonged stressors to which refugee communities are typically exposed. In a recent key critical review of the literature, Hynie (2018) concludes that.

G. Theisen-Womersley, *Trauma and Resilience Among Displaced Populations*,
https://doi.org/10.1007/978-3-030-67712-1_2

> historically, the focus of mental health research and interventions with these populations has been on the impact of pre-migration trauma. Pre-migration trauma does predict mental disorders and PTSD, but the post-migration context can be an equally powerful determinant of mental health. Moreover, post-migration factors may moderate the ability of refugees to recover from pre-migration trauma. (p. 297).

Research over the past decade is indeed starting to shift focus towards the impact of the post-migration environment on the mental health of refugees (Korup Kjærgaard & Koitzsch Jensen, 2018; Li et al., 2016). Unsurprisingly, this research has highlighted the importance of post-migration factors in predicting the maintenance of PTSD symptoms in resettled refugees—including unemployment, family separation, constant mobility and ongoing conflict in the country of origin (Lie, 2002; Schick et al., 2016). The respective impact of these potentially traumatic stress factors continues to be the subject of increased debate. Some scholars argue that exposure to extreme stressors such as war trauma or torture is the strongest predictor of PTSD, whilst others have argued that it is the impact of post-migration stressors upon resettlement in the host country (Song et al., 2015).

In this chapter, I present an overview of the literature examining the factors which influence trauma among refugee populations both pre-, peri- and post-migration. The trauma experienced by refugees during these three stages of migration has been referred to in the literature as the "triple trauma paradigm" (TTP), where "through each of these stages the refugee or asylum seeker experiences and re-experiences the traumatic events, events that vary during each stage and depend on the particular adverse circumstances and situations they confront" (Ringler-Jayanthan et al., 2020, p. 82). As useful as it is to highlight the factors characterising each phase of the migration journey, what we need to bear in mind (as we embark on this "mapping") is the interrelation of all of these factors. There is evidently a dynamic, complex and ongoing exchange between all of them—a point to which I return later on in the chapter.

Pre-migration

Given the very nature of the refugee experience, many refugees by definition have been exposed to a variety of traumatic experiences prior to leaving their country of origin—including trauma related to war and conflict, persecution, violence and torture experienced by themselves as well as loved ones. Among a sample of 420 refugees living in Sweden, Steel and colleagues (2016) found that 89% reported having experienced at least one traumatic experience prior to migration. Common sense would dictate that some of the most significant pre-migration factors related to PTSD would be that of exposure to wartime atrocities inherent to contexts of conflict—a hypothesis which has unsurprisingly been well documented in the literature (Bogic et al., 2012; Heeren et al., 2014; Morina et al., 2018). Several studies have indicated a robust dose–response relationship of trauma to the development of PTSD (Kartal & Kiropoulos, 2016; Mollica et al., 1998; Momartin et al., 2003; Silove, 1999; Silove et al., 1998; Steel et al., 2009).

Torture

Torture represents an extraordinary exception in the psychopathology field. Past torture is well documented to be a particularly triggering factor for PTSD It is consistently shown in the literature to be significantly and consistently associated with emotional distress, even years after the event (Carlsson et al., 2006; Hodges-Wu & Zajicek-Farber, 2017; Kira, 2010; Le et al., 2018; Liddell et al., 2017). This is particularly true in the case of prolonged exposure to multiple types of torture (Song et al., 2015, 2017). Research indicates that it is the perceived uncontrollable nature of, rather than the exposure to, torture, which most accurately predicts PTSD (Le et al., 2018; Liddell et al., 2017). The variety of complex psychological responses to torture, linked to higher prevalence of PTSD, include alterations in emotion regulation capacity (notably anger), impaired interpersonal processing, reduced perceptions of control, and identity loss (Liddell et al., 2017). The particularity of torture as pathogenic is linked to the fact that the act itself is taught, organized, elaborated, and perpetrated by humans against other humans (Sironi, 1999; Viñar, 2005a). It destroys the fabric of the social network of which we humans form an integral part. It disrupts our connection to all that make us human. Moreover, it is another human being who has deliberately constructed this unimaginable madness (Goguikian Ratcliff & Strasser, 2009; Viñar, 2005a).

Kirmayer and colleagues (2018) highlight the fact that it is the moral emotions (shame, guilt and humiliation) that are intently used to inflict the most damage in torture. Such moral emotions inevitably reflect the cultural systems of meaning:

> All forms of torture follow an affective logic rooted both in human biology and in local social and cultural meanings of experience. Understanding the impact of specific forms of torture on individuals requires knowledge of their learning histories, and of the personal and cultural meanings of specific kinds of violence. Exploring cultural meanings requires attention to over-arching discourse, embodied practices, and everyday engagements with an ecosocial environment (p. 84)

To reflect on the consequences of torture from an ecological, social and cultural perspective, they present a model of adaptive systems affected by torture (p. 87): Table 2.1

As indicated by the model, the psychopathologic disorder of the survivor cannot be reduced to the intrapsychic plane. It is not an individual act, but a social one. It does not only have individual consequences, but social, legal, and political ones for those who survive. It damages different spheres of an individual including body, personality, hope, aspirations for life, identity, integrity, belief systems, the sense of being grounded and attached to a family and society, autonomy, community relationships, and a sense of safety. It recreates a social order colored by suspicion, shame, and

Table. 2.1 Adaptive systems affected by torture

Adaptive system	Threats	Emotional reactions	Psychopathology	Interventions
Attachment	Separation from significant others, and culture	Anxiety Grief home sickness Nostalgia	Anxiety depression complicated grief	Re-connection with loved ones mourning creation of new bondss membership in social groups recreating community systems
Security	Uncertainty loss of control	Anxiety insecurity Hypervigi lance	Anxiety PTSD	Re-assert control over self and environment
Identity/role	Loss of social and occupational roles and status Misrecognition, identity	Powerlessness, shame and humiliation	Suicidality role confusion	Recognition of status and identity opportunities for meaningful action family interventions community membership human right protection social security
Justice	Sense of injustice, arbitrary violence Impunity	Anger, hostility lack of trust resentment bitterness	Traumatic anger Paranoia	Engagement trust redevelopment family trust redevelopment Truth and reconciliation human rights protection
Existential meaning	Loss of sense of coherence, purpose, and hope for future	Search for meaning	Alienation disengagement crisis of faith transgenerational transmission	Testimonial approach, telling one's story re-engagement in life projects linking with culture, community and religious traditions political activism

Adapted from Silove (1999,2007), Ekblad and Jaranson (2004), and Kirmayer et al. (2010)

secrecy (Barudy, 1989). Family disruptions, collective fear and community dysfunction and decomposition have all been noted in the literature as consequences of trauma (Barudy, 1989; Hodges-Wu & Zajicek-Farber, 2017). As noted by Liddell and colleagues (2017), General Comment 3 of the United Nations Committee Against Torture published on Dec 13, 2012 (which explains the signatory States' responsibilities under Article 14 of the UN Convention Against Torture and Other Cruel, Inhuman and Degrading Treatment or Punishment) is significant in that it explicitly recognises that the effects of torture extend beyond individuals to encompass their immediate families and dependents. These far-reaching effects may interact and manifest in complex and diverse ways, mediated by culture, gender and other aspects of the context of the torture survivor, the context of torture and the context of the recovery environment (Esala et al., 2018; Patel et al., 2014).

Migration

It is not only what is lost in leaving one's home but similarly *t*he migration experience itself which necessarily disrupts family and cultural systems and separations from the family and ethnic community, including stays in unsafe refugee camps during the migration process (Lambert & Alhassoon, 2015). Arriving in Europe, and often not necessarily to the country of their choice, some refugees arrive and are fighting to stay—yet some soon discover that things are not quite as expected and realise they must either go back or proceed to another destination (Gkionakis, 2016). Nathan (1986 as cited in Sturm et al., 2010) argues that the experience of migration is necessarily traumatic—as the "cultural envelope" can no longer hold traumatic, non-elaborated or psychically 'indigestible' experiences. In a multi-agency guidance note released in 2015 in collaboration with the UNHCR (MHPSS, 2015), the following factors related to the mental health of refugees and migrants during migration were observed and noted by a conglomerate of humanitarian aid agencies:

> Refugees and migrants who come to Europe often faced war, persecution and extreme hardships in their countries of origin. Many experienced displacement and hardship in transit countries and embarked on dangerous travels. Lack of information, uncertainty about immigration status, potential hostility, changing policies, undignified and protracted detention all add additional stress. Forced migration erodes pre-migration protective supports – like those provided by extended family – and may challenge cultural, religious and gender identities. Forced migration requires multiple adaptations in short periods of time. People - especially but not only - children, become more vulnerable to abuse and neglect. Pre-existing social and mental health problems can be exacerbated. Importantly, the way people are received and how protection and assistance is provided may induce or aggravate problems, for example by undermining human dignity, discouraging mutual support and creating dependency. (p. 3).

Among a cohort of 200 asylum seekers attending a centre run by *Médecins Sans Frontières* (2016) in Italy, 86.9% said that they experiences difficulties in post-migration life—difficulties which were significantly associated with a diagnosis of PTSD The most common difficulties in life during the asylum seeking period were found to be "the feeling of uncertainty and fear for the future" (18.8%), "concern for the family back home" (13.8%), "conflicts within the authorities" (11%), "fear of the asylum request being rejected" (8.8%), "the feeling of being neglected" (7.2%), "the inability to integrate and feel integrated"(7.7%), "prolonged waiting times for the [asylum] Commission's outcomes" (5.5%), "lack of daily activities" (3.9%), "a sense of loneliness and boredom" (2.2%) and, to a lesser extent, other difficulties such a widespread sense of injustice and feeling unable to control events.

This is a period which Métraux (1999a) has described as suspended or "mute" time, which he defines as "being absent from all temporality, the social time of [refugees] being also a waiting period, a suspended time, a time dissolved in the heart of an indeterminable parenthesis[1]" (p. 52), a temporary immobility which only either a forced expulsion, or a negative or positive response to the request for asylum would be able to end.

Requesting Asylum

The majority of research regarding forced migration and mental health has focused on refugees, with a more limited number of studies looking at asylum seekers. While there is a crucial difference in the legal status of refugees and asylum seekers, only few scholars have made a distinction between the two in examining risk factors for mental health problems (Georgiadou et al., 2018; Nakash et al., 2017). In general, the little research that exists does indeed attest to the impact of legal status on mental health, in particular prevalence rates of PTSD (Georgiadou et al., 2018). Among such scholars exploring this is Betty Goguikian Ratcliff (2016; Womersley et al., 2017). She identifies the period before and after being granted asylum as being two distinct periods in the psychological lives of migrants, noting that both stages involve substantial psychological stress, but for different reasons. She identifies the following stressors related to the period in which asylum is sought:

- Delays in the processing of asylum application
- Fear of repatriation
- Exclusion from the labor market
- Forced dependence on social welfare
- Loneliness, boredom
- Discrimination, marginalization
- Poor housing conditions
- Prolonged uncertainty, insecurity, lack of control.

[1] My own loose translation.

These factors are further confounded by unstable conditions wherein individuals may be forced into a rhythm of perpetual displacement. Many are moved from one center to another, experiencing delayed asylum procedures and poor living conditions in reception centers—often poorly accessible by public transport to main economic and social hubs. Left with a life in limbo, activities of social integration and personal development are hindered under such conditions. The longer one waits for asylum, the less likely one is to find employment (Hynie, 2018), and the higher the risk for psychopathology (Laban et al., 2004). Furthermore, a recent meta-review observed associations between length of stay in asylum centres and poor mental health (Korup Kjærgaard & Koitzsch Jensen, 2018).

Hauswirth and colleagues (2004) identify the following specific stressors related to the request for asylum:

- applying for asylum involves a submission of oneself to more powerful authorities, without necessarily have knowledge of the language and administrative functioning necessary to be able to keep a sense of control over key decisions.
- the seemingly random assignment to a place of residence, the obligation to to stay in a center, are all related to a loss of freedom and perceived control.
- access to the labour market is made difficult during this period because the individual is unable to guarantee the prospective employer a commitment in the long run because of its status.

A sense of de-individuation and diminishing feelings of self-worth and self-esteem may be exacerbated by the *"en masse"* treatment of migrants as they enter the host country. In research conducted among refugees and asylum seekers on the Greek island of Lesbos, Eleftherakos and colleagues (2018) noted that the "elimination of each individual's identity was quoted by many migrants while the response to questions regarding information about their cases or complaints regarding living conditions was usually answered with another insult." (p. 5). Maier and Straub (2011) unpack the psychological impact of this loss of identity: "through extreme trauma and forced migration, the [asylum seekers] seemed to be thrown back to a biographical 'zero' point from which they had to almost redefine their entire identity. The severity of their trauma and loss probably exceeded what any individual, social, cultural, and religious concept available could explain and integrate" (p. 243). Despite the fact that the majority of participants in their study attributed the main source of their current suffering to earlier traumatization, one third identified their actual living situation as the essential cause of their traumatic stress, more specifically the harsh conditions in the asylum-seekers camp which lead them to feel trapped, unconfident and with "a dark future" (p. 239).

It is not difficult to imagine that living with constant fear of authorities could similarly trigger old fears related to traumatic events experienced in the countries of origin as well as during the migration period. In examining trauma among asylum seekers on the island of Lesbos in Greece, research conducted by a team from *Médecins Sans Frontières* (Eleftherakos et al., 2018) noted that the majority of participants reported living in a context characterised by (a) a state of permanent emergency, (b) preoccupation with threats on present and future, and (c) absence of protective measures.

Such a state of existence, they argue, is related to the concept of continuous traumatic stress, a concept notably developed by South African researchers (Eagle & Kaminer, 2013) to describe the psychological impact of being continuously exposed to traumatic stressors over an extended period of time. Living under continual threat of repatriation thus serves to reinforce a compromised and precarious political, social and economic position which significantly influences mental health (Bogic et al., 2012; Heeren et al., 2014; Kirmayer, 2001; Porter & Haslam, 2005; Silove et al., 1998). Put simply, the fear does not end.

Given the factors mentioned above, it is therefore no surprise that an insecure residency status has been shown in the literature to be one of the strongest predictor of mental health disorders (Heeren et al., 2014; Hynie, 2018; Momartin et al., 2003; Morgan, Melluish, & Welham). As noted in a key review by Nickerson and colleagues (2018), such an insecure status associated with impaired interpersonal functioning and persistent worry and social withdrawal. These may in turn exacerbate PTSD and depression symptoms regardless of pre-migration trauma. Indeed, a convincing body of literature clearly attests to the fact that stressors associated with the process of seeking asylum contribute to elevated psychological distress, including PTSD symptomatology (Nickerson et al., 2018).

Prolonged Detention

In a comprehensive review on the impact of mandatory, indefinite detention on the mental health of asylum seekers, commissioned as part of the independent review of policies and procedures affecting the welfare of those held in immigration removal centres in the United Kingdom (Bosworth, 2016), the following conclusions were drawn:

- Literature from across all the different bodies of work and jurisdictions consistently finds evidence of a negative impact of detention on the mental health of detainees.
- The risk increases the longer detention persists.
- The mental health impact endures long after release.
- Causes identified in the literature include pre-existing trauma (including torture and sexual violence); pre-existing mental and physical health problems; and poor healthcare and mental health care services in detention.

Their findings are echoed elsewhere in the literature (Korup Kjærgaard & Koitzsch Jensen, 2018; Loizos, 2002; Mueller et al., 2011; Robjant et al., 2009). A similar comprehensive review by Silove and colleagues (2007) highlights that the substantial issues related to mental health and prolonged detention include restricted access to work, education, housing, welfare, health care services, abuse, untreated medical and psychiatric illnesses, suicidal behaviour, hunger strikes, and outbreaks of violence reported among asylum seekers in detention centres. Another meta-review of the literature further highlights extended period of time in asylum detention centres, and the number of relocations as significant factors impacting mental health (Korup Kjærgaard & Koitzsch Jensen, 2018).

Court Proceedings

Typically following the period of detention is the court proceeding, which risks being a traumatic event in and of itself. The recent findings of Schock and colleagues (2015) working at a centre for victims of torture in Germany, revealed the stressful impact of asylum interviews on refugees which lead to a significance increase in post-traumatic intrusions. They and other authors have hypothesised that a deliberate avoidance of thinking of traumatic events initially serves as a survival strategy during the migration period, yet may be ruthlessly undermined during the testimony phase of a court hearing, consequently fostering significant potential for re-traumatisation (Jakobsen et al., 2017; Nickerson et al., 2018; Rogers, Fox, & Herlihy, 2015; Turner, 1992; Turner, 2015).

There is also an increasing body of scientific evidence looking at the assumptions recorded by authorities in their asylum decisions and the psychological processes at play during the court proceeding. This literature suggests not only that there may be marked uncertainty in how to reach the correct determination but also that there is often the potential for bias against the person genuinely fleeing from trauma and persecution, with mental health problems negatively impacting on the credibility and consistency of their verbal accounts (Bögner et al., 2010; Herlihy & Turner, 2018; Linton, 2015; Mueller et al., 2011; Rogers et al., 2015; Schock et al., 2015; Turner, 1992; Turner, 2015). Bögner et al. (2010), for example, investigated factors related to the disclosure of personal sensitive information during asylum interviews and found that those with a history of exposure to traumatic events (in this study, namely sexual violence) reported more difficulties in disclosing personal information in a coherent manner. The catch-22, as Linton (2015) notes, is that an acceptable demeanour and coherent and credible story remains the basis of being granted asylum:

> Asylum seekers from oppressive regimes may have learned to distrust government officials and may be hesitant or frightened when speaking to authorities. Women in particular may have been taught not to make eye contact and not to reveal private details to strangers. These experiences and cultural norms may cause an applicant to look down, appear nervous and distrustful, sweat excessively, and hesitate during her hearing—all things that could lead an IJ to believe, based on her demeanour, that she is not telling the truth… Ironically, the fraudulent applicant is better situated to relate a detailed story with appropriate demeanour than the genuine applicant (p. 1085).

Paradoxically, trauma may decrease an asylum seekers' capacity to recount a coherent narrative of their lives—the very coherence needed for "credibility," for their claim to asylum to be believed (Herlihy & Turner, 2018). The high potential for asylum seekers not to be believed during the court proceeding and for their claim to be denied inevitably leads to a situation of increasing physical and psychological vulnerability. For victims of torture and other atrocities, both individual and collective, the responses of criminal and social justice systems in particular may also be importantly implicated in whether people transcend or continue to suffer the impact of traumatic stressors (Eagle, 2014).

Being Denied Asylum

As demonstrated by Mueller and colleagues (2011), failed asylum seekers showed as much severely affected mental health as pending and temporarily accepted asylum seekers. These are the trapped "invisible" (Sanchez-Mazas et al., 2011), coping with the daily threat of forced expulsion. Apart from the obvious physical, legal and material implications of not being granted refugee status, the psychological impact of the court proceedings, of not having one's story believed and subsequently being branded 'illegal,' is one of many inter-related factors negatively impacting on the mental health of the immigrant. As stated by Sturm et al. (2007):

> With migrant populations, we do not only have to work on loss, rupture and bereavement but also on the experience of feeling oneself 'outside humanity,' when the individual has lost confidence in others and may carry feelings of guilt and shame... The outcome of the asylum process is of major importance for the mental health of asylum seekers. It is linked to the recognition or not of the testimony (validation or not of experiences), the experience of being recognised as a victim of violence and injustice may be extremely supportive. At the same time, once the individual feels that he or she is in a secure place, they may be overwhelmed with traumatic memories or depressive feelings. Some experience guilt or shame in relation to those whom they have left behind. Others have to deal with the traumatic memories the current situation evokes (for example, not being granted asylum and fearing for the police, not having food or money or shelter… (p. 213-216)

The result is a loss of all one's bearings, a sense of absurdity, a misunderstanding. the situation in the face of doubts regarding the veracity of the abuse they suffered (Hauswirth et al., 2004).

Post-migration

Many stress factors related to seeking asylum mentioned above may indeed be alleviated by obtaining refugee status. However, after months or years of suspended and uncertain lives, this is a period where refugees are required to quickly adjust and integrate into their new environment. During this transition, many may lose access to benefits specifically allocated to asylum seekers (accommodation, social services, financial aid, etc.). As refugees, they are now expected to fully participate in a new sociocultural environment and locally reconstruct their lives, all the while maintaining their cultural identity. During this stage, new stressors specifically related to this stage of the migration journey may be encountered. Saechao and colleagues (2012), for example, identify six primary stressors during the post-migration phase: economic hardships, discrimination, acculturation due to language differences, enculturation, parenting differences, and finding suitable employment. Among one cohort of refugees diagnosed with PTSD, such stressors were deemed to impact 39% of sessions with treating clinicians (Bruhn et al., 2018). As noted by Goguikian Ratcliff (2009), a plethora of studies exist which convincingly demonstrate that psychological, social and cultural difficulties encountered in the host country after arrival have a more significant impact on mental health than pre-migration exposure to traumatic events.

Reception in the Host Country

Post-migration experiences, such as unemployment, insecure residency, fear of repatriation, and social discrimination have similarly been shown in the literature to be significantly correlated with mental problems in refugees (Bogic et al., 2012; Loizos, 2002; Tekin et al., 2016; Volkan, 2004; Watters, 2001). Volkan (2004) refers to the "Janus-face" (p. 14) reception of refugees by the host society, representing them as at once victims/heroes as well as diseased intruders. As numbers of migrants into Europe swell, attitudes harden with the transforming anti-migration political rhetoric that positions refugees as an economic and social threat. He argues that this serves to remodel refugees' self-representations as they struggle with the process of integrating the new culture with the old and with the "survivor guilt" of having left loved ones at home in danger in the country of origin.

In a recent review of the literature, Kartal and Kiripoulos (2016) note that the relationships between traumatic events, migration, and mental health outcomes upon arrival in the host country are complex and poorly understood. Acculturative stress within the sample of refugees they examined was associated with greater experiences of cultural loss and nostalgia. This loss itself was found to exacerbate PTSD symptoms. They suggest that the influence of post-migratory demands on mental health differs not only based on the individual's acculturation process alone. It also depends on the characteristics of the local context reflecting the acculturative preferences of the host society. The authors highlight these findings as a confirmation of Berry's (Berry, 1997, 2003; Sam & Berry, 2010) acculturation model which delineates the mechanisms through which the host society impacts on the acculturation process of refugees by imposing either encouraging or less desirable acculturative strategies (either encouraging or oppose ethnic diversity and participation in the larger society) which in turn influences mental health. This model has been confirmed elsewhere in the literature: multiple comparative studies examining correlations between the post-migration context and refugees from the same country of origin yet who have resettled in different countries convincingly demonstrate the significant effect of post-migratory factors on symptoms of PTSD Bogic and colleagues (2012) for example, assessed 854 war refugees from the former Yugoslavia having resettled across three countries. They found higher rates of PTSD to be significantly associated with migration-related stress and having a temporary resident permit. Similarly, Kartal and Kiropoulos (2016) assessed a sample of 138 Bosnian refugees resettled in both Austria and Australia. After controlling for age, sex, and exposure to traumatic events, acculturative stress associated with post-migratory experiences predicted severity of PTSD Acceptance of the host society matters.

Multiple Losses and Social Isolation

As summarized by Fox (Fox, 2018):

> They [refugees] have suffered unimaginable loss of family, friends, home, community, country and language. Once here, they find themselves subjected to poverty and discrimination as well as a loss of self-esteem, status and identity. Some demonstrate remarkable resilience and fortitude in facing psychological pain, dislocation and hardship…they remain in contact with a life force , a good internal object, that enables them to tolerate and endure these privations and losses. For some asylum seekers who are less resilient, it is the loss of contact with a supportive internal relationship that depletes their capacity for resilience, leaving them inadequately resourced to face and endure the realities of their situation. (p. 103)

In the process of migration, refugees suffer numerous losses, such as economic stability, familiar surroundings, and relationships that hinder their ability to thrive in their new place of settlement. The literature highlights one of the most powerful stressors experienced by refugees after arrival in the host country as being social isolation, typically associated with ongoing family separation, loss, and a breakdown in familiar social and community structures (Miller & Rasmussen, 2017; Nickerson et al., 2018; Schouler-Ocak et al., 2016). Among a cohort of refugees in Holland, 78% expressed an unmet need for company (Strijk et al., 2011). Among a cohort of refugees in Australia, such isolation emerged as a major predictor of PTSD and other mental health challenges (Chen et al., 2017). Perceived social support has been shown to serve as a significant moderator in the relationship between exposure to traumatic events and PTSD symptoms among asylum seekers (Nakash et al., 2017; Schweitzer et al., 2006). In a study among African asylum seekers in Israel, social support was associated with lower prevalence rates of PTSD (except in the case of extreme exposure to traumatic events where social support did not have a substantial impact) (Nakash et al., 2017).

As refugees struggle to maintain cultural identities and networks (Watters, 2001), such isolation brings the further risk of losing the "social capital" (Lecerof et al., 2015; Loizos, 2002; Tortelli et al., 2017) inherent to resources associated with economic status as well as social and professional identity. The loss of social capital, exacerbated by social discrimination and marginalization, has similarly been linked to poorer mental health outcomes (Brand et al., 2017).

Continual Exposure to Trauma

Research evidence suggests that refugees are continually exposed to multiple, sometimes extreme traumas such as torture, rape, or death of family members (Hollander et al., 2016; Kartal & Kiropoulos, 2016; Steel, 2001; Steel et al., 2009; ter Heide et al., 2016). In a recent analysis of all crimes reported across Switzerland from 2009–2012, Coutennier and colleagues (2016) discovered that cohorts exposed to civil conflicts/mass killings during childhood are on average 40 percent more prone to violent crimes than their co-nationals born after the conflict. Furthermore, their analysis showed that conflict exposed cohorts have a higher propensity to target victims from their own nationality. Rousseau and colleagues (1997) similarly found that the culture of origin radically modulated the relationship between the pre-migration experience and the developing post-migration universe of refugees—mediated through experiences of torture in countries of origin leading to increased levels of violence and social isolation subsequently perpetuated within the family post-migration. Indeed, continuous or sustained exposure to trauma has been found to create a life condition that increases risk of exposure to a multiplicity of types of traumatic events (ter Heide et al., 2016). Furthermore, there is substantial evidence in the literature that refugees suffering from PTSD in the aftermath of an initial trauma are vulnerable to increased PTSD symptoms after subsequently experiencing a new traumatic event or ongoing daily stressors (Schock et al., 2016).

Unemployment

Many consider the lack of employment to add further fuel to this fire: unemployment and unstable working conditions do not only present serious economic challenges, but have understandable negative consequences for social integration and psychological well-being (Kartal & Kiropoulos, 2016; Goguikian Ratcliff & Rossi, 2015; Schick et al., 2016; Silove et al., 1998). As noted by Du and Winter (2020), "not only does unemployment itself threaten one's identity and role in society, but the lack of recognition for one's skills and prior career path can lead to further losses of one's sense of self" (p. 39). Goguikian Ratcliff and colleagues (2014) allude to the phenomenon of 'deskilling' which they found to exist among refugee populations. They define this as a downgrade in terms of professional skills and educational levels of achievement recognised in the host country as compared to existing experiences in countries of origin. They attribute the phenomenon in part to restrictive institutional practices anchored in discriminatory legislation, institutional practices, and social representations of refugees. The difficulty in finding employment, deskilling, social isolation, and the significant differences between the pre-migration work expectations and encountered reality on the labor market upon arrival are likely to produce feelings of discouragement, injustice, self-deprecation, social and occupational worthlessness, and lack of satisfaction and, ultimately, are likely to harm mental health.

Referring to the psychological consequences of this lack of agency inherent to situations of unemployment, Holzkamp (2013) states:

> Each individual's existential orientation is a subjective aspect of the type and degree of her/his agency – that is, opportunities to act and constraints on those opportunities. Human suffering or, generally, any injury, including anxiety, has the quality of being exposed to and dependent upon other - directed circumstances, dissociated from possibilities of controlling essential, long-term conditions, i.e. constraints on possibilities to act… a real improvement in the subjective quality of my life is synonymous with enhanced influence over my objective life conditions – that is, with my opportunities for forming alliances, i.e. uniting with others. (pp. 20–21).

He continues to argue that 'by attempting to obtain some discretion to act through participating in power and utilizing the allowed leeway, one concurrently confirms and reinforces the conditions of one's own dependency.' (p. 24). The implication is that an insecure residency status dependant on being vouchsafed by the particular authorities could be rescind at any time and only serves to perpetuate unequal power relations and negate legitimate freedom to act. The impact is two-pronged: the lack of employment opportunities has inevitable socio-economic consequences which in turn affect mental health—on top of being potentially socially demeaning or devaluing which in turn affects self-worth (Hynie, 2018). A meta-analysis of 56 reports published from 1959 to 2002, representing 22 221 refugees, found that mental health status was worse among those living in institutional accommodation or with restricted economic opportunity (Porter & Haslam, 2005). Successful recovery from traumatic experiences depends to a large extent on the social, political and economic conditions and opportunities in the receiving country (Heeren et al., 2014).

Race-Related Trauma

A plethora of research has demonstrated the psychological impact of discrimination and racism experienced by migrants in general (Akhtar, 1999; Kartal & Kiropoulos, 2016; Goguikian Ratcliff et al., 2014). Visible minority status leads to more post-migratory psychosocial adversity (Hollander et al., 2016) and even more so when it comes as a surprisingly new and disorienting experience (Akhtar, 1999). Indeed, race-based traumatic stress has been demonstrated to be significantly related to trauma reactions (e.g., dissociation, anxiety, depression, sexual problems, and sleep disturbance), especially in instances where individuals have endorsed negative race-based experiences as stressful. This race-based traumatic stress model is based on empirical evidence from the racial discrimination, discrimination, race-related stress, and life-event research literatures. Empirical evidence has been generated in support of the construct and measurement of race-based traumatic stress (Carter et al., 2017). Research confirms that stigmatization (linked to discrimination and racism) is strongly associated with a higher prevalence of current and lifetime PTSD, a decreased likelihood of spontaneous remission and lower therapy success beyond the well-known effect of trauma load (Schneider et al., 2018).

This literature highlights how, especially among refugees, there are many subtle and complex stressors linked to race-based trauma with significant negative consequences for mental health. These stressors may be perpetuated by being forced to discover a new sense of identity, when many external factors indicate a person's "otherness." In considering the role of ethnic identity in post-migration acculturation in particular, Tummala-Nara (2007) highlights how racial trauma can have a profound impact on an individual's sense of self, identity formation, relationships with others, and perceptions of mental health care. She demonstrates how racially driven trauma poses distinct challenges to an individual's development of a positive identity by arguing that this type of trauma has the effect of dehumanizing one's sense of security in and identification with larger social structures. In other words, the experience of race-related trauma, such as misdiagnosis in mental health care systems, racism, and racially based violence on individual and group levels, has significant impact on individuals' sense of cultural and racial identity and trust in larger social structures. This is particularly true in interactions with professionals of institutions with little or no training in how to think or react in multicultural contexts (Goguikian Ratcliff & Rossi, 2015).

Language Proficiency

A key specific aspect of the process of acculturation identified in the literature is that of language, and the role of language proficiency in determining social identity and power relations (Bucholtz & Hall, 2005; Kartal & Kiropoulos, 2016; Norton, 2000; Silove et al., 1998). Unsurprisingly, therefore, language barriers have been shown significantly to affect refugee mental health in both qualitative and quantitative studies (Hynie, 2018). Many authors in the field of socio-linguistics refer to the use of language and semiotic practices in determining social positioning within interactions between migrants and host populations, looking to notions of "indexicality" to examine the relationship between words and their social meanings (Bucholtz & Hall, 2005). The influential role of language in social integration (and by extension, mental health) is not to be underestimated. As Norton (2000) notes:

> Relations of power in the social world impact on social interactions between second language learners and target language speakers. Language is not...a neutral medium of communication but is understood with reference to its social meaning. Identity construction must be understood with reference to relations of power between language learners and target language speakers. The very heterogeneity of society must be understood with reference to an inequitable structured world in which the gender, race, class and ethnicity of second language learners may serve to marginalize them. Subjectivity and language are ... mutually constituted. (p. 5)

Kartal and colleagues (2018) recently developed a mediation model to examine the relationship between exposure to traumatic events, host language acquisition and mental health among refugee communities. Their robust model convincingly demonstrates that the indirect pathway from trauma to mental health via language acquisition was significant for PTSD.

Gender

The literature indicates that while refugees of both genders are exposed to stressful events to a similar degree, twice as much women develop PTSD in response to these experiences (Alpak et al., 2015). Tekin and colleagues (2016), however, have noted that gender differences in PTSD prevalence may simply be a question of how trauma manifests: their study revealed that women with PTSD reported flashbacks, hypervigilance, and intense psychological distress due to reminders of trauma more frequently than men, whereas men with PTSD reported feelings of detachment or estrangement from others more frequently than women. Whether or not women experience *more* symptoms of PTSD, or whether they just experience it *differently* remains open to debate. However, the literature consistently highlights gender as a significant factor influencing the experiences and subsequent mental health status of asylum-seeking and refugee women. Firstly, women seeking asylum are less likely to be granted refugee status than men, given greater structural and cultural barriers in the asylum process (Hollander et al., 2016). Gogukian Ratcliff and colleagues (2014) further highlight the link between language proficiency, gender and mental health, noting that refugee women in particular find themselves at the cross-roads of multiple motives for discrimination such as gender, race, level of education and language proficiency. In theorizing the gendered nature of refugee women's experiences, Norton (2000) refers to the silencing that women experience within the context of larger patriarchal structures in society, exacerbated by a gendered access to the public world to which immigrant women in particular are limited (Norton, 2000). This powerlessness is inextricably linked to what Kiguwa and Hook (2004) term the "triple oppression" of women "in terms of race, class and gender" (p. 239). Among torture survivors in particular, gender has been shown as associated with severely impaired global functioning and poorer mental health including anxiety (Song et al., 2015).

Daily Stressors

Due to the very nature of the refugee experience, many typically encounter a myriad of chronic daily stressors in their host environment, including—for example—general and acculturation hassles. Such post-migration or displacement-related stressors have been observed to have a significant impact on the mental health of resettled refugees, compounding the dose–response relationship between past trauma and PTSD symptoms (Carswell et al., 2011). In a recent study conducted by Minihan and colleagues

(2018) among Australian refugees, living difficulties emerged as the most consistent predictor of PTSD symptomatology. Indeed, the impact of these daily stressors may extend over and above the effects of past trauma (Li et al., 2016; Miller & Rasmussen, 2014; Nickerson et al., 2018; Porter & Haslam, 2005; Schock et al., 2016; Song et al., 2015) – a phenomenon referred to by Keles and colleagues (2016) as the "above-and-beyond trauma effect" of such hassles. In a recent study on the impact of new traumatic or stressful life events on pre-existing PTSD in traumatized refugees, Schock et. al. (2016) discovered that, "contrary to our expectations, new stressful life events influenced the symptom course more than the experience of a new traumatic event." (p. 7, my emphasis). In their study, most of the mentioned stressors were related to an unsecure residence status and the related insecurity concerning their life and their future—as well as new or ongoing political unrest in their home county. Another study goes so far as to purport that individuals who are resettled longer may encounter a greater accumulation of daily stressors leading to a deterioration in mental health and increasing the predictability of PTSD (Kubiak, 2005).

Considering the Interrelation of Factors

It is clear that the road to recovery for refugees is a long and complicated one, and that the mental health needs of this population remain poorly understood. Many studies on traumatized refugees demonstrating the relationship of ongoing psychological impairment and overextending post-migration living conditions, even if formal safety is achieved (Bogic et al., 2012; Schick et al., 2016). In one example in the literature on mental health among resettled refugees in Switzerland, (Schick et al., 2016) participants in general showed remarkably poor integration, particularly in terms of labour market participation and language proficiency, and were subject to a high number of migration-associated living difficulties. This was despite comparably high education and long duration of residency in Switzerland typically over 10 years.

Although systematic research into the mental health of asylum seekers is in its infancy, there is growing evidence that salient migration stress facing asylum seekers adds to the effect of previous trauma in creating risk of ongoing posttraumatic stress disorder and other psychiatric symptoms (Silove et al., 2007, 2000). Once again, what is highlighted is the interplay of pre-migration and migration factors influencing mental health. This includes the physical and material hardships of the journey and poor treatment by authorities. Such difficulties encountered during migration risk perpetuating the structural violence, injustice and intolerance faced by asylum seekers in their countries of origin and once more during the asylum seeking process, thereby serving to reinforce physical and psychological vulnerability (d'Halluin, 2009; Fassin & d'Halluin, 2005).

Two key models highlight this interaction of factors influencing the mental health of refugees pre-, during and post-migration:

(1) Drožđek's (2015) model identifies factors of damage as well as resources during the pre-migratory phase, the period of forced migration and the period of resettlement. Furthermore, these are factors are mapped according to the ecological levels of the microsystem, the mesosystem, the exosystem and the macrosystem. Such a model thus incorporates the multiciplity of factors influencing mental health—including experiences of trauma as well as resilience.

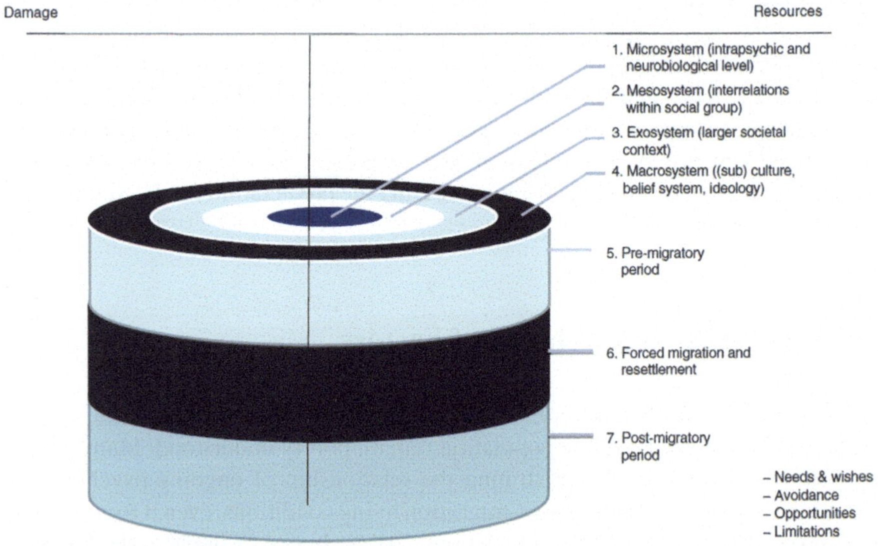

(2) Miller and Rasmussen's (2017) social ecological model similarly expands the view beyond the field's historical focus on premigration factors alone, by drawing attention to current stressors associated with the challenges of adapting to life in exile, or displacement-related stressors. They argue that such ecological conceptualisations of refugee distress show significantly greater predictive power than the more narrowly focused single-event trauma exposure model that has guided earlier research.

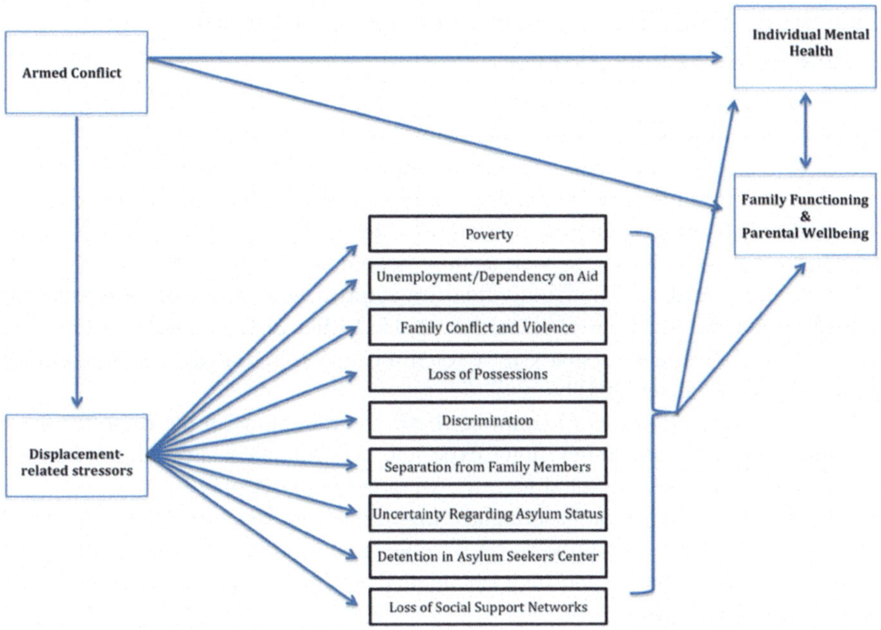

Such models, often based on the socio-ecological tradition of Bronfenbrenner (1986), conceptualise psychological distress associated with trauma as stemming not only from the violence and destruction of traumatic events such as war, but also from stressful life conditions linked to social and material conditions of everyday life following displacement.

The multiple stressors faced by refugees are continuous and interconnected—before fleeing home to after having spent years in a host country. Given this complex interplay of factors, it is questionable as to whether or not one could neatly separate the pre-migration, migration and post-migration periods as being distinct phases. The difficulties inherent to each of these speak among each other in a way which appears to be more circular than linear. Therefore, as useful as it is to "map" the factors affecting refugee mental health, one needs to move beyond such a static representation in our reflections. Let us consider the refugee who receives news of a beloved family member's passing back home in their country of origin, yet who is left with little resources to mourn the death outside of his familiar religious community. Let us consider the refugee whose experience with the police force upon arrival in Europe echoes similar experiences with the police force of her country of origin. It is exactly this dynamic complexity of human experiences of migration and mental health that needs to be considered, and which will be highlighted in the following two case studies.

Case Study One: Trauma Among Displaced Victims of Torture in Athens, Greece

The first case study is taken from my doctoral thesis, which involved two years of fieldwork in a centre for victims of torture run by *Médecins Sans Frontières* (Operational Centre Belgium), in partnership with local NGO Babel, in Athens, Greece. Here, individual refugee victims of torture were interviewed multiple times over the course of this fieldwork, as well as their accompanying psychologists, doctors, and community leaders. Their individual trajectories were analysed based on the ecological models noted above (Drožđek, 2015; Miller & Rasmussen, 2017). The case described here also appears in a scientific article published in *Intervention* (Womersley & Kloetzer, 2018b).

The case study allows us to examine these contradictions in the importance of the socio-legal environment in refugee experiences of trauma. Many cultural factors, such as a specific socio-political identity, were evidently at play for this particular individual. Furthermore, the case clearly highlights the impact of particular legal and medical institutional pathways on psychosocial recovery. It further offers the possibility of triangulating the data obtained from this individual participant, his doctor and psychologist.

Case Presentation

The case presented is a 30-year-old Indian asylum seeker of Sikh religion, whom I interviewed multiple times from 2016 to 2018. In 2007, he was arrested and tortured on numerous occasions, often for months at a time, due to his involvement as a Sikh political activist. He managed to escape from prison with the help of an uncle and arrived alone in Athens to seek asylum in September 2015. He was referred to the centre for victims of torture in June 2016, where his treating doctor describes 'a clear case of post-traumatic stress disorder', including symptoms of flashbacks and nightmares, at the first consultation. I first interviewed him in August 2016. From the very beginning of the very first interview, he highlighted his family's collective identity as Sikh political activists, with a long history of trauma across the generations:

> My father's, my father family and my mom's family – they are very, very connected with their religion […] from my mom's family, I have seen a lot of dead bodies. They were innocent and they were killed by the Indian government police and the secret services, because of that, because we were fighting for our freedom.

Over the course of the following four interviews, he described the psychological impact of the various methods of torture to which he was subjected in minute detail, including sexual abuse, his legs being 'ripped apart' the meta-tarsals in his feet being broken, as well as electrification:

> From the front, they were giving the electric shocks. They never give the scars on my body but they give me the scars on my personality. They give me the scars on my soul … lots of things from my mind has been wasted.

For the first 4 months after his arrival, he was living alone in a 30 m-squared hotel room in an old building recently repurposed to house asylum seekers. Alone, lost and scared of being recognised by other members of the Indian community, he barely left his apartment. At the end of August 2016, he was given an appointment for his asylum interview. However, the administrator responsible was not present on the day and he was given a new date for his interview in December. This seemed to symbolise a denial of his story, of his cultural identity as a Sikh political activist, of his very being. He explained that:

> During the interview, I want to be wearing a turban because during the interview I want to tell them that I am a part of the Sikh religion because of my religion, because of my race, I have been persecuted in my country.

This fear seemed to echo the past traumatic experience of being tortured, a fundamental part of which involved the torturers removing his turban and mocking his Sikh identity. He consulted a doctor and a psychiatrist at the centre, who wrote a medical report to add to his request for asylum. The report stated that he was suffering from PTSD, yet this was a concept unknown to him and he continued to refer to his psychological state as one of depression:

> P: "Mr. Psychologist doctor, he gave me the report. In that report, he has written that I'm in very big depression. Actually, I don't know if I'm in depression or not. I know only one thing, that my world is just only this room … I'm just killing my time here until I'm not getting my papers or they are not going to take my interview […]."
>
> Interviewer: 'Tell me about the psychiatrist you said that you're going to be seeing later."
>
> P: 'Why I'm seeing a psychiatrist – well, without any reason. . . In my dreams, I saw this police officer because in front of me, he was kicking my mom's stomach … I'm still having dark dreams …" Interviewer: "Is it helpful for you to see a psychiatrist?"
>
> P: "No, it's not- What he is going to do, I don't think he's going to help me in any way. The things that happened to me, what he wants to do, he's just speaking, and speaking, and speaking, and talking about things, nothing much … Why I am coming to the people here, to see the psychiatrist and the doctor, because then they will know that I'm also here. There are thousands and millions of refugees here. If were to come in here, I will be in front of their face, and they will be knowing about me."

The contradictions between his own explanatory model, and that of the psychiatrist, are striking. He reported not finding the consultations with the psychiatrist helpful, seeing little use in being required to 'talk about things'. Not only did he not agree with the PTSD diagnosis, he mistook it for a diagnosis of depression. There seemed to be little correlation between the words of the psychiatrist and the "scars of [his] soul." Despite continually being haunted by "dark dreams," his focus was on being "seen" as a refugee. Never having heard of a psychologist or psychiatrist before, he saw psychotherapy as a useful way to obtain this legal goal. Towards the end of 2016, his psychological condition deteriorated. Due to financial reasons, he was forced to move out of his small hotel room into shared accommodation. He accused his Pakistani roommate of spying on him. Psychotic symptoms started to emerge, including auditory hallucinations and paranoia. Many of the voices were those of authority figures, including the torturers in India and, rather tellingly, police officers, bureaucrats and judges in the asylum procedure in Greece. He was hospitalised as a result. When interviewed about his hospitalisation and the deterioration in symptoms, his psychologist stated:

> One voice said, 'You will be homeless you will be homeless,' and there is a possibility to be homeless. Or another voice said that, "They will not believe you they send you back to India," and that is true ... What he hears is normal, it's his fear.

His doctor similarly noted the potentially harmful effect of forced hospitalisation:

> Psychiatrists are not sure whether his post-traumatic stress disorder was that and only that or if he even before had some psychotic elements that now worsened. Hospitalization was difficult for him; it reminded him of prison. All the staff would kept visiting, bringing chocolates or to distract the prison-like atmosphere. I am worried about him, because he doesn't seem to respond to treatment that well ... It's not a good time for him generally, because first he found himself living in an apartment with Pakistanis. They could speak the language; he got afraid. They were having drinking, smoking and things like that; he got very scared. That was when things really got bad and he went to this hospital ... Then he heard from his relatives in India that his mother and father are in prison. His father is probably killed, because we hear from these relatives too, but he doesn't know. He knows that his father has disappeared in prison. The news that he receives about his mother is that she's in prison with an infected leg. She has nothing, just a rag to wipe the pus. That's what he knows about his mother. This is another stress factor. Another very stressing thing for him is that his interview got postponed till August. That made him really angry and frustrated. All these things add up.

She also noted the impact of his current reality on the process of diagnosis:

> I could see the face of the psychiatrist who at first said, 'You think the secret services of India are after you?' I could see the paranoia. Then [the patient] said his story. There he goes, Oh, oh, oh, oh. [laughter] This is not paranoia. This is real life.

Feedback loops

So what is "paranoia" and what is "real life?" To analyse the data, we draw on the concept of feedback or 'looping effects' (Kirmayer & Ramstead, 2016) defined by the authors as links in a causal chain "whereby individuals interpret and respond to their own symptoms with culturally varied coping strategies that may change the course of the illness, amplifying or reducing symptoms and distress" (p. 6). They argue that such socio-cultural feedback amplification extends beyond the individual to include a wider network of relationships and processes wherein the individual is embedded. We posit that such a series of "feedback loops" (which we define as a process whereby an effect is reinforced by its own influence on the process giving rise to it) impacted post-traumatic symptoms as well as the patient's self-representation of his own mental health status. A number of feedback loops may be identified on an individual, interpersonal, and social level, as illustrated by the following model:

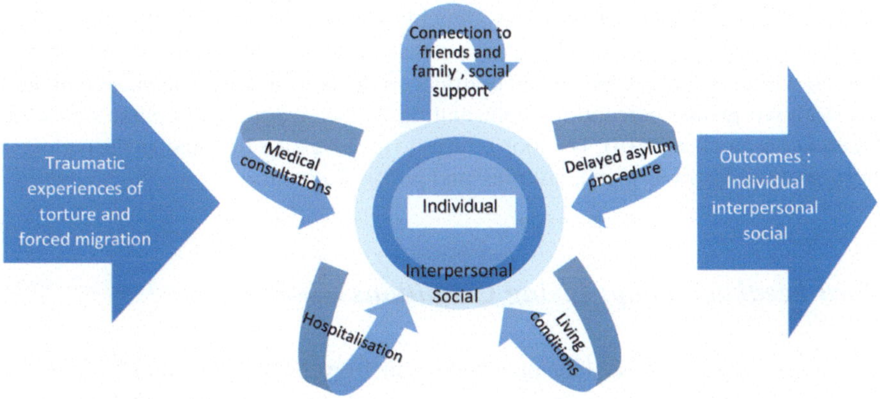

First Feedback Loop: Breakdown of Interpersonal Relations

The experience of being tortured is arguably a traumatic experience in and of itself. However, added to this is the fact that the patient is not the only member of his family to have been tortured. His father's presumed death and mother's alleged detainment and torture alludes to a traumatic experience extending far beyond that of the individual. Indeed, the torture of his family and subsequent forced migration, which he undertook alone, created traumatic ruptures in his interpersonal relationships and by extension, his broader social world. Paradoxically, such connections would have connected him to the very resources necessary to heal. These are both resources found on an interpersonal level in disclosure and sharing emotional experiences, and on a social level within secure group membership. Thus, a vicious cycle of isolation and disconnection is perpetuated, seemingly serving to exacerbate his fear. Furthermore, the disconnection cannot be considered as a "once-off" event, which occurred at a particular moment in the past: ruptures continue with each phone call bringing news from India.

Second Feedback Loop: Delayed Asylum Procedure

A long asylum procedure has been found in the literature to be associated with psychiatric disorders (Laban et al., 2004). For the patient, his insecure residency status increased uncertainty regarding his future as well as his ability to integrate, look for work, and create a life for himself. Waiting for his asylum interview, his fear was compounded by being in an irregular legal situation and the risk of being forced out of the country. This fear kept him from leaving his house and integrating into his new social environment. On an interpersonal level, this reduced opportunities for exchanges. On a social level, the delay arguably contributed to further disconnections in visibility, representation and the acknowledgement of the torture, which he had endured within broader, societal and political contexts, which were intricately linked to restorative justice perceptions contributing to the severity and course of PTSD (Maercker & Hecker, 2016). The loop returns to the level of individual, in the patients' questioning of his own social, cultural, and political identity.

Third Feedback Loop: Living Conditions

The delayed asylum procedure prevented him from having the right to look for work and find an apartment on his own. Without more financial, legal, or social resources and, thus, still dependant on state services as an asylum seeker, he was moved from his own hotel room to new accommodation. Sharing with Pakistanis whom he did not trust, his interpersonal resources were further compromised and his social world further limited by not being able to find work. Such conditions seem to have exacerbated the post-traumatic symptoms, with auditory hallucinations telling him that he would be homeless leading to his hospitalisation.

Fourth Feedback Loop: Hospitalisation and Interpersonal Encounters in Medical Consultations

His post-traumatic stress symptoms exacerbated, he was hospitalised. Again institutionalised, finding himself once more at the mercy of the state, it was perceived as a further enforced period of detention where he was subjected to bodily treatments against his will. It triggered memories of the past torture he endured. Furthermore, it positioned him in the role of patient leading him to question, whether he was "sick" or not. He was promised by the hospital staff that they would not inject him. They did. This deepened his sense of mistrust, paranoia, and isolation creating further interpersonal ruptures. His hospitalisation and numerous encounters with medical staff lead him to question his own status as "sick" or healthy, "normal" or abnormal. His psychologist explained:

> When I asked him what is his request and what is his reason and why he decide to visit psychologist, he said to me, 'I don't know, because of my doctor said to me that it's good for me. My psychiatrist said the same, my social worker said the same, a police man who stopped me said the same.' I asked him, 'Then what do you think, why do all this people propose to you to come and see the psychologist?' He said to me, 'I don't know, maybe they need a psychologist'.

On an interpersonal level, it speaks to the feelings of both shame and anger he expressed throughout the interviews in being seen as someone in need of psychiatric care. His doctor explained:

> He doesn't seem to understand it as an illness. He says that he feels abnormal, he feels wrecked; he says that he's not dangerous; that he is not crazy. Every time I say to him, 'These voices is just a symptom of a disease that will go away eventually,' he doesn't seem to listen.

Such discrepancies between his own explanatory model for his symptoms and that of others around him had an impact on his interpersonal relationships. They seemed only to reinforce his solitude. Here, it is worth returning once more to his stated reason for attending consultations with the psychologist and psychiatrist as highlighted above. It is not because he seems himself as a patient. It is for visibility and recognition.

It is so that "they will know that I am also here."

As illustrated by the case of this particular individual, post-migration factors encountered in Europe, including delayed asylum trials and poor living conditions, had a substantial impact on post-traumatic symptoms among the refugee victims of torture in the study. These symptoms were never static but in a continual state of flux, in dynamic interaction with the socio-cultural environment.

Case Study Two: Self-immolation Among an Asylum Seeker in Switzerland

In April 2016, Armin,[2] an asylum seeker in a village of Switzerland, set himself alight in the public square of the town, one of a few cases reported across Europe. He performed the act following a denied request for asylum and was saved by bystanders. Here, I present the results of two qualitative interviews which I conducted with Armin, his translator and his roommate following the incident. The case study also appears in a scientific article published in *Frontiers in Psychiatry* (Womersley & Kloetzer, 2018a).

The Self-immolation of Armin

Armin is an asylum seeker from North Africa who arrived in Switzerland in September 2014. He had been imprisoned in his country of origin in 2008 after having physically attacked a judge in an attempt to gauge out his eyes. This incident occurred during a court case involving a land dispute wherein the judge ruled against his favour. In prison, he began engaging in hunger strikes to protest against the conditions. After serving six years out of a 20-year sentence, he managed to escape and make his way to Europe.

---

[2]Name changed in line with standard ethical protocols and the recommendations of the Ethics Review Committee.

Upon his arrival in Switzerland, he was transferred to multiple reception centres where he would go on hunger strike for eight days at a time to protest against the reception conditions. He describes, "sleeping on the sofa with eight people living and breathing in the same room." The situation become unbearable for him to such an extent that he began sleeping in the bathroom. He was subsequently transferred to a private apartment with he shared with an Eritrean refugee. He began using marijuana and cocaine "because it helped me to forget my problems," and was arrested by the police for shoplifting whilst intoxicated. He also started grinding up paracetamol and selling it as cocaine—using the money to send back to his mother. In November 2015, he heard news of his eleven-year old daughter drowning to death in his country of origin.

After having waited for 23 months for the results of his second asylum application, he attempted to leave Switzerland by asking to annul his asylum application. He boarded a train heading for Germany. However, due to the fact that his fingerprints were already registered, he was prevented from leaving the country. In November 2015, he heard news of his sole remaining child, his 12-year old son, being killed. It was during the same time that he heard of the fact that his application for asylum had been refused, a decision which he decided to appeal. According to his personal file, he attempted suicide in February 2016 following an argument with his doctor and was sent to a psychiatric hospital. Upon returning to his apartment, he received the second negative response to his request for asylum, with a deadline to leave Switzerland by the 7th of July.

On April 20th, the morning of the self-immolation, his roommate reports that the police came to his apartment at five o'clock in the morning looking for drugs. According to his roommate, he was detained at the police station until 11:00 a.m., whereupon he was released and returned home for lunch. His roommate describes his mood as being "calm and quiet" during the meal. Thereafter, he headed to the town's biggest public square with a can of petrol in his bag. In his words, "I was very very angry and very… I poured the petrol onto myself and the people stopped me…I found that there was no other solution but death and that's why I took the petrol and a lighter and set myself alight." According to newspaper reports, passers-by heard him screaming incoherently in Arabic and rushed to pour water over him to extinguish the flames.

The incident was poorly reported in the media and few if any public statements were made on behalf of any of the institutions working with asylum seekers. The little that was reported focused mainly on applauding the quick-thinking actions of the citizens and local fire brigade in putting out the fire. One newspaper report concluded that the act did not seem to have been of a political nature. Little was said by the community of asylum seekers and refugees themselves living in the town. The following day, roughly 70 people congregated in a demonstration in solidarity. There was no report of this demonstration in the local media. It was as though a veil of silence shrouded the incident. Armin ended up in intensive care for a month with severe burn injuries, and seven weeks later was subsequently transferred to a psychiatric hospital.

Analysis

The first interview I conducted with him was at this psychiatric hospital, with the assistance of a translator. Upon meeting him, the first words he said were, "We find ourselves in a country where we are considered terrorists ...we need to unite." He stated that he planned to go to Geneva the following day to visit the head office of Al Jazeera, the international news network. He wanted to be interviewed to tell people that "the prison of my people in Africa is better than the prison here...I want to explain to my people what Switzerland actually is." From the first interview, what Armin immediately highlights is wanting to "show" and "explain" to people the dire reality of his situation, for his suffering to be seen. It is the need for social recognition.

He went on to describe a life without meaning: an endless and empty repetition, a wordless nothing:

> There's nothing to do in the apartment. You eat, you drink, you sleep, you eat, you drink, you sleep, you eat, you drink, you sleep. There is nothing.

There appears to be a striking absence of connection to Others mentioned in his speech. The endlessness is repetitive; past and future are circular, not linear. He continues the conversation by reflecting on his initial arrival to Switzerland, where he was housed in a reception centre for asylum seekers staying:

> for 8 months sleeping on the sofa and not on my bed where 8 people lived and breathed in the same room

Armin found the physical proximity to the other living, breathing people unbearable, resulting in him leaving the communal room and isolating himself. He continued the interview by explaining this:

> Armin: I slept in the toilets. I slept in the toilets! 15 nights I slept in the toilets!
>
> Translator: Why?
>
> Armin: I took my mattress and went to sleep in the toilets!
>
> Translator: Why?
>
> [silence]

His silence is striking. There are no words to describe this disconnection, this descent into nothingness. He explained that the centre for him had been.

> An open prison. It's the place where you return to no matter in which direction you go. So long as there are no offers of work, no internship for mutual benefit, there is no future here

Once again, time is represented in a circular fashion, not a linear one. No matter the direction, there is a return to this same place of nothingness. Any hope for a future is linked to "mutual benefits"—in other words, a dialogue with an Other who could serve to recognise him, to assist him in creating future plans. In the absence of this Other, Armin remains disconnected not only from society but from his own future; "there are inexplicable events, life is unendurable, and ... justice is a mirage" (Geertz, 1993, p. 108 as cited in Tankink & Richters, 2007).

He continued.

> I set myself on fire because I didn't have any will to live. I found myself in a situation without future, without anything and therefore a worthless person, like this cup...without future, without anything, like this cup. I am like this cup. No future for me, no work, no marriage, no learning.

In this discussion, Armin asserts that there is no future here for him, which he relates to the lack of work or professional training. This seems to be for him both an "entry ticket" to normal life, and a way to overcome suffering. It is not only the economic security of a job which he has lost, but the social security of connection to Others and the recognition of himself as a valued member of society—without which he is "worthless," something less than human.

He believes there to be no possible life for himself in Europe, there is "no work," "no school," "no marriage," "no future." He states the reason for having committed suicide as being "I need to have work, to do something." Elsewhere, it has been argued that the process of forced migration risks creating an "a-temporal space," a transitional and disconnected period wherein experiences, skills, connections acquired and built in the past are rendered inaccessible (Métraux, 1999), as are any clear perspectives on the future. A consequence of such overwhelming episodes is that the experience seems dissociated—isolated in one's consciousness (Zittoun & Sato, 2018).

Poignantly, he concludes this interview by saying:

> Yes, I went to death[3]

The second interview, similarly conducted in the presence of a translator, occurred once Armin had been released from the psychiatric hospital. He began by saying:

> I came to Switzerland, but Switzerland wasn't my destination. In my mind, there were other destinations like France, Italy, England, but I was stopped.

His words imply a sense of being stuck, of thwarted dreams and ambitions for the future. He is overwhelmed by the reality of the situation, in rude contrast to what he imagined for his life:

> Armin's words (spoken by his interpreter): After 9 days, I went back home but I encountered the same problems of solitude, there is nothing to do, there is no solution but death. I thought there was no solution but death, and for this reason, I brought petrol and a lighter and I set myself fire.
>
> Interpreter: Why did you choose that way?
>
> Armin: So that people know. I did it so that people could be made aware, to stop despising people like me, to know that all people are equal.
>
> And so far, nothing happens. I stay home, I... I eat, I drink, I sleep. There is nothing. There is no future in Switzerland. No future. I got married, my wife died, my two children died. There is nothing. (translation and exchange in Arabic)
>
> Interpreter: I told him that we were here with him. He told me there is nothing. The dog here is better treated than me."
>
> Armin: In this case, is it not better to die?

[3]In the translation from French into English, the words may be translated either as "I surrended to death" or "I went to death".

Further on in the interview, he continued:

> I'm not happy with my life, I do this and that, I do some terrible things, I sell drugs, I take cannabis, things like that and I'm unable to find a solution - not for me nor for my family …I want to live like other people. I don't consider what I have to be a life. I am not living. (…) I am a shirt and walking trousers, not a human being.

An underlying sentiment of shame pervades his speech: he is ashamed of being someone who sells drugs, ashamed of not being able to support his family and make them proud. The mystifying dualism of this shame is that it is at once an isolating, intimately intra-psychic phenomenon seeking concealment, yet remains deeply embedded in a visual and public interpersonal space where the self is violently and unexpectedly exposed to the critical gaze of the Other (Womersley et al., 2011). The source of shame can therefore never be completely in the self or in the Other, but is a rupture of what Kaufman (1989) calls the "interpersonal bridge" (p. 22) binding the two. It is a disconnection and consequent lack of social recognition which underlies this shame.

Armin comments on the act of self-immolation in relation to his negative evaluation of his own life and thwarted expectations of living a normal life, a "human" life. The feelings expressed seem to be the same: injustice, solitude, sadness, emptiness, uselessness, all worsened by a perceived lack of hope in a better future. Here, time is a circular, wordless nothing. His act is defined explicitly as communicative, a direct call for social recognition:

> I did it so that people could be made aware, to stop despising people like me, to know that all people are equal.

Continuing the interview, he paused and stated, "I don't know. Maybe I'm mad." It is impossible to grasp the full meaning behind these words. At face value, Armin seems to be considering whether or not he is indeed suffering from a psychiatric disorder, as stated by the many professionals with whom he has been in contact in Switzerland. However, throughout the two interviews we conducted with him, we are left with the impression that, for the most part, he appears to be contesting this very idea. Indeed, his words seem to reflect a resistance to the fact that he is a psychiatric patient in the face of others telling him that he is "mad."

Concluding Remarks

Although he finds himself cast out of the networks of humanity—having lost his family, his friends, his cultural homeland, his work, he justifies his act as a will to communicate his situation and humanity to other human beings. For Stolorow (2011), being plunged into such singularity and solitude may paradoxically bring about an enhancement of "resoluteness" (p. 45). In such a state, the individual returns from the publicness of "they" to a more authentic and steadfast sense of self and purpose, which may lead to authentic "Being-toward-death." In his own words, "Yes, I went to death." However, on analysing his motives for committing the act, it is evident that it goes beyond a simple desire to commit suicide. The self-stated reasons for him having committed the act highlight both the socio-political conditions in which he finds himself, as well as an internal psychological state of despair. This echoes the work of Biggs (2008), who highlights the paradox that, in many cases, the act serves as both an escape and a protest.

Based on this hypothesis, considering the act "as escape" would arguably be indicative of suicidal ideation possibly linked to psychological factors of depression including a sense of helplessness and despair—in his own words "having no will to live." Armin continues this reflection on his "situation without future" in which he finds himself. Not only does he perceive a life without future, he perceives a life where "dogs are treated better than me" and he is no better than "a cup". He sees himself without a future and, most significantly, he connects this state to the lack of relationship with a social Other—in other words, his relationship to the network of human society which places him in the position of less-than-human, outside of social recognition.

In the apparent absence of social recognition, Armin found himself "a worthless human." Cast outside of the containment of human plurality as a result of a myriad of political and social mechanisms of exclusions, we hypothesize that his act of self-immolation serves as both an escape and a protest, both a "relational striving" for "being-in-the-world,"—profoundly embedded in an intersubjectively constitutive context, and a "being-toward-death" (Stolorow, 2011). Is the act both a significant indicator of deep psychological distress and despair, as well as an attempt to restore a connection to the world of the living? We argue that the utterance is at once disruptive and engaging, destructive and constructive, a conflict and a collaboration, a death instinct towards destruction but a "destruction as the cause of coming into being" (Spielrein, 1994). To quote Armin himself, it is at once a "yes, I went to death" as well as an "I want to live like other people."

When he placed himself in the most public space of a Swiss town and set himself alight "to show that all men are equal," it was an attempt to overcome trauma, social isolation and lack of social recognition, a co-constructed inquiry to begin to try and put symbolic expression to experience (Rosenbaum, 2016). A "social interaction in its own right" (Rasool & Payton, 2014), it represents an attempt to restore interaction. As such, it is a way of metaphorically construing and narrating experience; a compelling narrative enjoining others to take action (Kirmayer & Ramstead, 2016). This is an utterance, a communicative act with the consequent potential to promote agency and civic engagement (Yang, 2011) which demands a response from the addressee, the Other. It demands and forces social recognition.

The brutality of such acts leave the public with little choice but to be disrupted and engaged as an "addressee"—whether voluntarily or not. In such moments, 'the public sphere can no longer turn a blind eye to its privileged bodies' (Habermas, as cited in Cho, 2016), "the audience is not allowed to simply demonstrate 'distant compassion' but rather they are encouraged to engage and self-reflect about local injustices and activism within their own vicinities." (Bhimji, 2015, p. 100). This self-immolation was a powerful communicative act that utilized self-inflicted violence as a means of forcing social recognition, both a personal and political action.

References

Akhtar, S. (1999). *Immigration and identity: Turmoil, treatment, and transformation.* Northvale, N.J.: Jason Aronson.

Alpak, G., Unal, A., Bulbul, F., Sagaltici, E., Bez, Y., Altindag, A., Dalkilic, A., Savas, H. A. (2015). Post-traumatic stress disorder among Syrian refugees in Turkey: a cross-sectional study. *International Journal of Psychiatry in Clinical Practice, 19*(1), 45–50.

Barudy, J. (1989). A programme of mental health for political refugees: Dealing with the invisible pain of political exile. *Social Science & Medicine, 28*(7), 715–727.

Berry, J. W. (1997). Immigration, acculturation, and adaptation. *Applied Psychology, 46*(1), 5–34.

Berry, J. W. (2003). Conceptual approaches to acculturation. In K. M. Chun, P. B. Organista, & G. Marín (Eds.), *Acculturation: Advances in theory, measurement, and applied research* (pp. 17–37). Washington D.C.: American Psychological Association.

Bhimji, F. (2015). Collaborations and performative agency in refugee theater in Germany. *Journal of Immigrant and Refugee Studies, 1,* 1–23.

Biggs, M. (2008). dying for a cause—Alone? *Contexts, 7*(1), 22–27.

Bogic, M., Ajdukovic, D., Bremner, S., Franciskovic, T., Galeazzi, G. M., Kucukalic, A., et al. (2012). Factors associated with mental disorders in long-settled war refugees: Refugees from the former Yugoslavia in Germany, Italy and the UK. *The British Journal of Psychiatry, 200*(3), 216–223.

Bögner, D., Brewin, C., & Herlihy, J. (2010). Refugees' experiences of home office interviews: A qualitative study on the disclosure of sensitive personal information. *Journal of Ethnic and Migration Studies, 36*(3), 519–535.

Bosworth, M. (2016) *The impact of immigration detention on mental health: a literature review.* Criminal Justice, Borders and Citizenship Research Paper No. 2732892. Retrieved from https://papers.ssrn.com/sol3/papers.cfm?abstract_id=2732892. On the February 11, 2020.

Brand, T., Samkange-Zeeb, F., Ellert, U., Keil, T., Krist, L., Dragano, N., et al. (2017). Acculturation and health-related quality of life: Results from the German National Cohort migrant feasibility study. *International Journal of Public Health, 62,* 1–9.

Bronfenbrenner, U. (1986). Ecology of the family as a context for human development: Research perspectives. *Developmental Psychology, 22*(6), 723–742.

Bruhn, M., Rees, S., Mohsin, M., Silove, D., & Carlsson, J. (2018). The range and impact of postmigration stressors during treatment of trauma-affected refugees. *The Journal of Nervous and Mental Disease, 206*(1), 61–68.

Bucholtz, M., & Hall, K. (2005). Identity and interaction: A sociocultural linguistic approach. *Discourse Studies, 7*(4–5), 585–614.

Carlsson, J. M., Mortensen, E. L., & Kastrup, M. (2006). Predictors of mental health and quality of life in male tortured refugees. *Nordic Journal of Psychiatry, 60*(1), 51–57.

Carswell, K., Blackburn, P., & Barker, C. (2011). The relationship between trauma, post-migration problems and the psychological well-being of refugees and asylum seekers. *International Journal of Social Psychiatry, 57*(2), 107–119.

Carter, R. T., Johnson, V. E., Roberson, K., Mazzula, S. L., Kirkinis, K., & Sant-Barket, S. (2017). Race-based traumatic stress, racial identity statuses, and psychological functioning: An exploratory investigation. *Professional Psychology: Research Practice, 48*(1), 30–37.

Chen, W., Hall, B. J., Ling, L., & Renzaho, A. M. (2017). Pre-migration and post-migration factors associated with mental health in humanitarian migrants in Australia and the moderation effect of

post-migration stressors: Findings from the first wave data of the BNLA cohort study. *The Lancet Psychiatry, 4*(3), 218–229.
Cho, Y. C. (2016). The art of self-concretization as a necropolitical embodiment: The self-immolation of Chun Tae-il. *Quarterly Journal of Speech, 102*(1), 21–40.
Copping, A., Shakespeare-Finch, J., & Paton, D. (2010). Towards a culturally appropriate mental health system: Sudanese-Australians' experiences with trauma. *Journal of Pacific Rim Psychology, 4*(01), 53–60.
Couttenier, M., Preotu, V., Rohner, D., & Thoenig, M. (2016). *The violent legacy of victimization: Post-conflict evidence on asylum seekers*, Crimes and Public Policy in Switzerland.
Crepet, A., Rita, F., Reid, A., Van den Boogaard, W., Deiana, P., Quaranta, G., et al. (2017). Mental health and trauma in asylum seekers landing in Sicily in 2015: A descriptive study of neglected invisible wounds. *Conflict and Health, 11*(1), 1.
d'Halluin, E. (2009). La santé mentale des demandeurs d'asile. *Hommes et migrations. Revue française de référence sur les dynamiques migratoires* (Vol. 1282, pp. 66–75).
de Arellano, M. A., & Danielson, C. K. (2008). Assessment of trauma history and trauma-related problems in ethnic minority child populations: An INFORMED approach. *Cognitive and Behavioral Practice, 15*(1), 53–66.
Drožđek, B. (2015). Challenges in treatment of posttraumatic stress disorder in refugees: Towards integration of evidence-based treatments with contextual and culture-sensitive perspectives. *European Journal of Psychotraumatology, 6,* 24750.
Drožđek, B., Noor, A. K., Lutt, M., & Foy, D. W. (2003). Chronic PTSD and medical services utilization by asylum seekers. *Journal of Refugee Studies, 16*(2), 202–211.
Du, B., & Witmer, J. (2020). Loss of possessions, identity, and sense of self. In J. Kottler, S. Banu, & S. Jani (Eds.), *Handbook of refugee experience: Trauma, resilience, and recovery* (pp. 35–42). San Diego, California: Cognella.
Eagle, G. (2014). From evolution to discourse: Key conceptual debates in the history and study of traumatic stress. *Psychology in Society, 47,* 1–20.
Eagle, G., & Kaminer, D. (2013). Continuous traumatic stress: Expanding the lexicon of traumatic stress. *Peace and Conflict: Journal of Peace Psychology, 19*(2), 85.
Eleftherakos, C., van den Boogaard, W., Barry, D., Severy, N., Kotsioni, I., & Roland-Gosselin, L. (2018). I prefer dying fast than dying slowly, how institutional abuse worsens the mental health of stranded Syrian, Afghan and Congolese migrants on Lesbos island following the implementation of EU-Turkey deal. *Conflict and Health, 12*(1), 38.
Esala, J. J., Vukovich, M. M., Hanbury, A., Kashyap, S., & Joscelyne, A. (2018). Collaborative care for refugees and torture survivors: Key findings from the literature. *Traumatology, 24*(3), 168–185.
Fassin, D., & d'Halluin, E. (2005). The truth from the body: Medical certificates as ultimate evidence for asylum seekers. *American Anthropologist, 107*(4), 597–608.
Georgiadou, E., Zbidat, A., Schmitt, G. M., & Erim, Y. (2018). Prevalence of mental distress among Syrian refugees with residence permission in Germany: A registry-based study. *Frontiers in Psychiatry, 9,* 393.
Gkionakis, N. (2016). The refugee crisis in Greece: Training border security, police, volunteers and aid workers in psychological first aid. *Intervention, 14*(1), 73–79.
Goguikian Ratcliff, B. (2009). Conclusion: Pour une clinique plus sociale du traumatisme et de l'exil. In B. Goguikian Ratcliff, & O. Strasser (Eds.), *Clinique de l'Exil : Chroniques d'une Pratique Engagée* (p. 185–196). Georg.
Goguikian Ratcliff, B. (2016, June 23–24). Asylum process and psychological distress: A two waves temporal pattern? Paper presented at the Second Annual Conference of the NCCR—On the Move. Neuchâtel, Switzerland.
Goguikian Ratcliff, B. G., & Rossi, I. (2015). Santé mentale et sociétés plurielles. *Alterstice-Revue Internationale De La Recherche Interculturelle, 4*(2), 3–12.

Goguikian Ratcliff, B., & Strasser, O. (2009). Clinique de l'Exil. Chroniques d'une pratique engagée. In G. Thésée, N. Carignan, & P. Carr (Eds.), *Les Faces Cachées de l'Interculturel: De la Rencontre des Porteurs de Cultures* (pp. 29–31). L'Harmattan.
Goguikian Ratcliff, B., Bolzman, C., & Gakuba, T. (2014). Déqualification des femmes migrantes en Suisse: Mécanismes sous-jacents et effets psychologiques. *Alterstice, 4*(2), 63–76.
Hauswirth, M., Canellini, A. M., & Bennoun, N. (2004). Un improbable refuge. Les répercussions sur la santé mentale des procédures en matière d'asile. *Psychothérapies, 24*(4), 215–222.
Heeren, M., Wittmann, L., Ehlert, U., Schnyder, U., Maier, T., & Müller, J. (2014). Psychopathology and resident status–comparing asylum seekers, refugees, illegal migrants, labor migrants, and residents. *Comprehensive Psychiatry, 55*(4), 818–825.
Herlihy, J., & Turner, S. (2018). Legal and ethical considerations related to the asylum process. In N. Morina, & A. Nickerson (Eds.), *Mental Heath of refugee and conflict-affected populations* (pp. 305–324). Springer.
Hodges-Wu, J., & Zajicek-Farber, M. (2017). Addressing the needs of survivors of torture: A pilot test of the psychosocial well-being index. *Journal of Immigrant & Refugee Studies, 15*(1), 71–89.
Hollander, A.-C., Dal, H., Lewis, G., Magnusson, C., Kirkbride, J. B., & Dalman, C. (2016). Refugee migration and risk of schizophrenia and other non-affective psychoses: cohort study of 1.3 million people in Sweden. *BMJ, 352*, i1030.
Holzkamp, K. (2013). *Psychology from the Standpoint of the Subject: Selected writings of Klaus Holzkamp (edited by Ernst Schraube and Ute Osterkamp)*. London: Palgrave Macmillan.
Hynie, M. (2018). The social determinants of refugee mental health in the post-migration context: A critical review. *The Canadian Journal of Psychiatry, 63*(5), 297–303.
Jakobsen, M., Meyer DeMott, M. A., Wentzel-Larsen, T., & Heir, T. (2017). The impact of the asylum process on mental health: A longitudinal study of unaccompanied refugee minors in Norway. *BMJ open, 7*(6).
Kartal, D., & Kiropoulos, L. (2016). Effects of acculturative stress on PTSD, depressive, and anxiety symptoms among refugees resettled in Australia and Austria. *European Journal of Psychotraumatology, 7*(1), 28711.
Kartal, D., Alkemade, N., & Kiropoulos, L. (2018). Trauma and mental health in resettled refugees: Mediating effect of host language acquisition on posttraumatic stress disorder, depressive and anxiety symptoms. *Transcultural Psychiatry, 56*(1), 3–23.
Kaufman, G. (1989). *The psychology of shame: Theory and treatment of shame-based syndromes*. Springer.
Keles, S., Idsøe, T., Friborg, O., Sirin, S., & Oppedal, B. (2016). The longitudinal relation between daily hassles and depressive symptoms among unaccompanied refugees in Norway. *Journal of Abnormal Child Psychology, 1*, 1–15.
Kiguwa, P., & Hook, D. (2004). Feminist critical psychology in South Africa. *Self, Community and Psychology, 7*, 1–38.
Kira, I. A. (2010). Etiology and treatment of post-cumulative traumatic stress disorders in different cultures. *Traumatology, 16*(4), 128.
Kirmayer, L. J. (2001). Cultural variations in the clinical presentation of depression and anxiety: Implications for diagnosis and treatment. *Journal of Clinical Psychiatry, 62*, 22–30.
Kirmayer, L. J., & Ramstead, M. J. (2016). Embodiment and enactment in cultural psychiatry. In C. Durt, T. Fuchs, & C. Tewes (Eds.), *Embodiment, enaction, and culture: Investigating the constitution of the shared world* (pp. 397–422). Cambridge, MA: MIT Press.
Kirmayer, L. J., Kienzler, H., Afana, A. H., & Pedersen, D. (2010). Trauma and disasters in social and cultural context. *Principles of Social Psychiatry, 2*, 155–177.
Kirmayer, L. J., Ban, L., & Jaranson, J. (2018). Cultural logics of emotion: Implications for understanding torture and its sequelae. *Torture Journal, 28*(1), 84–100.
Korup Kjærgaard, T., & Koitzsch Jensen, N. (2018). Post-migratory risk factors and asylum seekers' mental health. *International Journal of Human Rights in Healthcare, 11*(4), 257–269.
Kubiak, S. P. (2005). Trauma and cumulative adversity in women of a disadvantaged social location. *American Journal of Orthopsychiatry, 75*(4), 451–465.

Laban, C. J., Gernaat, H. B., Komproe, I. H., Schreuders, B. A., & De Jong, J. T. (2004). Impact of a long asylum procedure on the prevalence of psychiatric disorders in Iraqi asylum seekers in The Netherlands. *The Journal of Nervous and Mental Disease, 192*(12), 843–851.

Lambert, J. E., & Alhassoon, O. M. (2015). Trauma-focused therapy for refugees: Meta-analytic findings. *Journal of Counseling Psychology, 62*(1), 28.

Lecerof, S. S., Stafström, M., Westerling, R., & Östergren, P.-O. (2015). Does social capital protect mental health among migrants in Sweden? *Health Promotion International, 31*(3), 644–652.

Le, L., Morina, N., Schnyder, U., Schick, M., Bryant, R. A., & Nickerson, A. (2018). The effects of perceived torture controllability on symptom severity of posttraumatic stress, depression and anger in refugees and asylum seekers: A path analysis. *Psychiatry Research, 264,* 143–150.

Liddell, B. J., Nickerson, A., & Bryant, R. A. (2017). Clinical science and torture survivors' rights to rehabilitation. *The Lancet Psychiatry, 5*(2), 101–103.

Lie, B. (2002). A 3-year follow-up study of psychosocial functioning and general symptoms in settled refugees. *Acta Psychiatrica Scandinavica, 106*(6), 415–425.

Linton, R. (2015). A Presumption of disclosure: Towards greater transparency in asylum proceedings. *Seattle UL Rev, 38,* 1069–1139.

Li, S. S., Liddell, B. J., & Nickerson, A. (2016). The relationship between post-migration stress and psychological disorders in refugees and asylum seekers. *Current Psychiatry Reports, 18*(9), 82.

Loizos, P. (2002). Misconceiving refugees. In R. Papadopoulos (Ed.), *Therapeutic care for refugees. No place like home* (pp. 41–56). Karnac

*Médecins Sans Frontières (*M.S.F.) (2016). *Neglected Trauma—Asylum seekers in Italy: An analysis of mental health distress and access to healthcare.* Rome, Italy. Retrieved from https://www.msf.org/sites/msf.org/files/neglected_trauma_report.pdf. On the February 12, 2020.

Maercker, A., & Hecker, T. (2016). Broadening perspectives on trauma and recovery: A socio-interpersonal view of PTSD. *European Journal of Psychotraumatology, 7,* 29303.

Maier, T., & Straub, M. (2011). My head is like a bag full of rubbish: Concepts of illness and treatment expectations in traumatized migrants. *Qualitative Health Research, 21*(2), 233–248.

Métraux, J.-C. (1999a). Au temps du silence, la nosographie reste muette. Le syndrome post traumatique en question. In F. Maqueda (Ed.), *Traumatisme de guerre. Actualités cliniques et humanitaires.* (pp. 41–66). Paris Hommes et Perspectives.

Miller, K., & Rasmussen, A. (2014). War experiences, daily stressors and mental health five years on: Elaborations and future directions. *Intervention, 12,* 33–42.

Miller, K., & Rasmussen, A. (2017). The mental health of civilians displaced by armed conflict: An ecological model of refugee distress. *Epidemiology and Psychiatric Sciences, 26*(2), 129–138.

Minihan, S., Liddell, B. J., Byrow, Y., Bryant, R. A., & Nickerson, A. (2018). Patterns and predictors of posttraumatic stress disorder in refugees: A latent class analysis. *Journal of Affective Disorders, 232,* 252–259.

Mollica, R., McInnes, K., Poole, C., & Tor, S. (1998). Dose-effect relationships of trauma to symptoms of depression and post-traumatic stress disorder among Cambodian survivors of mass violence. *The British Journal of Psychiatry, 173*(6), 482–488.

Momartin, S., Silove, D., Manicavasagar, V., & Steel, Z. (2003). Dimensions of trauma associated with posttraumatic stress disorder (PTSD) caseness, severity and functional impairment: A study of Bosnian refugees resettled in Australia. *Social Science and Medicine, 57*(5), 775.

Morina, N., Akhtar, A., Barth, J., & Schnyder, U. (2018). Psychiatric disorders in refugees and internally displaced persons after forced displacement: A systematic review. *Frontiers in Psychiatry, 9,* 433.

Mueller, J., Schmidt, M., Staeheli, A., & Maier, T. (2011). Mental health of failed asylum seekers as compared with pending and temporarily accepted asylum seekers. *The European Journal of Public Health, 21*(2), 184–189.

Nakash, O., Nagar, M., Shoshani, A., & Lurie, I. (2017). The association between perceived social support and posttraumatic stress symptoms among Eritrean and Sudanese male asylum seekers in Israel. *International Journal of Culture and Mental Health, 10*(3), 1–15.

Neace, R. T., Thaier, C., & Nasir, S. (2020). Understanding refugees: A complex discussion. In J. Kottler, S. Banu, & S. Jani (Eds.), *Handbook of refugee experience: Trauma, resilience, and recovery* (pp. 9–20). California Cognella Academic Publishing: San Diego.

Nickerson, A., Liddell, B., Asnaani, A., Carlsson, J., Fazel, M., Knaevelsrud, C., Morina, N., Neuner, F. Newnham, E., & Rasmussen, A. (2018) Trauma and mental health in forcibly displaced populations: an International Society for Traumatic Stress Studies Briefing Paper. ISTSS, Chicago. Retrieved from https://istss.org/getattachment/Education-Research/Briefing-Papers/Trauma-and-Mental-Health-in-Forcibly-Displaced-Pop/Displaced-Populations-Briefing-Paper_Final.pdf.aspx. On the February 12, 2020.

Norton, B. (2000). *Identity and language learning: Gender, ethnicity and educational change.* Harlow, England: Pearson Education.

Patel, N., Kellezi, B., & Williams, A. (2014). Psychological, social and welfare interventions for psychological health and well-being of torture survivors. *Cochrane Database of Systematic Reviews 2014, 11* (Art. No.: CD009317).

Porter, M., & Haslam, N. (2005). Predisplacement and postdisplacement factors associated with mental health of refugees and internally displaced persons: A meta-analysis. *JAMA, 294*(5), 602–612.

Rasool, I. A., & Payton, J. L. (2014). Tongues of fire: Women's suicide and self-injury by burns in the Kurdistan Region of Iraq. *the Sociological Review, 62*(2), 237–254.

Ringler-Jayanthan, E., Neibich-Gianni, M., Brubaker, D., & Naranjo, F. (2020). Integrating trauma-informed care in providing services for refugees and asylum seekers. In J. Kottler, S. Banu, & S. Jani (Eds.), *Handbook of refugee experience: Trauma, resilience, and recovery* (pp. 82–91). San Diego, California: Cognella.

Robjant, K., Hassan, R., & Katona, C. (2009). Mental health implications of detaining asylum seekers: Systematic review. *The British Journal of Psychiatry, 194,* 306–312.

Rogers, H., Fox, S., & Herlihy, J. (2015). The importance of looking credible: The impact of the behavioural sequelae of post-traumatic stress disorder on the credibility of asylum seekers. *Psychology, Crime and Law, 21*(2), 139–155.

Rosenbaum, P. J. (2016). How self-harmers use the body as an interpretive canvass. *Culture & Psychology, 22*(1), 128–138.

Rousseau, C., Drapeau, A., & Corin, E. (1997). The influence of culture and context on the pre- and post-migration experience of school-aged refugees from Central America and Southeast Asia in Canada. *Social Science and Medicine, 44*(8), 1115–1127.

Saechao, F., Sharrock, S., Reicherter, D., Livingston, J. D., Aylward, A., Whisnant, J., et al. (2012). Stressors and barriers to using mental health services among diverse groups of first-generation immigrants to the United States. *Community Mental Health Journal, 48*(1), 98–106.

Sam, D. L., & Berry, J. W. (2010). Acculturation when individuals and groups of different cultural backgrounds meet. *Perspectives on Psychological Science, 5*(4), 472–481.

Sanchez-Mazas, M., Efionayi-Mäder, D., Maggi, J., Achermann, C., Schaer, M., Escoda, R. I., & Coumou-Stants, F. (2011). *La Construction de l'Invisibilité: Suppression de l'Aide Sociale dans le Domaine de l'Asile.* Geneva: IES.

Schick, M., Zumwald, A., Knöpfli, B., Nickerson, A., Bryant, R. A., Schnyder, U., et al. (2016). Challenging future, challenging past: The relationship of social integration and psychological impairment in traumatised refugees. *European Journal of Psychotraumatology, 7*(1), 28057.

Schneider, A., Conrad, D., Pfeiffer, A., Elbert, T., Kolassa, I. T., & Wilker, S. (2018). Stigmatization is associated with increased PTSD risk and symptom severity after traumatic stress and diminished likelihood of spontaneous remission–A study with East-African conflict survivors. *Frontiers in Psychiatry, 9,* 423.

Schock, K., Rosner, R., & Knaevelsrud, C. (2015). Impact of asylum interviews on the mental health of traumatized asylum seekers. *European Journal of Psychotraumatology, 6,* 26286.

Schock, K., Böttche, M., Rosner, R., Wenk-Ansohn, M., & Knaevelsrud, C. (2016). Impact of new traumatic or stressful life events on pre-existing PTSD in traumatized refugees: Results of a longitudinal study, *7,* 32106

Schouler-Ocak, M., Wintrob, R., Moussaoui, D., Villasenor Bayardo, S. J., Zhao, X.-D., & Kastrup, M. C. (2016). Background paper on the needs of migrant, refugee and asylum seeker patients around the globe. *International Journal of Culture and Mental Health, 9*(3), 216–232.

Schweitzer, R., Melville, F., Steel, Z., & Lacherez, P. (2006). Trauma, post-migration living difficulties, and social support as predictors of psychological adjustment in resettled Sudanese refugees. *Australian and New Zealand Journal of Psychiatry, 2*(40), 179–187.

Silove, D. (1999). The psychosocial effects of torture, mass human rights violations, and refugee trauma: Toward an integrated conceptual framework. *The Journal of Nervous and Mental Disease, 187*(4), 200–207.

Silove, D., Steel, Z., McGorry, P., & Mohan, P. (1998). Trauma exposure, postmigration stressors, and symptoms of anxiety, depression and post-traumatic stress in Tamil asylum-seekers: Comparison with refugees and immigrants. *Acta Psychiatrica Scandinavica, 97*(3), 175–181.

Silove, D., Steel, Z., & Watters, C. (2000). Policies of deterrence and the mental health of asylum seekers. *JAMA, 284*(5), 604–611.

Silove, D., Austin, P., & Steel, Z. (2007). No refuge from terror: The impact of detention on the mental health of trauma-affected refugees seeking asylum in Australia. *Transcultural Psychiatry, 44*(3), 359–393.

Sironi, F. (1999). *Bourreaux et victimes: Psychologie de la torture.* Odile Jacob.

Song, S. J., Kaplan, C., Tol, W. A., Subica, A., & de Jong, J. (2015). Psychological distress in torture survivors: Pre-and post-migration risk factors in a US sample. *Social Psychiatry and Psychiatric Epidemiology, 50*(4), 549–560.

Song, S. J., Subica, A., Kaplan, C., Tol, W., & de Jong, J. (2017). Predicting the mental health and functioning of torture survivors. *The Journal of Nervous and Mental Disease, 206*(1), 33–39.

Spielrein, S. (1994). Destruction as the cause of coming into being. *Journal of Analytical Psychology, 39*(2), 155–186.

Steel, Z. (2001). Beyond PTSD: Towards a more adequate understanding of the multiple effects of complex trauma. In C. Moser & D. Nyfeler (Eds.), *Traumatiserungen von Flüchtlingen und Asyl Schenden: Einflus des politischen, sozialen und medizinischen Kontextes* (pp. 66–84). Zurich: Seismo.

Steel, Z., Chey, T., Silove, D., Marnane, C., Bryant, R. A., & Ommeren, M. V. (2009). Association of torture and other potentially traumatic events with mental health outcomes among populations exposed to mass conflict and displacement: A systematic review and meta-analysis. *JAMA, 302*(5), 537–549.

Steel, J., Dunlavy, A., Harding, C., & Theorell, T. (2016). The psychological consequences of pre-emigration trauma and post-migration stress in refugees and immigrants from Africa. *Journal of Immigrant and Minority Health, 19*(3), 1–10.

Stolorow, R. D. (2011). *World, affectivity, trauma.* New York: Routledge.

Strijk, P. J., van Meijel, B., & Gamel, C. J. (2011). Health and social needs of traumatized refugees and asylum seekers: An exploratory study. *Perspectives in Psychiatric Care, 47*(1), 48–55.

Sturm, G., Baubet, T., & Moro, M. R. (2007). Mobilising social and symbolic resources in transcultural therapies with refugees and asylum seekers: The story of Mister Diallo. In B. Droždek & J. Wilson (Eds.), *Voices of trauma: Treating psychological trauma across cultures* (pp. 211–231). New York: Springer.

Sturm, G., Baubet, T., & Moro, M. R. (2010). Culture, trauma, and subjectivity: The French ethnopsychoanalytic approach. *Traumatology, 16*(4), 27–38.

Tankink, M., & Richters, A. (2007). Silence as a coping strategy: The case of refugee women in the Netherlands from South-Sudan who experienced sexual violence in the context of war. In B. Droždek & J. Wilson (Eds.), *Voices of trauma: Treating psychological trauma across cultures* (pp. 191–210). New York: Springer.

Tekin, A., Karadağ, H., Süleymanoğlu, M., Tekin, M., Kayran, Y., Alpak, G., & Şar, V. (2016). Prevalence and gender differences in symptomatology of posttraumatic stress disorder and depression among Iraqi Yazidis displaced into Turkey. *European Journal of Psychotraumatology, 7,* 28556.

ter Heide, F. J. J., Mooren, T. M., & Kleber, R. J. (2016). Complex PTSD and phased treatment in refugees: A debate piece. *European Journal of Psychotraumatology, 7*(1), 28687.
Tortelli, A., Sauzé, D., & Skurnik, N. (2017). Capital social, santé mentale et immigration. *Annales Médico-Psychologiques, Revue Psychiatrique, 175*(6), 573–576.
Tummala-Narra, P. (2007). Conceptualizing trauma and resilience across diverse contexts. *Journal of Aggression, Maltreatment & Trauma, 14*(1–2), 33–53.
Turner, B. (1992). *Regulating bodies: Essays in medical sociology.* London: Routledge.
Turner, S. (2015). Refugee blues: A UK and European perspective. *Psychotraumatology, 6*(1), 29328.
Van Ommeren, M., de Jong, J. M., Sharma, B., Komproe, I., Thapa, S. B., & Cardeña, E. (2001). Psychiatric disorders among tortured bhutanese refugees in nepal. *Archives of General Psychiatry, 58*(5), 475–482. https://doi.org/10.1001/archpsyc.58.5.475.
Viñar, M. N. (2005). La spécificité de la torture comme source de trauma. *Revue Française De Psychanalyse, 69*(4), 1205–1224.
Volkan, V. D. (2004). From hope for a better life to broken spirits: An introduction. In J. P. Wilson & B. Drožđek (Eds.), *Broken spirits: The treatment of traumatized asylum seekers, refugees, war and torture victims* (pp. 7–12). New York: Brunner Mazel/Routledge.
Watters, C. (2001). Emerging paradigms in the mental health care of refugees. *Social Science and Medicine, 52*(11), 1709–1718.
Weine, S., Kuc, G., Eldin, D., Razzano, L., & Pavkovic, I. (2001). PTSD among Bosnian refugees: A survey of providers' knowledge, attitudes and service patterns. *Community Mental Health Journal, 37*(3), 261–271.
Womersley, G., & Kloetzer, L. (2018). This is not paranoia, this is real life: Psychosocial interventions for refugee victims of torture in Athens. *Intervention, 16*(2), 95.
Womersley, G., & Kloetzer, L. (2018). Being through doing: The self-immolation of an asylum seeker in Switzerland. *Frontiers in Psychiatry, 9,* 110.
Womersley, G., Maw, A., & Swartz, S. (2011). The construction of shame in Feminist reflexive practice and its manifestations in a research relationship. *Qualitative Inquiry, 17*(9), 876–886.
Womersley, G., Kloetzer, L., & Goguikian Ratcliff, B. (2017). Mental Health Problems Associated with Asylum Procedures of Refugees in European Countries [Press release]. Retrieved from https://nccr-onthemove.ch/highlights-2/highlights-2-5-2/. On the February 13, 2020.
Zittoun, T., & Sato, T. (2018). Imagination in adults and the aged person. In T. Zittoun & V. P. Glăveanu (Eds.), *Handbook of imagination and culture* (pp. 187–208). New York, NY: Oxford University Press.

Chapter 3
Prevalence of PTSD Among Displaced Populations—Three Case Studies

As explored in chapter two, displaced populations face a myriad of traumatic events, throughout the migration process. It comes as no surprise than, that two landmark, systematic meta-reviews found prevalence rates among refugee populations of **40%** (Turrini et al., 2017) and **30.6%** (Steel et al., 2009) respectively. Another meta-review noted that PTSD prevalence rate among first generation migrants in general and refugees/asylum seekers ranged from **9 to 36%** compared with reported prevalence rates of 1–2% in the general population (Close et al., 2016). There is evidence that these high prevalence rates of PTSD persist several years after displacement, both in countries of settlement and refugee camp contexts (Bogic et al., 2015; Kaltenbach et al., 2018; Nickerson et al., 2018). Prevalence rates of PTSD reported in displaced populations screened using the Harvard Trauma Questionaire (HTQ) in particular, include **45.5%** among earthquake survivors in Wenchuan China (Kun et al., 2009), **37.2%** among Cambodian refugees living on the Thai–Cambodian border camps (Cardozo et al., 2004), **29.3%** among populations living in conflict-ridden southern Lebanon (Farhood et al., 2006), and **11.8%** among displaced Guatemalans living in Chiapas, Mexico (Sabin et al., 2003).

This chapter will present prevalence rates of PTSD noted among displaced populations in three independent studies I conducted in collaboration with colleagues in South Africa, Iraq, and the Philippines respectively.

- A study in South Africa with *Médecins Sans Frontières*, which I conducted among refugees and asylum seekers from other African countries who fled to displaced camps after a flare-up of xenophobic violence occurred in Durban, revealing a prevalence rate of PTSD of **85%**.
- A study in Iraq with the Free Yezidi Foundation, which I conducted among displaced Yezidi communities in the context of an internal evaluation of the Free Yezidi Foundation's mental health intervention, revealing a prevalence rate of PTSD of **82%**
- A study in the Philippines with the Global Initiative for Stress and Trauma Treatment (Gist-T), I conducted in collaboration with colleagues among displaced

G. Theisen-Womersley, *Trauma and Resilience Among Displaced Populations*,
https://doi.org/10.1007/978-3-030-67712-1_3

communities affected by the recent conflict in Marawi in the context of a mental health needs assessment, revealing a prevalence rate of PTSD of **78%**.

In the first two case studies, The **Harvard Trauma Questionnaire (H.T.Q.)** was used as a screening instrument due its recognised cultural sensitivity in assessing highly traumatised populations (Mollica et al., 1992, 1998; Shoeb et al., 2007). PTSD in this case is defined according to a scoring algorithm previously described by the Harvard Refugee Trauma Group on the basis of DSM IV diagnostic criteria (Association, 1980; Mollica et al., 1992). In the third case study, the **Posttraumatic Stress Disorder Checklist (PCL-5)** was used as a screening instrument to assess the prevalence rate of PTSD Developed in 1990 at the National Center for PTSD, the PCL comprises 17 items corresponding to the PTSD symptom criteria in the *Diagnostic and Statistical Manual of Mental Disorders* (American Psychological Association (APA), 2013), and is one of the most widely used self-report measures of posttraumatic stress disorder (PTSD) (Blevins et al., 2015). The instrument been revised to include new symptoms and to conform to the DSM's four-factor conceptualization of PTSD and its corresponding symptom clusters: re-experiencing, avoidance, negative alterations in cognition and mood, and increased arousal and reactivity (Ashbaugh et al., 2016). In all studies, the aim of assessing the prevalence rate of PTSD was to identify and highlight the mental health needs of this particular population, to develop a culturally-appropriate intervention programme as well as to enrich advocacy campaigns for their humane treatment by state and non-governmental organizations alike.

Case Study One: Durban, South Africa

In April 2015, following an upsurge in violent xenophobic attacks throughout the country, displacement camps were set up to house roughly 7,500 foreign nationals seeking refuge in Durban, KwaZulu-Natal. *Médecins Sans Frontières* (MSF) were among the actors intervening in the camp by providing the population with basic medical care and psychosocial support. The majority if displaced individuals in the camp were refugees and asylum seekers from the Democratic Republic of Congo and Burundi who choose to remain in the camps: stating that they cannot return home to their countries of origin safely due to fear of persecution and that they fear returning to the South African communities from which they fled, in many cases after experiencing significantly violent attacks on themselves and their property. The people remaining in the displacement camps represent a population which has been exposed to multiple traumatic events—both in their countries of origin and more recently in South Africa—and were therefore presumed to be at risk of experiencing symptoms of post-traumatic stress. As part of a package of psychosocial care offered by MSF in the displacement camps, I conducted a study of post-traumatic stress symptoms among a convenience sample of refugees in order to explore the extent of the psychological trauma among this particular population, to reflect on the relevance of a PTSD diagnosis within this particular cultural setting and to offer relevant treatment. The case described here also appears in a chapter of a book entitled "Post-traumatic stress responses among refugees following xenophobic attacks in Durban, South Africa" first published by InScience Press (Womersley et al., 2016).

Method

After obtaining authorization from the local municipality and campsite managers, men and women—all of them foreign nationals from the DRC or Burundi—were approached by myself on site at three displacement camps.

Results

27 participants completed the Harvard Trauma Questionnaire. The results of questions 1–16 of part 4 of the HTQ were subsequently noted and scored. The mean score was 2.87. Participants included 12 women, out of which all 12 (100%) met diagnostic criteria and 15 men, out of which 12 (80%) met diagnostic criteria. When questioned about the traumatic event which participants had either experienced, witnessed or heard about, the majority referred to events which had taken place in their country of origin, as well as the recent xenophobic attacks. 22 participants (81%) reported experiencing or witnessing conflict, murder, torture and/or sexual violence. All participants had been in the camp for at least 7 weeks after the xenophobic violence. For all participants, the traumatic symptoms reported were related to events which had happened in their countries of origin, exacerbated by the xenophobic violence and experiences of being in a refugee camp.

Participants rated the items of the HTQ on a scale of 1–4. A score of 1 indicates 'not at all', 2 indicates 'a little,' 3 indicates 'quite a bit' and 4 indicates 'extremely.' The mean results of these scores are indicated below:

	Item	Mean score	Standard deviation
1.	Recurrent thoughts or memories of the most hurtful or terrifying events	3.11	0.89
2.	Feeling as though the event is happening again	3.41	0.75
3.	Recurrent nightmares	2.37	1.21
4.	Feeling detached or withdrawn from people	3.00	1.11
5.	Unable to feel emotions	2.48	1.25
	Feeling jumpy, easily startled	3.00	0.92
7.	Difficulty concentrating	2.78	0.93
8.	Trouble sleeping	3.04	0.94

(continued)

(continued)

	Item	Mean score	Standard deviation
9.	Feeling on guard	3.19	0.89
10.	Feeling irritable or having outbursts of anger	3.07	0.87
11.	Avoiding activities that remind you of the traumatic or hurtful event	2.85	1.67
12.	Inability to remember parts of the most traumatic or hurtful events	1.93	1.11
13.	Less interest in daily activities	2.96	1.06
14.	Feeling as if you don't have a future	3.15	1.06
15.	Avoiding thoughts or feelings associated with the traumatic or hurtful experience	2.41	1.15
16.	Sudden emotional or physical reaction when reminded of the most hurtful or traumatic events	3.34	0.83
Total mean		3.34	

There were no statistically significant outliers in terms of the mean response to individual items ($p < 0.05$). However, it must be noted that the mean response of items 3, 5, 12 and 15 fell below 2.5. This suggests that participants reported not being strongly affected by recurrent nightmares, an inability to feel emotions, an inability to remember part of the most traumatic or hurtful event in their lives or a sense of avoiding thoughts or feelings associated with the traumatic or hurtful experience. In general, participants reported being fully aware and emotionally responsive to the traumatic events which they had experienced or witnessed. The highest mean response to an individual item was to item number 2 (mean score = 3.4). This item refers to a feeling that the event is happening again. When questioned, the majority of participants explained that the recent xenophobic attacks which they had experienced or witnessed in South Africa had triggered traumatic memories or flashbacks of events from which they had had to flee in their country of origin. The greatest standard deviations were for item 3 ('recurrent nightmares,' std dev = 1.21), 5 ('unable to feel emotions,' std dev = 1.25) and 11 ('avoiding activities that remind you of the hurtful or traumatic event,' std dev = 1.67).

Case Study Two: Yezidis in Iraq

Yezidism arguably remains one of the most oppressed religions in Iraq, with the population historically confronted by many attempts at genocide. In the summer of 2014, fighters tore into Kurdish northern Iraq and committed attacks against the Yezidi under the black banner of Islamic State. They took more than 7000 people hostage, killing around 5000, mainly men (Mohammadi, 2016). Although men were mostly killed, women and girls were kidnapped, taken a hostage, raped and used or traded as sex slaves. For many, these catastrophic events lasted for years. These atrocities have left many survivors displaced and affected by trauma. Furthermore, the deep-rooted trauma is collective: 3500 women and 1200 children are still held captive by Islamic State. Indeed, recent research on socioecological mental health and psychosocial support (MHPSS) interventions suggests that individuals may suffer from posttraumatic stress through the impact of the disaster on their community, even if not directly exposed (Wind & Komproe, 2018). Little research has been conducted on experiences of trauma among this population. The detrimental effect of the torture, sexual abuse and genocide of this population remains largely unaddressed (Hoffman et al., 2018). One study estimates the prevalence of post-traumatic stress disorder (PTSD) among Yezidis seeking refuge in Turkey at **43%** (Tekin et al., 2016), with women being more frequently affected than men. Another preliminary study assessed both PTSD and complex post-traumatic stress disorder (CPTSD) among female Yazidi former captives residing in post-ISIS camps. The results indicated that **50.9%** women had probable CPTSD, while 20.0% had probable PTSD (Hoffman et al., 2018). A few more studies confirm this alarmingly high prevalence of trauma among the Yezidi population (Ceri et al., 2016; Gerdau et al., 2017; Nasıroğlu & Çeri, 2016).

The Free Yezidi Foundation (FYF) women's centre is situated in the Duhok province of the Kurdistan Region of Iraq. This centre offers psychological interventions for women who suffered in captivity and eventually escaped, as well as those who were never captured but were displaced by attacks and whose entire families are now homeless and jobless. The centre, inside the Khange IDP camp, serves all the women in the camp, including women who have escaped ISIS captivity. The facility at present features a counselling/recreation room, an art corner, a computer lab, a classroom area (for teaching English, Arabic, Women's Rights, Kurdish and Yezidi culture and history), a sewing room and an outdoor garden. The project collaborates with over 20 non-governmental and governmental actors in Kurdistan to coordinate MHPSS responses. Furthermore, FYF is also active in global advocacy for genocide recognition and more resources to Yezidi survivors. An essential part of the programme focuses on addressing the significantly high levels of trauma in the community.

This specific MHPSS intervention, informed by the mental health pyramid alluded to in the Inter-Agency Standing Committee (IASC) guidelines,[1] targets three levels of interventions—the level of the individual, the level of the group (of service users) and the level of the wider community. Broadly, the intervention is informed by empirically validated trauma treatment interventions, which include principles of psychoeducation, and stabilisation techniques based on trauma processing therapies such as Eye Movement Desensitization and Reprocessing (EMDR) Therapy (Eichfeld et al., 2018). This includes pilot projects implementing group EMDR Group Traumatic Episode Protocol (GTEP) therapy under the clinical supervision of international experts. Individual and group therapy is offered by the project psychologists. Intake interviews are held with each service user to allocate them to appropriate groups or to refer them to individual therapy according to their specific mental health needs.

[1] https://www.who.int/mental_health/emergencies/IASC_guidelines.pdf.

Group sessions draw on techniques of emotional regulation, grounding and stabilisation tools and skills—and are complemented by further extra activities, such as art, exercises, games, role playing, singing and dancing. Furthermore, 13 service users have been trained as lay counsellors to provide psychological first and second aid, and work under the supervision of the project psychologist. Part of this community work includes facilitating psychoeducation workshops to raise the community's awareness on trauma and its impact on psychological wellbeing, and conducting community sensitisation/awareness sessions. For example, with the input of the lay counsellors, cultural mediators and the art teacher, a toolbox was created, which included pictures and text (in Arabic and Kurdish), demonstrating reactions to trauma and loss as well as basic stabilisation techniques. The case described here also appears in a scientific article published in *Intervention* (Womersley & Arikut-Treece, 2019).

Method

In the context of an internal evaluation, Yezidi women, service users of the FYF, were screened before starting and after completing the programme using the WHO-5 well-being scale—among the most widely used questionnaires assessing subjective psychological well-being with demonstrated clinimetric validity (Topp et al., 2015). For further quantitative data on the prevalence of trauma among the population, the Harvard Trauma Questionnaire (HTQ) was used due its recognised cultural sensitivity in assessing highly traumatised populations (Mollica et al., 1992, 1998; Shoeb et al., 2007). It has been validated for assessing PTSD in Iraqi refugees in particular (Shoeb et al., 2007). PTSD was defined according to a scoring algorithm previously described by the Harvard Refugee Trauma Group on the basis of DSM-IV diagnostic criteria (APA, 1980; Mollica et al., 1992). A client satisfaction questionnaire was completed by service users in individual psychotherapy upon completion of the programme in June.

Results: Topline Findings

- 37 out of 54 individuals from a convenience sample of displaced Yezidi community in Khanke **(69%)** met the diagnostic criteria for PTSD
- This suggests a substantially high prevalence rate of PTSD among the Yezidi community in general, compared to other displaced populations exposed to conflict globally **(estimated at 31%).**
- Average score among 16 service users of **2.81** in February (**81%** of service users met diagnostic criteria for PTSD)
- Average score among 19 service users of **2.4** in June (**45%** of service users met diagnostic criteria for PTSD)
- A **15% decrease in post-traumatic symptoms**

- A **44% decrease in service users meeting diagnostic criteria for PTSD**
- The cohort started with a rate of PTSD higher than the general Yezidi population of Khanke (69%), yet dropped below this average after having completed the programme

WHO-5

Service users of the FYF were screened pre- and post-programme using the WHO-5. Out of 200 women attending the programme, 170 completed the pre-test and 113 the post-test. The lower number of women completing the post-test was due to the logistical challenges of having all participants available for testing in the particular week of evaluation. The average pre-test score was 12.35 (49%, n = 170), and the average post-test score was 22.56 (90.24%, n = 113). This represents an 83% increase in self-reported wellbeing among service users who have completed the programme. The pre-test score was found to be lower in comparison to general population studies conducted in Denmark, where the mean score was found to be 14 (Bech et al., 2003; Ellervik et al., 2014), yet substantially higher upon completion of the programme.

When WHO-5 is used for the screening of depression, a cut-off score of $\leq$ 10 is used (Topp et al., 2015). At baseline, 45% of participants in this sample fell below this cut-off score, meeting diagnostic criteria for depression upon entering the programme. Service users of the project were screened using the HTQ upon entering the project and again upon graduating from the programme. The baseline prevalence rate of PTSD was **81.25%,** with an average score of 2.81. Upon completing the programme, the prevalence rate of PTSD was 45%, with an average score of 2.4. This represents a decrease in service users meeting diagnostic criteria for PTSD of 45%. Despite this, the symptoms decreased on average by only 15%. This suggests that there may be a sub-population who continued to meet the diagnostic criteria for PTSD (without any reduction in symptoms) and who continued to need psychotherapeutic support.

Harvard Trauma Questionnaire

	Item	Mean score: February 2018	Mean score: June 2018	Percentage increase/decrease
1.	Recurrent thoughts or memories of the most hurtful or terrifying events	2.8	3.2	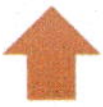 12%

(continued)

(continued)

	Item	Mean score: February 2018	Mean score: June 2018	Percentage increase/decrease
2.	Feeling as though the event is happening again	2.6	2.5	−6%
3.	Recurrent nightmares	3	2.4	−23%
4.	Feeling detached or withdrawn from people	2.7	2.4	−12%
5.	Unable to feel emotions	2.4	1.9	−18%
6.	Feeling jumpy, easily startled	3.4	3.1	−10%
7.	Difficulty concentrating	3	2	−33%
8.	Trouble sleeping	2.8	1.6	−41%
9.	Feeling on guard	2.5	2.1	−14%
10.	Feeling irritable or having outbursts of anger	3	2.6	−12%
11.	Avoiding activities that remind you of the traumatic or hurtful event	3.3	2.7	−18%
12.	Inability to remember parts of the most traumatic or hurtful events	2.5	2.2	−12%
13.	Less interest in daily activities	2.7	2.1	−20%

(continued)

(continued)

	Item	Mean score: February 2018	Mean score: June 2018	Percentage increase/decrease
14.	Feeling as if you don't have a future	2.3	2.7	19%
15.	Avoiding thoughts or feelings associated with the traumatic or hurtful experience	3.1	2.7	–13%
16.	Sudden emotional or physical reaction when reminded of the most hurtful or traumatic events	2.9	2.2	–23%
Total mean		2.8	2.4	–15%

It is interesting to note that, despite a clear reduction in symptoms of trauma globally, there was an increase in symptoms related to question 14 of 19% (feeling as if you don't have a future). This may not necessarily relate directly to symptoms of PTSD but could be more related to the ongoing sociopolitical and economic environment in which the population finds themselves, including poor material living conditions and prospects for the future.

There was similarly a 12% increase in self-reported "recurrent thoughts or memories of the most hurtful or terrifying events." Given the overall reduction in post-traumatic symptoms, this is an anomaly. A full understanding of the reason for this increase is beyond the scope of this paper. It would be interesting to explore the reason behind this through qualitative interviews. As has been suggested in literature on refugee mental health (Steel et al., 2016), one hypothesis could be the reduction in dissociative symptoms associated with trauma leading to service users being more able to think about or remember the events—the relatively safer space of the camp in general, and the project in particular, allowing them to confront these thoughts and memories.

The most significant improvement in symptoms was a 41% decrease in having trouble sleeping, and a 33% decrease in having difficulty concentrating. The overall decrease in symptoms may be attributed to a variety of factors—including as a reflection of the efficacy of the MHPSS intervention in reducing symptoms, as well as the simple fact of time having passed because the traumatic events experienced by the population as they were forced to flee their homes.

Case Study Three: Marawi, Philippines

On 23 May 2017, affiliated militants of the Islamic State (IS), including the Maute and Abu Sayyaf Salafi jihadist groups, launched an attack on the Philippine government security forces in Marawi, Mindanao, the country's largest Muslim-majority city. It was a planned effort to establish an 'IS province' in the Philippines. Government troops took an unexpected five months to liberate Marawi, at a cost of near-total destruction of the old city and displacement of some 350,000 citizens (who became 'internally displaced persons', or IDPs), plus more than 1,000 dead. Then, on 22 December 2017, tropical storm Tembin (known as Vinta in the Philippines) struck Mindanao Island and turned another 100,000 people, already living in the IDP reception areas following the violence, into new IDPs, and also added several hundred dead.

The recent Marawi crisis is not an isolated traumatic incident or event. Rather, it reveals a context and pattern of deeply engrained complex trauma dating back generations, related to:

- Historical and intergenerational trauma
- Intra-familial trauma, including *Rido*
- Endemic political violence
- Violent extremism
- Sexual Gender-Based Violence (SGBV)
- Natural disasters
- History of forced evacuations/displacement.

Furthermore, the current context is characterised by long waiting lists for resettlement, the impossibility for many to return to their homes, increased reports of SGBV and of young women sent away to Manila and elsewhere to earn money as commercial sex workers, rising tension among IDPs and host communities, and a risk of compassion fatigue among host communities and even engaged humanitarian actors. All of this increases the risk of polarisation and violent extremism. This is a critical consideration for the mental health of this community, given the role that exposure to complex trauma may play in the cycle of violence, abuse and aggression.

Method

In response to these events, I was part of a five-member team from the Global Initiative for Stress and Trauma Treatment (GIST-T), in consultation with EMDR Philippines, Philippines Psychiatric Association, Nonviolent Peaceforce (NP) and World Bank Manila, conducted a needs assessment to understand the psychosocial impact of the recent crises in Marawi on the affected population—individuals, families, and local communities. The team was composed of Rolf Carriere, Dr. Derek Farrell, Fr. Cornelio Jaranilla, Dr. Sushma Mehrotra, and myself. The aim was to gather first-hand information from IDPs, review the state of current psychological services available, identify unmet mental health needs, and propose immediate and medium-term ways to strengthen capacity of mental health professionals and paraprofessionals to provide appropriate treatment.

The team interviewed some 120 people, including 80 IDPs for psychometric screening using eight standardized instruments (in four Evacuation Centres and as 'Homestays'). Others interviewed were 20 humanitarian workers, eight teachers, three psychiatrists and two military commanders. Focus Group Discussions were held with an additional 30 local actors closely associated with the events. The rapid assessment, conducted over a five-day period with the help of four interpreters speaking English, Maranao, Bisaya, and Tagalog, limited itself to parts of the two Lanao provinces. Given these cultural/linguistic challenges, time restrictions and geographical limitations, the results cannot claim to be representative of the whole community. Even so, involvement of local partners allowed the mission access to a wide range of key stakeholders and to a surprising depth of people's emotions and experiences of violence, abuse and aggression.

Results

- **Nearly half (49%)** of the IDPs screened for anxiety with the GAD-7 could be diagnosed with ***severe*anxiety** warranting a specialist referral to a psychiatrist.
- **Nearly half (46%)** of the IDPs screened for depression with the PHQ9 could be diagnosed with ***severe*depression** warranting initiation of pharmacotherapy and psychological treatment.
- The population of adults who were screened have been exposed to a high number of adverse events in childhood, such as abuse, neglect, violence, and poverty. The average individual screened had been exposed to around three different adverse events in their childhood.
- **78%** of the IDPs screened for PTSD with the PCL-5 meet the criteria for **PTSD**.

In terms of prevalence rates of PTSD in particular, the focus of this chapter, the more detailed results of the PCL-5 was as follows:

PCL-5 Scores per Cluster (*N*= 80)

PCL-5	Mean
Criterion *A*	100%
Cluster *B* (1)	2.5
Cluster *C* (1)	2.54
Cluster *D* (2)	2.06
Cluster *E* (2)	2.29
Total mean	**45.19**

(continued)

(continued)

PCL-5	Mean
μ	15.66
Cut-off score	33
Meeting DSM-5 criteria for PTSD	**77.5%**

The results indicate that 100% of participants reported being exposed to death, threatened death, actual or threatened serious injury, or actual or threatened sexual violence through direct exposure, witnessing the trauma, learning that a relative or close friend was exposed to a trauma—diagnostic criterion A of a PTSD diagnosis according to the DSM-5 (Association, 2013). 77.5% met the diagnostic criteria for PTSD.

Conclusion

Significant limitations of all three case studies include the convenience sampling and the small sample size taken by convenience. Meta-analyses of prevalence studies have indicated that small studies have much higher prevalence than the apparent true prevalence (Terhakopian et al., 2008). Another limitation is potential self-reporting bias. Perceived secondary gain for being considered psychologically impacted by the events may have included, for example, the perceived hope of improved access to social, medical, psychological and legal services in all three cases. To minimise the impact of this bias, all participants were clearly informed of the fact that responses to the questionnaire would in no way impact treatment by state mechanisms or NGOs.

Despite this, the prevalence rates of **85, 82** and **78%** across these three vastly different contexts are remarkably similar. This is even more remarkable given the fact that they are significantly more than those reported in other long-term refugee populations screened using the HTQ noted above—typically noted as being somewhere between 11.8% (Sabin et al., 2003) and 45.5% (Kun et al., 2009). The results of these case studies indeed attest to the alarmingly high rates of trauma among the displaced populations. Furthermore, they highlight the substantial impact of the political, legal and sociocultural environment on both the prevalence of trauma as well as processes of psychosocial rehabilitation.

It is possible that the high prevalence rate of traumatic stress response symptoms reported could be partly attributed to the current significant levels of environmental stress and insecurity. All three contexts were that of ongoing displacement in a situation of crisis. In all three communities—the trauma was not necessarily linked to one specific catastrophe, but a series of traumatic incidents facing the population collectively. In all three cases, the situation remained unstable—communities often living in appalling conditions, meeting a hostile reception by host communities, and remaining unsure as to whether or not they'd be able to return home. In all three cases, the trauma linked to the precarious nature of this ongoing displacement was not the only trauma affecting the community. It was on the back of multiple traumas dating back generations. Trauma was related to not only direct exposure to human rights violations and other atrocities leading to the displacement itself (in other words, the "headline events") but compounded variables related to.

- Multiple losses (home, family members, possessions, socioeconomic status)
- Fear of ongoing attacks
- Breakdown of the family unit (due to loss, separation and family members seeking refuge abroad)
- Poverty
- Gender roles being threatened due to men losing employment opportunities
- Poor living conditions in the camps (including cramped living quarters)
- Feeling "trapped" in the camps
- Uncertain futures
- Ethnic discrimination.

Trauma across all three contexts was shown to be related to collective and historic trauma experienced on a community level. For many, the uncertainty as to whether or not their loved ones were alive or dead appears to have complicated the mourning process. Many individuals across all contexts reported feeling as though they are "frozen" in the liminal space of displacement, unable to start on the important and necessary work of grieving. Furthermore, hope that loved ones may still be alive is a double-edged sword—keeping many stuck on a perpetual loop of acute and intense pain, unable to proceed along the emotional journey of mourning.

The prevalence rates of trauma is presented here in this chapter in terms of percentages, in neat figures. Yet trauma is irrevocably collective, symbolic, and deeply political. Can this "dynamic" nature of trauma—the complex inter-relation of factors across multiple levels—truly be measured by instruments such as the HTQ and PCL-5? Is PTSD a valid diagnostic entity? Can it adequately capture the economic, social, and political landscape? Is it culturally relevant? Is it useful—for whom and for what? Yes—high prevalence rates of PTSD were noted among displaced populations in the case studies explored here in this chapter. Yes, we need to be shocked by these figures. They bear witness to deep suffering. Yes, it is important that we take stock of the real challenges people report facing. Yes, the trauma is real, it is there. However, I would argue that we also need to look "beyond" this diagnosis—which in the contexts noted above seemed to have little or no meaning for the communities affected. In the following chapter, I explore some of these questions by providing examining the politicized history of PTSD, the criticisms levelled against it, and the way in which it is understood and used by various actors—including health professionals working with displaced populations across the E.U.

References

American Psychiatric Association. (1980). *Diagnostic and Statistical Manual of Mental Disorders* (3rd ed). American Psychiatric Association.

American Psychiatric Association. (2013). *Diagnostic and Statistical Manual of Mental Disorders* (5th ed.). American Psychiatric Association.

Ashbaugh, A. R., Houle-Johnson, S., Herbert, C., El-Hage, W., & Brunet, A. (2016). Psychometric validation of the English and French versions of the Posttraumatic Stress Disorder Checklist for DSM-5 (PCL-5). *PloS one, 11*(10), e0161645.

Bech, P., Olsen, L. R., Kjoller, M., & Rasmussen, N. K. (2003). Measuring well-being rather than the absence of distress symptoms: A comparison of the SF-36 Mental Health subscale and the WHO-Five well-being scale. *International Journal of Methods in Psychiatric Research, 12*(2), 85–91.

Blevins, C. A., Weathers, F. W., Davis, M. T., Witte, T. K., & Domino, J. L. (2015). The posttraumatic stress disorder checklist for DSM-5 (PCL-5): Development and initial psychometric evaluation. *Journal of Traumatic Stress, 28*(6), 489–498.

Bogic, M., Njoku, A., & Priebe, S. (2015). Long-term mental health of war-refugees: A systematic literature review. *BMC International Health and Human Rights, 15,* 29.

Cardozo, B. L., Talley, L., Burton, A., & Crawford, C. (2004). Karenni refugees living in Thai-Burmese border camps: Traumatic experiences, mental health outcomes, and social functioning. *Social Science and Medicine, 58*(12), 2637–2644.

Ceri, V., Özlü-Erkilic, Z., Özer, Ü., Yalcin, M., Popow, C., & Akkaya-Kalayci, T. (2016). Psychiatric symptoms and disorders among Yazidi children and adolescents immediately after forced migration following ISIS attacks. *Neuropsychiatrie, 30*(3), 145–150.

Close, C., Kouvonen, A., Bosqui, T., Patel, K., O'Reilly, D., & Donnelly, M. (2016). The mental health and wellbeing of first generation migrants: A systematic-narrative review of reviews. *Globalization and Health, 12*(1), 47.

Eichfeld, C., Farrell, D., Mattheß, M., et al. (2018). Trauma stabilisation as a sole treatment intervention for post-traumatic stress disorder in Southeast Asia. *Psychiatric Quarterly, 90,* 1–26.

Ellervik, C., Kvetny, J., Christensen, K. S., Vestergaard, M., & Bech, P. (2014). Prevalence of depression, quality of life and antidepressant treatment in the Danish General Suburban Population Study. *Nordic Journal of Psychiatry, 68*(7), 507–512.

Farhood, L., Dimassi, H., & Lehtinen, T. (2006). Exposure to war-related traumatic events, prevalence of PTSD, and general psychiatric morbidity in a civilian population from Southern Lebanon. *Journal of Transcultural Nursing, 17*(4), 333–340.

Gerdau, I., Kizilhan, J. I., & Noll-Hussong, M. (2017). Posttraumatic stress disorder and related disorders among Female Yazidi Refugees following Islamic state of Iraq and syria attacks—A case series and mini-review. *Frontiers in Psychiatry, 8,* 282

Hoffman, Y. S., Grossman, E. S., Shrira, A., Kedar, M., Ben-Ezra, M., Dinnayi, M., et al. (2018). Complex PTSD and its correlates amongst female Yazidi victims of sexual slavery living in post-ISIS camps. *World Psychiatry, 17*(1), 112.

Kaltenbach, E., Schauer, M., Hermenau, K., Elbert, T., & Schalinski, I. (2018). Course of mental health in refugees–a one year panel survey. *Frontiers in Psychiatry, 9,* 352.

Kun, P., Chen, X., Han, S., Gong, X., Chen, M., Zhang, W., & Yao, L. (2009). Prevalence of post-traumatic stress disorder in Sichuan Province, China after the 2008 Wenchuan earthquake. *Public Health, 123*(11), 703–707.

Mohammadi, D. (2016). Help for Yazidi survivors of sexual violence. *The Lancet Psychiatry, 3*(5), 409–410.

Mollica, R., Caspi-Yavin, Y., Bollini, P., Truong, T., Tor, S., & Lavelle, J. (1992). The Harvard trauma questionnaire: Validating a cross-cultural instrument for measuring torture, trauma, and posttraumatic stress disorder in Indochinese refugees. *The Journal of Nervous and Mental Disease, 180*(2), 111–116.

Mollica, R., McInnes, K., Poole, C., & Tor, S. (1998). Dose-effect relationships of trauma to symptoms of depression and post-traumatic stress disorder among Cambodian survivors of mass violence. *The British Journal of Psychiatry, 173*(6), 482–488.

Nasıroğlu, S., & Çeri, V. (2016). Posttraumatic stress and depression in Yazidi refugees. *Neuropsychiatric Disease and Treatment, 12,* 2941.

Nickerson, A., Liddell, B., Asnaani, A., Carlsson, J., Fazel, M., Knaevelsrud, C., Morina, N., Neuner, F. Newnham, E., & Rasmussen, A. (2018) *Trauma and mental health in forcibly displaced populations: an International Society for Traumatic Stress Studies Briefing Paper.* ISTSS, Chicago. Retrieved from https://istss.org/getattachment/Education-Research/Briefing-Papers/Trauma-and-Mental-Health-in-Forcibly-Displaced-Pop/Displaced-Populations-Briefing-Paper_Final.pdf.aspx. On February 12, 2020.

Sabin, M., Cardozo, B. L., Nackerud, L., Kaiser, R., & Varese, L. (2003). Factors associated with poor mental health among Guatemalan refugees living in Mexico 20 years after civil conflict. *JAMA, 290*(5), 635–642.

Shoeb, M., Weinstein, H., & Mollica, R. (2007). The Harvard trauma questionnaire: Adapting a cross-cultural instrument for measuring torture, trauma and posttraumatic stress disorder in Iraqi refugees. *International Journal of Social Psychiatry, 53*(5), 447–463.

Steel, Z., Chey, T., Silove, D., Marnane, C., Bryant, R. A., & Ommeren, M. V. (2009). Association of torture and other potentially traumatic events with mental health outcomes among populations exposed to mass conflict and displacement: A systematic review and meta-analysis. *JAMA, 302*(5), 537–549.

Steel, J., Dunlavy, A., Harding, C., & Theorell, T. (2016). The Psychological Consequences of Pre-Emigration Trauma and Post-Migration Stress in Refugees and Immigrants from Africa. *Journal of Immigrant and Minority Health, 19*(3), 1–10.

Tekin, A., Karadağ, H., Süleymanoğlu, M., Tekin, M., Kayran, Y., Alpak, G., & Şar, V. (2016). Prevalence and gender differences in symptomatology of posttraumatic stress disorder and depression among Iraqi Yazidis displaced into Turkey. *European Journal of Psychotraumatology, 7,* 28556.

Terhakopian, A., Sinaii, N., Engel, C. C., Schnurr, P. P., & Hoge, C. W. (2008). Estimating population prevalence of posttraumatic stress disorder: An example using the PTSD checklist. *Journal of Traumatic Stress, 21*(3), 290–300.

Topp, C. W., Østergaard, S. D., Søndergaard, S., & Bech, P. (2015). The WHO-5 well-being index: A systematic review of the literature. *Psychotherapy and Psychosomatics, 84*(3), 167–176.

Turrini, G., Purgato, M., Ballette, F., Nosè, M., Ostuzzi, G., & Barbui, C. (2017). Common mental disorders in asylum seekers and refugees: Umbrella review of prevalence and intervention studies. *International Journal of Mental Health Systems, 11*(1), 51.

Wind, T. R., & Komproe, I. H. (2018). Closing the gap between disaster mental health research and practice: Evidence for socio-ecological mental health interventions through multilevel research. *Intervention, 16*(1), 5.

Womersley, G., & Arikut-Treece, Y. (2019). Collective trauma among displaced populations in Northern Iraq: A case study evaluating the therapeutic interventions of the Free Yezidi Foundation. *Intervention, 17*(1), 3.

Chapter 4
Beyond PTSD

> It is necessary not to give way to the social demand to 'psychiatrise' this problem, but instead to preserve it as a human problem and a political problem of an enormous scale rather than reducing it to a health problem, this being a perverse trick which makes the establishment feel comfortable. (Viñar, 2005b, p. 322)

PTSD as a disorder was first introduced as a diagnosis by the American Psychiatric Association (American Psychiatric Association (APA), 1980) in the DSM III in 1980, with interest in it booming to such an extent thereafter that it was referred to in mass media as "the disorder of the 1990s" (Marsella et al., 1996). There was equally a rapid international diffusion of the concept from its conception, including a politically-driven mobilization of this concept to highlight the suffering of refugees coming into Europe in the late twentieth century (d'Halluin, 2009). Referring to the now ubiquitous use of the word "trauma," Laqueur (2010) notes: "having once been relatively obscure, it is now found everywhere: used in the New York Times fewer than 300 times between 1851 and 1960, it has appeared 11,000 times since" (p. 19). Beyond the field of mental health, this category has also imposed itself in the social world: in public spaces, as a mode of intelligibility of individual and collective experiences related to dramatic events, and in action as a form of response to these situations (d'Halluin et al., 2004). It is a "sexy diagnosis" (Struwe, 1994, p. 319) However, despite its popularity and dominance in Western cultural discourse as an integral part of our collective conscious (Summerfield, 1996), PTSD has had a much longer and complex history (Andreasen, 2010; d'Halluin, 2009; Fisher, 2014; Larrabee et al., 2003; Summerfield, 2001).

Disputes over the legitimacy of the diagnosis, particularly during the period leading up to its codification as a disorder in the DSM-III, are well documented in the social science literature (Eagle, 2014; Fisher, 2014; Herman, 1997; Young, 1995). Andreasen (Andreasen, 2010), for example, highlights how the roots of the diagnosis as a construct as well as its popularity has been inextricably linked to post-war experiences of predominantly white male American soldiers:

> Because World War II brought together psychiatrists from all over the world and from all over the United States, it became clear that they could differ in training, conceptual framework, and in approaches to diagnosis and treatment. A consensus developed that some standardization was needed, and this challenge led to the creation of the first diagnostic manual, developed

G. Theisen-Womersley, *Trauma and Resilience Among Displaced Populations*,
https://doi.org/10.1007/978-3-030-67712-1_4

> by the Veterans' Administration. This provided an incentive to the American Psychiatric Association (APA) to develop its own manual: the first Diagnostic and Statistical Manual of the APA, or DSM-I, which appeared in 1952. This manual included a category called gross stress reaction… The first revision of this manual, DSM-II, was published in 1968. Without any explanation, the diagnosis of gross stress reaction was omitted. The most plausible explanation for the omission is that the concept was closely linked to warfare and combat, and DSM-II was written in a peaceful era (p. 68).

It was notably with this work with veterans of the Vietnam combat in the 1960s that the trauma mental health movement can really be said to have begun. These socio-political forces and trends drove the rise in the popularity and salience of discourses of trauma—including the political momentum produced by the Vietnam Veteran's associations and the anti-war movement of the United States who were seeking recognition of the damages of conflict (Eagle, 2014; Herman, 1997). This later expanded to include female survivors of sexual assault (Burgess & Holmstrom, 1974; Foa & Kozak, 1986; Koss & Harvey, 1991). Another significant wave of interest in the category of PTSD similarly occurred in the nineties, where a surge of humanitarian actors drew on the concept. They used it not only to inform their emergency medical interventions but also as a way to testify to the suffering of populations in the developing world. Indeed, this application of PTSD was fundamental in the formation a new language of political denunciation of the dramas humanitarian actors encountered in the field (d'Halluin et al., 2004). The stage was similarly set for the modern era of research into trauma among refugee populations in particular, with the first studies being conducted among South East Asian refugees—for example Cambodian survivors of the Khmer Rouge (Mollica et al., 1992, 1998). PTSD thus has been "glued together by the practices, technologies, and narratives with which it is diagnosed, studied, treated and represented and by the various interests, institutions, and moral arguments that mobilised these efforts and resources" (Young, 1995, p. 5). Today, the burgeoning interest in PTSD among refugee populations continues to shape the humanitarian field.

Models of Trauma: Conflicting Theoretical Traditions

Since the 1950s, two main positions on trauma have been articulated (Andreasen, 2010; Eagle, 2014). The first position (the "neurobiological school"), represented by thinkers such as Selye (1950, 1956), emphasized how environmental stressors set into motion certain physiological reactions mediated through the nervous and the hormonal systems. Selye coined the term "stress" in the 1950s and hypothesized that physiological reactions to stressors within the environment are mediated by the hypothalamic–pituitary–adrenal (HPA) axis. Within this medical model, the HPA axis is generally considered as a healthy and functional system but maladaptive and physically debilitating under continued exposure to extreme stress. The second position (the "psychological school") was rooted in psychodynamic theory. It considered responses to stress from a more subjective and context-specific perspective by emphasizing the role of the unconscious and of repressed childhood memories in how individuals respond to stressors within their environment.

These two conceptual frameworks, the neurobiological and the psychological, continue to set the stage for debates in the field of traumatology regarding the cross-cultural applicability of PTSD as a diagnostic construct. Is PTSD a universal construct? What is the same and what is different across cultures? Scholars falling predominantly into the "neurobiological school" point to the scientific evidence, particularly neurobiological studies, which have documented that affect regulation and right hemisphere alterations in brain functioning are indeed universal (Schore, 2003). They refer to the stable and consistent neurobiological pattern of changes involving the hyper arousal of the sympathetic nervous system such as the augmentation of the acoustic startle reflex, sleep abnormalities and changes in the H-P-A axis (Marsella, 2010; Marsella et al., 1996). This position highlights neurobiological/physical responses to trauma. These are responses not based on conscious or deliberate meaning, but which go directly to the nervous system as an automatic or "primitive" response based on evolutionary tactics for threat detection and survival (Eagle, 2014; Foa & Kozak, 1986).

In contrast to the neurobiological position, many theorists falling into the second "psychological" school of thought have argued that the location of trauma within a psychiatric/neurobiological paradigm neglects the broader socio-political context. They question the applicability of categories that structure Western psychological discourse, arguing that a diagnostic understandings of traumatic symptoms do not give careful attention to the notion that people's ways of seeing the world, their assumptions, and the discourses available to them, inform the meaning which is attributed to trauma. In short, current discourses on trauma are simply inadequate to grasp the complexity of how different human beings in different cultures respond to terrifying events (Bracken, 2001, 2002; Fisher, 2014; Janoff-Bulman, 1985; Kirmayer et al., 2010; Staeuble, 2004; Summerfield, 2001; Tummala-Narra, 2007; Wasco, 2003; Young, 1995). According to Eagle (2014), seen from within this psychodynamic perspective:

> Formulation of trauma impact requires careful exploration of the manner in which the individual describes the traumatic event and their response to it, including for example, the language they deploy, emphases, omissions, affective tone, and fantasy material; with a view to uncovering pre/unconscious associations to the trauma and the way in which intrapsychic constellations have shaped and/or mapped onto the experience. A strongly ideographic approach is maintained in which trauma impact can only be fully appreciated with a careful personal history taking, formulation of personality constellation and dynamics, and attention to unconscious as well as conscious meanings. (p. 9)

This relativistic and individualistic model is in clear contradiction of the "biological" model of psychiatry which seeks to re-position psychiatry as a medical specialty replete with well-defined disorders with identifiable symptomatology and treatment protocols (Marsella, 2010).

A third school of thought, based on the cognitive tradition, recognises that PTSD involves specific cognitive and behavioural responses mediated by forms of learning and memory, as well as processes of recall and narrative elaboration that are regulated by the personal as well as socio-cultural meaning of the traumatic events (Kirmayer, 2001). The respective fields of ethnopsychiatry in the French tradition (Afana et al., 2010; Aroche & Coello, 2004; Georges Devereux, 1967; Fassin, 2000; Moro, 1992; Nathan, 1986; Sironi, 1999), transcultural psychology (Moro & Baubet, 2013), and medical anthropology (Kleinman, 1978) are among the disciplines which have long criticised the use of PTSD as a nosological category—considering it to be the result of dialogue among different actors who create normative models to explain and treat suffering relating to trauma. Much criticism from the field of medical anthropology, for example, calls attention to the exclusion of alternate illness presentations related to trauma and a neglect of the role of contextual factors in the emergence and characteristics of psychopathology (Lewis-Fernández & Aggarwal, 2013). This, they argue, leads to a pathologization of reactions to trauma in part to determine social, cultural, and administrative acknowledgments and consequences.

On reflecting these different theoretical positions, Eagle (2014) wryly notes that "reading the traumatic stress literature (or at least a substantial proportion of it) it is sometimes difficult to comprehend that writers are describing the same phenomenon" (p. 47). She refers to Laqueur's (2010) observation that trauma is much of a moral as it is a medical category, and to Fassin and Rechtman's (2009) suggestion that trauma is a "floating signifier that denotes any number of ills which have the name" (p. 19). She concludes: "thus on the one hand we have the validity of traumatic stress ultimately tied to its location in neurophysiology or anatomy, and on the other, a suggestion that traumatic stress is to some extent a discursive or epiphenomenal construction with political and strategic effects. It is difficult to see how these positions might be reconciled" (p. 47).

Fisher (2014) similarly examines this debate and postulates that both the "biological" and "psychological" interpretations of PTSD may be true. He concludes that biopsychic realities, identified through biomedical knowledge structures, do indeed underlie the PTSD construct while the manner in which the disorder manifests is equally informed and shaped by the cultural meanings and perceptions attached to trauma. In other words, he views the disorder from within a "social diagnosis" framework which presumes that individuals contribute to the creation of a diagnosis which is inextricably linked to political, economic, cultural and social factors. His argument is linked to social constructionist critiques of medical diagnoses in general, as outlined in depth by Brown (1995) and others such as Goguikian Ratcliff and Rossi (2015) and Turner (1992) who have opened up a sociological debate about illness and advocate for attention to be paid to the individual social experience, language and symbols in order to deconstruct politically charged diagnostic categories and definitions. These ideas are based on Foucealdean (Foucault, 1988) principles of social constructionism which emphasize the role of language, definition-making, symbols and structures in psychiatric "illness" experiences and actions regarding the body, necessarily situated within personal, dyadic and group levels. Such a paradigm would imply that a thorough, integrative understanding of the multiple dimensions of each context is needed (Weine et al., 2002). As such, it is rooted in wider Foucauldian critiques of the way in which the production of academic and professional psychology has led to the "governing of the soul"—through a range of "technologies of subjectivity" that regulate human behaviour, often in ways that sustain deeply problematic power relations (Campbell & Cornish, 2014).

What Is "Trauma"?

One particular point of criticism highlighted is the fact that PTSD by its very definition requires a "traumatic" event to have taken place, which in itself relies on the subjective experience of the individual and subsequent cognitive appraisal of the event. The very first criterion required to meet the diagnosis, known as "Criterion A" according to the DSM-V (APA, 2013) is an "exposure to actual or threatened death, serious injury, or sexual violence" (p. 271). Thus, an explicit causal mechanism is built into its very diagnostic criteria. This is inherently related to the socio-political and historical context in which the diagnosis was developed. Indeed, the experience of war has been a central element in the search for relatively delineated traumatic events, such as a robbery, disaster, or traffic accident, mainly stemming from the second half of the twentieth century, when the psychological aftermath of World War II was being explored (ter Heide et al., 2016). As such, it was heavily based on assumptions of an otherwise "benign universe" being disrupted by a concrete isolatable event.

The reality, however, is not as simple. Not all trauma experiences relate solely to isolated events in the context of an otherwise stable environment. There are many ethical and clinical challenges associated with being able to identify a clear and discrete event as being "traumatic" required by its very definition for PTSD to be diagnosed. According to Maier and Straub (2011), the causal attribution of symptoms to a single traumatic event inherent to diagnosing PTSD represents the prevailing biomedical concept of illness, yet is certainly also one of the most significant shortcomings of psychotraumatology. Are the same events necessarily experienced as "traumatic" by everyone? What components determine whether an event is subjectively perceived as "traumatic" or not? Questions remain about the common elements underlying the diverse experiences of people across the world, and critics of a unifying model of PTSD therefore challenge the assumption that the same responses to a stressor would manifest across a multiplicity of events and contexts (Kirmayer et al., 2010; Momartin et al., 2003; Tummala-Narra, 2007). These critics view the context of trauma as shaping and in turn being shaped by worldview, cultural norms and constructions of society and individual victims. Trauma is therefore not a disembodied construct linked to a discrete event but a cultural and historical construction (Drožđek & Wilson, 2007). As Silove (1999) notes, it is possible that the significance and meanings underlying trauma experiences are more important than the concrete details of discrete events in determining risk to PTSD Considered from this perspective, PTSD is not a consequence of trauma but of the interaction between trauma and culture, specifically trauma experienced within an individualized western context (Bracken, 2002).

Recent research has highlighted substantial differences in the ways in which people experience ongoing trauma as opposed to those who have experienced a discrete traumatic event (Nicolas et al., 2015). PTSD, however, does not take into account the nature of the trauma—the near dead, horror, fear, the unthinkable, the unspeakable—in other words, the "trauma story" which may be experienced both singularly and collectively (Maqueda, 2005). For people whose lives are characterized by ongoing hardship, often shaped by discrimination, poverty and other current and future dangers, traumatic events may fall within a continuum of suffering and may not be singled out or experienced with the same precision as the definition of PTSD appears to demand (Eagle, 2014). Furthermore, individuals with a trauma history rarely experience only a single traumatic event but rather are likely to have experienced several episodes of traumatic exposure (Cloitre et al., 2009). In many countries around the world, conflict is not an abnormal situation of short duration but rather a *"fait connu"* (Summerfield, 1996, p. 33), influencing all aspects of political, socio-economic and cultural relations in a society. As such, extreme trauma owing to torture and war is both an individual and collective process that refers to and is dependent on a given social context, marked by its intensity, extremely long duration and interdependency between the social and the psychological dimensions (Becker et al., 1990).

In a study conducted by Maier and Straub (2011) among a sample of refugee patients in a health clinic in Zurich, they noted that many of their patients complained more about their current living conditions than they did about earlier trauma:

> Many patients perceived their (then) current suffering not as a consequence of identifiable traumatic events, but as a delayed consequence of their earlier lives under inhuman conditions. This concept is much broader than just the impact of a torture experience or war scene, and it comprises the impact of longer periods of life characterized by a constant threat, a general and complete negation of the values of humanity, and permanent feelings of helplessness (p. 235).

They continue:

> No participant mentioned a mono-causal concept of illness; none of the patients believed that a single traumatic event, or even a single experience of torture, was an adequate cause to provoke his or her symptoms. Therefore, the academic concept of PTSD (i.e., identifiable traumatic events directly provoking pathological symptoms) seems to have had limited explanatory value for these patients. However, many of the interviewees gave meaningful testimonies regarding how they lived over long periods of time under inhuman conditions of war and oppression… If their explanatory models had to be situated in the area between biological, psychological, and social concepts, they tended to relate mainly to social and psychological categories (p. 244).

Several studies on refugees and asylum seekers have confirmed this clinical impression (Silove, 1999; Silove et al., 1998; Van Ommeren et al., 2001). In their intriguingly titled paper, 'Is life stress more traumatic than traumatic stress?,' Gold et al. (2005) studied traumatic events among four hundred and fifty-four college undergraduates and found that those who reported a traumatic event which met the diagnostic criteria for DSM displayed *fewer* symptoms of PTSD then those who had not been exposed to a traumatic event meeting diagnostic criteria. This finding highlights the current debate regarding whether or not to remove "Criterion A" from the diagnosis of PTSD, a criterion which appears to reflect political or moral imperative alongside scientific/diagnostic considerations (Eagle, 2014). In a seminal paper on the topic, Brewin et al. (2009) argue that PTSD's "dependence on the etiological criterion is now more of historical interest rather than practical importance."

The notion of prolonged exposure to trauma as potentially resulting in a "complex PTSD" pathology was first developed by Herman (1992)—and has since become an integral concept in the literature examining the complex and prolonged traumatic experiences of refugee communities (Drožđek et al., 2003; Mollica et al., 1998; Momartin et al., 2003; Schweitzer et al., 2006). The notions of "cumulative trauma" first developed by Khan (1977), "complex PTSD" developed by Herman (1992, 1997), "extreme trauma" developed by Becker (1990) and 'Continuous Traumatic Stress' introduced by those offering psychological services to political activists during the repressive apartheid years in South Africa (Eagle, 2014; Eagle & Kaminer, 2013), were all constructs developed to conceptualize trauma as having been accumulated over time through exposure to repeated stressors within the environment.

Becker (2004) defines extreme trauma thus:

> Extreme traumatisation is an individual and collective process that refers to and is dependent on a given social context; a process that is marked by its intensity, its extremely long duration and the interdependency between the social and the psychological dimensions. It exceeds the capacity of the individual and of social structures to respond adequately to this process. Its aim is the destruction of the individual, of his sense of belonging to society and of his social activities. Extreme traumatisation is characterized by a structure of power within the society that is based on the elimination of some of its members by other members of the same society. The process of extreme traumatisation is not limited in time and develops sequentially. (p. 5).

Considering trauma thus as a process, elements of temporality are highlighted, as is the continual interaction of the person with their environment in a given social and historical context. What is particularly interesting in these conceptualisations is the highlighting of the socio-political context and power dynamics at play in influencing the mental health of whole populations. Indeed, considering the 'elimination of some of its members by other members of the same society' referred to in the definition is pertinent both to situations of conflict as well as to societal dynamics at play for refugee communities attempting to integrate into host societies and facing possible discrimination.

The concept of cumulative trauma similarly incorporates dimensions of time and the interactive relationship between an individual and his/her ecological surroundings into the discussion regarding trauma, thereby transforming the event (traumatic experience) into a process over the individual's entire life trajectory (Drožđek et al., 2020; Khan, 1977). The concept of continuous traumatic stress (Eagle & Kaminer, 2013) likewise developed in opposition to existing conceptualizations of traumatic stress which retained the assumption that traumatic experiences have occurred in the past. This is due to the fact that many patients living in apartheid South Africa faced the realistic prospect of future victimization and were often living under precarious circumstances, including moving from one potential place of refuge to another. As such, the concept is intended to more accurately capture the "experiences and impact of living in contexts of realistic current and ongoing danger" (Eagle & Kaminer, 2013, p. 85). It does this by taking into account the context of the stressor conditions, the temporal location of the stressor conditions, the complexity of discriminating between real and perceived or imagined threat, and the absence of current external protective systems by the state.

Complex PTSD, in comparison, refers not to trauma having accumulated over time specifically, but is used more to describe severe cases PTSD with comorbidity (dissociation, depression, substance abuse, personality disorders etc.). It is not recognized as a discrete disorder in psychiatric classifications (Drožđek, 2015b). However, the topic has gained new impetus in recent years, with an official complex PTSD diagnosis has been proposed for inclusion in the 11th version of the International Classification of Diseases (Maercker et al., 2013; Nickerson et al., 2016; Silove et al., 2017; ter Heide et al., 2016). The clinical definition of complex trauma[1] has gone virtually unchanged since its conception, with the ISTSS guidelines for complex PTSD speaking of "exposure to repeated or prolonged instances or multiple forms of interpersonal trauma, often occurring under circumstances where escape is not possible due to physical, psychological, maturational, family/environmental, or social constraints" (Cloitre et al., 2012, p. 4). Many refugees, almost by definition, meet these definitions. They have left their country of origin because of persecution, war, or organised violence. There is some preliminary evidence for the validity of Complex PTSD as a diagnostic construct among highly traumatised refugees emerging in the literature (Nickerson et al., 2016; Silove et al., 2017)—yet a plethora of research shows that refugees are more likely to meet a regular PTSD diagnosis or no diagnosis than a complex PTSD diagnosis, and that prevalence of complex PTSD in refugees is relatively low compared to that in survivors of childhood trauma (ter Heide et al., 2016). As such, the literature raises many questions regarding the clinical relevance and utility of both a simple and complex PTSD diagnosis among refugee communities.

Conflicting Concepts of Trauma

If PTSD were to exist between individuals and not only in them, the construct not only would be incapable of understanding the phenomenon but would also influence the appearance of the illness, treatment strategies (Becker, 1995). We need to see beyond narrow western constructs illness at the level of the individual (Nickerson et al., 2011). This is particularly true of researchers and clinicians working within

[1]Note that there is a distinction between complex trauma and complex PTSD., with complex trauma referring to complex traumatic experiences, and complex PTSD. to complex posttraumatic symptoms (Ford et al., 2009; ter Heide et al., 2016).

collectivist[2] communities wherein individuals rely more heavily on larger family systems and where mental health is typically seen to be more linked to a broader socio-cultural context (Droždek & Wilson, 2007; Tang, 2007). As Tang (2007) notes: "cultures differ regarding their dominant ideas about the ontology of self as well as relationship between self and others, between self and the universe, and between life and death." (p. 129).

From an historical perspective, cultures have been conceptualized as falling into two categories: the individualistic (guilt) and the collectivist (shame) cultures (Droždek & Wilson, 2007). In other words, in more typically Westernized societies, the emphasis is on guilt. Self-esteem, and the general moral judgement of behaviour, is based on individual competition. In more collectivist societies, the emphasis is on shame linked to (a lack of) cooperative behaviour. In simplistic terms, shame is based on the judgement of the other, guilt is based on our own moral judgement of our behaviour. Shame is external (located interpersonally), guilt is internal (located intrapersonally). Shame affects our entire sense of self, guilt is a judgement on specific behaviour. Tankink and Richters (2007), for example, refer to communities in South Sudan. Here, they noticed that research participants were framing their sense of identity from a collective perspective. In other words, they were presenting a more "family self"—an identity inherently based on relational models. Even the experiences of the self were described as being located on an intersubjective plane, rather than an intrapersonal one.

Bracken (2001) reflects on this individualistic versus collectivist cultural debate in the field of traumatology, similarly arguing that PTSD as a diagnosis is too heavily focused on a western understanding of illness as situated within an individual, neglecting the social or familial context. He quotes the reflection of Jenkins (1996) in her work with Salvadorian refugees:

> Because traumatic experience can also be conceptualized collectively, person-centred accounts alone are insufficient to an understanding of traumatic reactions. In addition to the social and psycho-cultural dynamics surrounding any traumatic response, the collective nature of trauma may be related to what was ... referred to as the political ethos characterizing an entire society (Jenkins, 1996, p. 177).

and Summerfield's work with Nicaraguan refugees:

> Western diagnostic classifications are problematic when applied to diverse non-Western survivor populations. The view of trauma as an individual-centred event bound to soma or psyche is in line with the tradition in this century for both Western bio- medicine and psychoanalysis to regard the singular human being as the basic unit of study" (Summerfield, 1997, p. 150).

Current thinking around responses to trauma shares the same fundamental assumptions with mainstream psychiatry in remaining too focused on an individualistic and positivist agenda, based on a split between 'inner' mind, which can be

---

[2]A note on terminology: I am aware that any easy division of societies into 'Western' and 'non-Western', 'individualistic' and 'collectivist' or 'developed' 'developing' is false to the complexity of the contemporary globalized world. My use of these terms does not mean that I am endorsing any sort of strong social or cultural classification (Patrick Bracken, 2001).

investigated scientifically, and the "outside" world (Bracken, 2001). This "reductionist discourse" locates the experience of distress solely within the intrapsychic realm of the individual, defining subjective experiences of trauma in terms of "illness, recovery, and broken brains"—a master narrative arguably unrepresentative of each individual's lived subjective experience (Adame & Knudson, 2007, p. 157).

Thus, it is evident that an individual's response to trauma necessarily be embedded within a socio-cultural context. Furthermore, one could further problematize this individual versus collectivist dichotomous split by acknowledging the fact that it is not only individuals themselves who face traumatic events, but indeed entire communities. Eagle (2014) refers to notions of collective or historical trauma whereby whole groups of people carry a sense of common persecution or victimization:

> The idea of historical trauma is associated most strongly with the history of first nation people in America and the genocidal violence to which they were subjected. Collective trauma is the term that tends to be used about the response of groups of South Africans subject to a brutal apartheid and colonial history, as well as about the response of groups of Jewish people to the Holocaust. Such trauma may be understood to be transmitted intergenerationally via both conscious and unconscious mechanisms, such that those of generations post those directly victimized nevertheless carry the experience of trauma within themselves. In some respects identity and collective trauma come to be intertwined. Such conceptualizations of trauma may encompass a somewhat broader definition of traumatic stressors including not only relations of oppression that threaten actual survival of the group, but also more ideological forces that threaten the eradication of cultural or group identity. In this framework racism, xenophobia or fundamentalisms based on oppression may be understood to produce collective traumatisation. (p. 13)

She suggests that persons may be traumatised at multiple levels including collective/social, personal/physical and role identity levels, and that which of these levels is most salient at a particular point in time will be dependent both on life history and current environment. This point is no more pertinent to bear in mind than in the case of refugee populations, often faced with a plethora of traumatic events on a collective level.

The Problem of Pathologization

In a recent paper, Droždek and colleagues (2020) have highlighted the "hidden" long-term impact of war and violence, including "dissociative states, attachment problems, personality changes, guilt, shame, rage, identity issues, moral injury, substances abuse, damaged core beliefs, and bodily sensations linked to stress activation." (pg. 1)—difficulties not adequately captured by a PTSD diagnosis. The PTSD diagnosis has been criticized for its failure fully to account for all of the changes and co-morbid clinical presentations that are common among people who have experienced prolonged exposure to potentially traumatizing events (Friedman & Marsella, 1996; Kirmayer et al., 2010; Steel, 2001; Wilson & Droždek, 2004). The existence of the stressor criterion (Criterion A) implies a unique relationship between trauma and PTSD, yet trauma is also associated with an increased prevalence of other disorders, most commonly depression, generalized anxiety disorder (GAD), panic disorder, and increased substance use (Brewin et al., 2009). Not only is it "too little" in accounting for all responses to trauma, it also "too much" in prescribing symptomatic responses which are not necessarily found among different populations across the world. In a meta-review of the literature, Hinton and Lewis-Fernandez (2011) found significant cross-cultural variability which cannot be ignored, including the salience of avoidance/numbing symptoms (far more common among western populations and which Bracken (2001) argues is a specifically westernized postmodern construct), the role of the interpretation of trauma-caused symptoms in shaping symptomatology, and the prevalence of somatic symptoms which were generally found to be more common among culturally diverse samples. Maier and Straub (2011) observed the following among a sample of refugee patients diagnosed with PTSD:

> Whether they suffered from flashbacks and nightmares, general anxiety, sleeplessness, irritability, chronic pain, or depression, the participants considered the symptoms to not be specific indications of any particular disorder, but merely general expressions of distress. The symptoms, although very discomforting, did not seem to be sufficiently mysterious or confusing to the participants to make them repeatedly search for (medical) explanations and clarification. (p. 239).

Wilson (2004, 2005 as cited in Drožđek & Wilson, 2007) has discussed the unique nature of trauma archetypes and trauma complexes and suggests that the experience of trauma is both universal and archetypal for the human species yet with specific manifestations of trauma complexes informed by culture. According to him, PTSD does not take into account the whole spectrum of the post-traumatic change, including core belief changes, dissociative moments, ruptures in the growth and development of the personality or other comorbid disorders such as depression, substance use and somatization, a view endorsed by many others in the field (Drožđek & Wilson, 2007; Kirmayer et al., 2010; Marsella, 2010; Marsella et al., 1996).

According to Wilson and Drožđek (2007):

> Posttraumatic syndromes involve a broad array of phenomena that include trauma complexes, trauma archetypes, posttraumatic self-disorders and posttraumatic alterations in core personality processes (e.g. the five factor model), identity alterations (e.g. identity confusion) and alterations in systems of morality, beliefs, attitudes, ideology and values. The experience of psychological trauma can have differential effects to personality, self, and developmental processes, including the epigenesis of identity within culturally-shaped parameters …given the capacity of traumatic events to impact adaptive functioning, including the inner and outer world of psychic activity, it is critically important to look beyond simple diagnostic criteria such as PTSD to identify both pathogenic and salutogenic outcomes as individuals cope with the effects of trauma on their lives. (p. 371)

It would seem that the diagnosis of PTSD is simply inadequate to capture this vast range of responses. As Hinton and Lewis-Fernández (2010, 2011) note, even within the strict frame of the DSM, traumatic exposure can lead to multiple syndromes, including acute stress disorder and adjustment disorder, as well as major depression, panic disorder, and dissociative identity disorder. Such criticisms raise legitimate concerns surrounding the shortcomings of the diagnosis in capturing the full range of human experiences in the aftermath of trauma. These criticisms hold true if viewed from the more narrow perspective of a clinical or "medical diagnosis" paradigm even before one widens the frame to consider broader social-constructionist criticisms of diagnoses in general.

Looking beyond the frame of the DSM, Young (Young, 1995) suggests that the diagnosis is just one part of a dynamic process of individual adaptation to adversities in life and shouldn't be considered as merely a diagnostic entity in and of itself. In his interactive model of individual reaction to trauma within a socio-cultural context, Chemtob (1996, as cited in Drožđek & Wilson, 2007) also describes responses to trauma as an inevitable interaction of the universal aspects of reactions to trauma and violence with the culture-bound reactions and the personal history of the trauma victim. Scientific research on PTSD, however, has been criticized for remaining badly skewed towards the study of psychopathology rather than on the growth, self-transformation, and resilience often observed among survivors of trauma (Roberto & Moleiro, 2016; Tummala-Narra, 2007; Wilson & Drožđek, 2007).

Criticism of the Use of PTSD as a Diagnosis Among Refugee Communities

Papadopoulos (2002b) notes how the predominant way in which refugees are viewed today is in terms of trauma theories, stating that "although there are numerous and varied theories about the related themes of conflict, violence, power, identity, ethnicity, trauma, etc., it seems that there is unanimity about one prevailing belief that according to which almost everybody affected by war experiences and political oppression is traumatised." (p.26). Despite this prevailing belief, the relevance of diagnosing PTSD among refugee populations has been criticized by scholars such as Summerfield (1996), Haans et al. (2007), Mattar (2011) and Sturm (2010). They highlight the limitations of western clinicians attempting to apply this medicalized construct among ethnically diverse populations with questionable relevance, as a result of having fallen into the "myth of sameness" (Young, 2004 as cited in Lindy et al., 2007).

According to Papadopoulos (Papadopoulos, 2002b), the "refugee trauma" discourse (p. 26), is a linear concept which implies a clear causal relationship between external events and intrapsychic consequences. As such, it ignores systematic complexities such as the relational nature of the event's impact among family, community, and ethnic group members, as well as the effects of the wider societal discourses which colour the meaning, emphasis and quality of events and experiences. Kirmayer (in introducing Drožđek & Wilson, 2007), similarly notes that:

> PTSD is a limited construct which captures only part of the construct of violence, ignoring issues of loss, injustice, meaning and identity that may be of greater concern to the traumatised individuals and to their families. A clinical focus on the symptoms of distress that presented by the refugee, survivor or victim may draw away from contexts that define their identities and possibilities. As time wears on, the salient concerns for survivors become less focused

> on the meaning of the past than the realities of the present, and possibilities for the future. For refugees, this shift in temporal perspective underscores the crucial importance of their place in host societies. (p.vi)

A significant criticism of the PTSD diagnosis noted by Hinton and Lewis-Fernández (2011) involves its dangerous potential for medicalizing human suffering; that is, for reducing the social and moral implications of traumatizing events, such as war or genocide, to a strictly professional, even biological, set of consequences. Thus, by emphasizing the "reality" of PTSD as a universal biopsychological category, a focus on PTSD may have unintentionally and paradoxically helped decrease social and moral responsiveness to these events. As Herman (1997) argues, this is another way for the political and social reality causing traumatic events to be denied or pushed out of our collective conscious. This would be particularly true, for example, in cases of war, which typically terrorizes and destroys entire communities, including social networks and collective identities. In such instances, it is likely that even those who have survived personal atrocities would deem their injuries to be social and political rather than psychological (Summerfield, 1996).

A very obvious but often neglected point is that not all refugees are traumatised. Recent research suggests that, despite a substantially higher prevalence rate of mental health disorders noted among the population, most refugees are not suffering from mental disorders and most appear recover to recover from distress related to experiences of migration within a year of arrival in the host country (Hynie, 2018). As stated by Summerfield (1996, 1999) in his extensive critique of trauma programmes and other psychosocial interventions of international NGOs: all refugees need social justice, and just some need psychological treatment. He criticizes the assumptions underpinning much humanitarian work informed by western models of trauma. These assumptions, he argues, reflect "a globalization of western cultural trends towards the medicalization of distress" (p. 1449). Marsella (2010), another ardent critic of the use of PTSD in humanitarian settings, quotes Wessels:

> In emergency situations, psychologists hired by NGOs or UN agencies often play a lead role in defining the situation, identifying the psychological dimensions of the problems, and suggesting interventions.... Viewed as experts, they tacitly carry the imprimatur of Western science and Western psychology, regarded globally as embodying the highest standards of research, education, training, and practice. ... Unfortunately, the dynamics of the situation invite a tyranny of Western expertise. The multitude of problems involved usually stems not from any conspiracy or conscious intent but rather from hidden power dynamics and the tacit assumption that Western knowledge trumps local knowledge. ... Local communities have specific methods and tools for healing such as rituals, ceremonies, and practices of remembrance. Since they are grounded in the beliefs, values, and traditions of the local culture, they are both culturally appropriate and more sustainable than methods brought in from the outside (Wessells, 1999, pp. 274-275).

Refugees are thus placed in the role of passive victims, their own choices, traditions, survival strategies and competencies ignored, and the role of Western "experts" and their technology in the field of mental health exaggerated (Summerfield, 1996).

To illustrate the cultural imperialism inherent in the imposition of psychological knowledge, Summerfield (1996), provides the example of the conflict in Rwanda in the 1990s which lead to many international NGOs implementing "psychosocial interventions." One of these interventions included an evaluation of the "knowledge learnt" about trauma by refugees—raising the interesting question of whose knowledge is being prioritised in a context where the local language, Kinyarwanda, does not include a direct translation of the word for "stress." He has been vociferous in his condemnation of this approach which, in his view, pigeonholes refugees as suffering from PTSD but pays scant attention to their own perceptions and interpretations of distress and their choices in terms of treatment (Summerfield, 1996, 1999; Watters, 2001). Losi (2002) is another ardent critic of humanitarian interventions focused on PTSD, arguing that it leads to a reductive assessment of the refugees plight, victimization and a shift in the interpretation (and understanding) of the refugees' experiences, where the reasons for their exile are no longer socio-political but belong to a more neutral, "technical" dimensions. He demonstrates how this de-contextualization of the lived experience of refugees leads to languages and concepts being lost and replaced by medical jargon and obscure terms. Simply put, imposing pre-packaged "universal" interpretations, definitions, tools, and approaches to human psychological suffering does not bring them the help they need. According to Watters (2001) a useful way of conceptualising the needs of refugees may be through the construction of a Maslowian hierarchy of needs wherein humanitarian interventions attend initially to needs relating to physical well-being, such as food and shelter and safety, before "higher-level" needs relating to psychological wellbeing are attended to.

In short, diagnosing an individual with PTSD may serve as a form of western cultural imperialism (Steel, 2001). The act denies the resilience of survivors (Marlowe, 2010) and serves to reinforce existing imbalances of power between Western "expert" and "victim-patient" (Summerfield, 1996). As stated by Pupavac (2002):

> Internationalization and professionalization of adversity, indigenous coping strategies are thus not merely demeaned and disempowered. The community itself is pathologized as dysfunctional and politically delegitimized (pg. 493).

A narrow preconception of refugees as invariably damaged, weak or scarred, manifest through the use of a diagnosis of PTSD, may have unintended negative consequences for refugee populations by minimizing strengths and positive adaptation mechanisms (Afana et al., 2010; Marlowe, 2010; Papadopoulos, 2002b; Sturm et al., 2010). Tummala-Nara (2007) explores the notion of "collective resilience" and post-traumatic growth and adaptation among various culturally diverse populations, noting that the research continues to be defined by predominantly middle-class North American and European values based on individualistic principles which "fail to consider the interdependence of individual capacities, salient attributes of family and community, and/or larger cultural belief systems" (p. 34). In response to this criticism, it must be noted that the notion of Post-Traumatic Growth (PTG) has begun to grow into a burgeoning field in the literature on cross-cultural responses to trauma (Calhoun & Tedeschi, 2014; Copping et al., 2010; Drožđek & Wilson, 2007; Knaevelsrud et al., 2010; Marsella, 2010; Tankink & Richters, 2007; Tedeschi & Calhoun, 2004; Tummala-Narra, 2007; Wagner et al., 2007), defined as significant beneficial change in psychosocial well-being, beyond previous levels of adaptation, psychological functioning, or life awareness. This growth includes changes in self-perception, interpersonal relationships and life philosophy (Wagner et al., 2007). More recently, key authors in the field have added the notion of sociocultural influences in their model of PTG—including both proximal family and community as well as the wider (distal) sociocultural environment in general (Calhoun & Tedeschi, 2014; Copping et al., 2010).

The diagnosis of PTSD also neglects to consider the fact that different reactions or non-reactions to trauma—not matching those prescribed by PTSD—may indeed serve as a defensive and adaptive survival mechanism for individuals who may not have the "luxury" of allowing the experience of psychological distress to impede the urgent and daily task of surviving. Refugees from Mozambique and Ethiopia, for example, have been reported in the literature as saying that an active process of forgetting is a culturally normative method used to overcome difficulties (Summerfield, 1996). In such a context, judging individuals according to a predetermined list of symptoms which are either "present" or "absent" is strikingly simplistic.

The Instrumentalisation of the Diagnosis Among Asylum Seekers

As succinctly highlighted by Drožđek (Droždek et al., 2020),

> Nowadays, the PTSD diagnosis is often a prerequisite for the survivor's access to specialized treatment services and for obtaining legal recognition or financial compensation when exposed to violence. However, some survivors do not meet all necessary criteria for the PTSD diagnosis, particularly not in the long term. Therefore, they run the risk of being misdiagnosed, inadequately helped or undertreated, and may remain legally unrecognized and unprotected (p. 1).

A significant criticism of PTSD as a diagnostic construct highlighted within the literature relates to its political use as a tool providing evidence of "damage" in order for individuals to claim quite concrete benefits. Fisher (2014), for example, explores the skewed and often confusing incentive structure for soldiers in the American military to claim a diagnosis of PTSD for obvious secondary gain. Among refugee populations more specifically, such a diagnosis may open the door for access to care (Brown, 1995) or assist the asylum-seeking process. However, this political use brings significant risk as well as potential benefits. d'Halluin (2009) convincingly demonstrates the dangers inherent in this contentious relationship between immigrant, medicine and social security by arguing that multiple investigations and abundant political discourses relating to the 'safety' of welcoming refugees into Europe or not began with psychiatrists in the 1970s and continues to this day. The result, she concludes, is that the diagnosis has ultimately become a 'pre-requisite' for validating the experiences of migrants, reifying and reducing these experiences by placing them within an exclusively psychiatric paradigm. Furthermore, she argues, by pathologizing asylum seekers, mental health damages inherent to this population have been used in anti-immigration public discourse to highlight security issues related to refugees as a damaged, diseased 'other'. As such, PTSD as a political tool has indeed been used to limit and control the influx of migrants. A worrying trend she observes by using the example of France is the way in which the supposedly poor mental health of refugees has similarly been used to justify limiting their right to work in host countries, adding further fuel to a disempowering, victimizing fire. It also serves to detract attention away from the structural violence inherent in the asylum seeking procedure of host countries to which many asylum seekers are exposed—a colonization of intimate psychic spaces in a manner of speaking.

For asylum seekers and their lawyers, the medical certificate, including evidence of PTSD, is an "open sesame" (Fassin & d'Halluin, 2005, p. 600); for officials and judges it is a piece of evidence among others; and for both it is an innovation in governmentality. This labelling of asylum seekers is supported by a system in which tabulation of numbers with psychiatric labels forms a crucial basis for the mobilisation of broader social supports (Watters, 2001) and a new form of the transnational administration of people (Fassin & d'Halluin, 2005). It risks tearing individuals away from the potential protection of their own resilience as well as from their community's traditional means of coping with trauma (Losi, 2002). As Papadopoulos (2002b) argues, in our efforts to express our justified condemnation of the individuals, groups and policies that lead to political oppression and crimes against humanity, we offer as 'proof' the fact that people have been 'traumatised' by these despicable actions. In doing so, we ignore all psychological considerations of how people process experiences and, unwittingly, we end up doing violence to the very people we want to help through psychologizing the political dimensions of human suffering.

In terms of Article 1, Chapter 1 of the Geneva Convention of 1951, a refugee is defined as being someone with a "well-founded fear of being persecuted for reasons of race, religion, nationality, membership of a particular social group or political opinion." The word "fear" here is of particular interest as it implies that a refugee is defined by his or her psychological response to events, not to the events themselves. This discursive shift away from a wider understanding of the political context from which refugees may be fleeing, towards a narrower and more medicalized concept of such refugees as suffering from PTSD, may also lead to the moral disqualification and criminalization of unsuccessful asylum seekers who are not found to be "traumatized" (Sturm et al., 2010). According to Summerfield (1996) such a politically loaded use of PTSD indeed leads to "absurd" (p. 14) situations whereby victims of torture and other atrocities fear not being believed unless they can 'check off the tick list of symptoms' required to be diagnosed with PTSD He notes that it would be terribly ironic if the survivors of trauma felt that their best chance of getting any help was to position themselves in the role of victim and diminish their knowledge, their anger at injustice and their resilience.

This poses a dilemma for health professionals working with asylum seekers. They may in fact be seen as agents of de-culturalisation and de-politicisation in that they transfigure the refugees' accounts of atrocities into individualised pathology—a process refugees themselves may not be averse to as it may be the only avenue available to secure wider legal and welfare benefits. Fassin and d'Halluin (2005) quote the June 2002 newsletter of the organization Primo Levi which aptly asks, "does one need a paper to prove torture?" The authors state:

> For immigrants, the poor, and more generally, the dominated – all of whom have to prove their eligibility to certain social rights – [the individual body and mind] has also become the place that displays the evidence of truth…asylum seekers are more and more submitted to the evaluation of their physical sequels and psychic traumas, as if their autobiographical accounts were not sufficient… Medical authority progressively substitutes itself for the asylum seekers' word. In this process of objectification, it is the experience of the victims as political subjects that is progressively erased (p. 597).

They argue that the medical certificate is detached from the lived experience of the victims of persecution, attempting a process of objectification through expert's words and thus desubjectifying individual narratives. A health professional they interviewed is quoted as saying that "by issuing certificates, we're busy judging who's guilty and who's innocent. What situation are we in? We're neither experts nor jurists" (p. 601). Another explains: "it is part of a programme designed to destructure and depersonalize the individual" (p. 602). This highlights the multitude of challenges often posed to health professionals, torn between the "moral demand" for PTSD to be diagnosed at the risk of influencing the therapeutic relationship, which by definition is less based on 'truth funding' and more on an exploration of the subjective experience of the individual. For many professionals who find themselves on the horn of this dilemma: "it is their burden and their duty to testify" (p. 604). The other health professionals interviewed by the authors similarly perceived the gap between the meaning that potentially traumatic acts can have for the people who were subjected to them and the "semantic reduction" (p. 603) of the clinical examination and medical report.

Despite the potential damage caused to the individual by the use of a PTSD diagnosis, there are instances where it can be used in the service of marginalized individuals or groups. Drawing up a certificate is a way of validating the violent acts and traumatic events to which the individual has been subjected—not only are people listened to, it is a recognition that the suffering has been seen. It thus carries a deeply symbolic value. Eagle (2014) refers to research conducted by Foster, Davis and Sandler (1987, as cited in Eagle, 2014) on the impact of torture and detention of political activists in apartheid South Africa which was used to substantiate that individuals have been subject to terror or traumatizing conditions, thereby placing moral pressure on the Nationalist government; as well as the mental health evaluations of political refugees that corroborate their need to escape ongoing brutality from repressive regimes (Steel et al., 2009). Furthermore, within the asylum seeking procedure itself, a recognition of trauma may assist judges and other decision makers in recognizing and being more attentive to the difficulties asylum seekers may have in verbalising and constructing their case as a result of a compromised mental state which "may impede the applicant's ability to testify in a manner that appears direct, specific, and emotionally appropriate" (Linton, 2015, p. 1085).

As Steel (2001) notes, making use of the PTSD diagnosis may present a double-edged sword. On the one hand, it may serve as an acknowledgement of the deep pain experienced by survivors of trauma and assist in getting the required help. On the other, it risks becoming a trendy 'catch-all' diagnosis open to various forms of political abuse or manipulation. What is needed is not a complete throwing of the metaphorical baby out with the bathwater, but a more nuanced and sophisticated appreciation of trauma in its various forms, an understanding which is less politically motivated and which more accurately reflects the lived experiences of individual survivors of traumatic events—including diagnostic constructs and tools which serve the best interests of those genuinely in need.

Conclusion

One could deconstruct the very notion of "PTSD" by breaking it up into its various linguistic constituents (Post, Traumatic, Stress and Disorder) in order to summarize some of the major criticisms cited above which have been levelled against it. The first word, "Post," refers to a discrete event of the past, thus denying the mental health impact of any ongoing factors of stress based on current economic, political and social hardships faced by refugee populations. The second word, "Traumatic," is problematic insofar as whether an event is perceived to be 'traumatic' or not is in part influenced by the individual's subjective perception of the event, in turn significantly informed by socio-cultural and historical context. The third word, "Stress" implies a specific reaction to the event based on a pre-determined range of psychological symptoms, thereby neglecting the wide variety of possible reactions an individual may have to a traumatic event. The fourth word, "Disorder," necessarily pathologises this reaction, placing it at the level of the individual and squarely within the framework of a Westernised medical discourse.

By framing trauma in clinical and psychiatric terms, PTSD has the power to legitimise certain forms of victimhood, victimization and suffering. It is not a politically nor socially neutral construct. Rather, notions of who exactly qualifies as a "victim of trauma" are structurally, ideologically, and discursively located (Eagle, 2014). Such a conceptualisation of trauma, than, situates suffering within specific social and historical context. Through creating "victims" or "survivors," it has the power to direct attention away from sociopolitical sources of suffering, towards a sense of damage and entitlement. By ignoring the quintessential soiocultural and political dimensions of this suffering, we restrict the individual to the role of patient-victim, rather than recognising them as an active participant in their recovery, and an active participant within their community (Van Der Kolk, 2015). Briefly put, PTSD risks pathologising responses to situations (including armed conflict and torture) which are primordially sociopolitical in nature—rather than a normal reaction to abormal events (Métraux, 1999). Yet, in general, psychometric scales measuring prevalence rates of PTSD based on self-reported symptoms tend to give inflated prevalence estimates, particular in post-conflict or crisis settings, because of the risk of conflating adaptive distress reactions with psychopathology (Ventevogel & Faiz, 2018).

What these critiques highlight, then, is an awareness of the social construction of this diagnostic category, which necessarily needs to be understood within a particular historical and cultural context, including administrative dimensions implying certain rights and treatment (d'Halluin, 2009). As argued by Brinkmann (2017),

> The most powerful tool to mediate our understanding of suffering today has arguably become the psychiatric diagnoses, serving as a widespread "language of suffering." ...to the extent that psychiatry's "language of suffering" permeates different parts of modern life, this specific understanding of mental illness and distress is likely to affect the ways we approach, treat and think about our problems. (pp. 1–2).

There is therefore a strong ethical case for taking a cautious approach to the application of PTSD as a psychiatric category among refugee populations, who come with a plethora of diverse histories, cultural traditions, definitions and understandings of self, economic priorities and health seeking behaviours (Bracken et al., 2016).

In summary: research identifies that refugees often meet the criteria for diagnoses such as PTSD, but that symptoms present as part of complicated constellations of problems for which there is no consensus regarding treatment approaches. Diagnostic labels may well be useful in drawing attention to problems and the need for support and intervention. However, confusion about the suitability of psychosocial interventions indicates that the kinds of problems experienced by people from refugee backgrounds are not necessarily well understood within the current mental health diagnostic nomenclature of universalized individualistic labels. As d'Halluin (2009) demonstrates in her analysis of psychiatric models used among migrant populations in France in the twentieth century, such universalist models of mental health developed after the second World War have rejected a priori any notion of singularity, or of ethnic or cultural differences in the manifestation of pathologies.

A more sophisticated, nuanced and culturally sensitive understanding of refugee trauma, merging clinical, psychological, anthropological, and epidemiological perspectives, is needed. As argued by Neace et al. (2020), "anything less than this level of nuance should be treated with suspicion, especially when the dialogue is focused around creating a special class of people, a trend which seems to dominate public and partisan political discourse" (p. 9). Therefore, in the following chapter, I continue these reflections by reviewing the literature exploring how cultural variations in ways of life and social contexts shape the embodied experience of trauma.

Case Study

To explore diverse representations of trauma (and PTSD in particular), I compare the way in which trauma is understood and described by refugees (in interviews with victims of torture in Athens) to how it is understood and described by health professionals (in 43 interviews I conducted among psychiatrists and psychologists from thirteen different countries across the E.U., all of whom work with refugee populations). A specific focus will be on the ways in which a diagnosis of PTSD is contested, appropriated, and used strategically for different purposes.

The transcriptions of these interviews were analysed by noting all the references made to PTSD or representations of trauma. An average of 3.7 of these representations was identified for each participant, 65% of them being spontaneous representations formulated by the participants during the interview, and 35% being direct answers to the researcher's question. These representations were collected, and a thematic analysis conducted on the content. Three major themes emerged which highlighted participants' statements falling along a continuum between (1) a complete, non-critical acceptance of a PTSD diagnosis, (2) making use of a nuanced, individualized and context-dependent diagnosis of PTSD, and (3) criticizing and problematizing the diagnosis.

Representations of Trauma Among Refugee Victims of Torture in Athens

The majority of refugee beneficiaries interviewed appeared to contest the medicalised notion of PTSD with which they had been diagnosed. When referring to their subjective experiences of trauma, they drew upon a variety of diverse cultural representations of suffering (explanatory models) and idioms of distress to explain their subjective experiences of trauma. To analyse this, I examined every instance in the interview transcripts that these individuals referred to PTSD and what it meant for them. Four main themes emerge:

(1) Fear
I'm tortured, I'm always afraid. [It] is not [an] illness
Trauma is somebody with many difficulties and fear. It is somebody without a calm state of mind. It is fear to be killed.

(2) Excess thought or thinking, rumination
I have many thoughts... I was "afraid", my mind is full of many things
I'm sick because I think a lot. It also affects my body. If you think too much, you fall sick

(3) Collective suffering
The problem of my family is the shock
I feel the pain of my family, the wounds on the body, and the heartache

(4) Spiritual suffering or "low morale"
This is when your morale is not at a 100%
In this case, the morale is not good

The first participant describes torture as something one "has." This is in direct contradiction to the idea that trauma is an event one has experienced. It is rather metaphorically represented as being internalized: the event has become part of him and what he is. The immediate consequence is the constant fear is feels. He absolutely rejects the idea that he is sick—his fear is related to the torture he experienced. According to him, it is clearly not a medical condition.

For one refugee, the trauma he experiences is not only his but related to the "shock" of the entire family. This contradicts the inherently individual narrative of PTSD The idea is similarly reflected in the words of participant 5, who feels "the pain of my families." This more collectivist representation of trauma has similarly been noted researchers and clinicians working within collectivist communities wherein individuals rely more heavily on larger family systems; here, mental health is typically seen to be more linked to a broader socio-cultural context (Adame & Knudson, 2007; Bracken, 2001; Drožđek & Wilson, 2007; Maercker & Hecker, 2016; Tang, 2007). As Tang (2007) notes, "cultures differ regarding their dominant ideas about the ontology of self as well as relationship between self and others, between self and the universe, and between life and death" (p. 129). Tankink and Richers (2007) give the example of South-Sudanese research participants who did not experience themselves so much as an individual in the Western sense of the term, but more as having a "family self" based on relational models where experiences are considered more within the intersubjective realm of the group rather than on an individual, intrapsychic level.

Another refugee's representation of trauma as "I'm sick because I think a lot. It also affects my body" reflects the idea of the mind and body being connected. However, inherent to his model appears to be the separation of a "medical" illness (the body being sick) and a psychiatric diagnosis or mental illness (the mind being sick) of which he makes no mention. In other words, according to his explanatory model, "too much thinking" lead to physical suffering. He refers to an illness in the body—which somehow bypasses any mention of a mental or psychiatric illness.

Representations of Trauma Among Medical Professionals Across Europe

The above representations of trauma emerging in interviews with refugee victims of torture often seem to be in contradiction with those emerging in interviews with health professionals working with refugee populations across Europe. In reflecting on the use of a PTSD diagnosis for refugees, many health professionals stated, for example:

> They don't understand that they have it, let's say. They do not realise that something is wrong with them, umm, but we're trying to show them how, show them how they can realise that they, they will suffer from that

> sometimes they say, uh, you know, um, magic, like spell, like 'somebody put a spell on me and they want to destroy my life' or 'they want to, because they don't like me so they put a spell on me and they want my money so they put a spell on me and because of that that I have this thinking and this insomnia and many many of things.' They don't understand the

psychology, that they have a, because of some event that happened before or some stress or something

Somebody who comes and is experiencing what we might consider an 'obvious' case of post traumatic stress... I try to explain [it] to them

Most of them suffer from [PTSD]

The words "they don't understand" reflect a recurring discourse among professionals that PTSD was something to be "understood." Refugees need it to be "explained" to them. Implicit therein is an unequal distribution of power related to western knowledge: it is the victim of torture diagnosed with PTSD who needs to "understand" the diagnosis from the perspective of a westernised, medical model of distress. The medical team ultimately hold the "true" knowledge. A diagnosis of PTSD was "obvious." "Most" had it. This "internationalisation and professionalisation of adversity" (Pupavac, 2002) enforcing "the asymmetry of the therapeutic relationship" (Wang, 2016) has been criticised in the literature as a form of "cultural imperialism" (Steel, 2001a) serving to reinforce existing imbalances of power between Western 'expert' and 'victim-patient' (Bracken et al., 2016; Summerfield, 1996; Watters, 2001).

However, the privileging of western psychiatric knowledge was not necessarily always the case. The majority of health professional's discourse reflects a certain ambivalence in the face of such contradictions, which appear to range on a continuum from complete and unproblematic acceptance of the category of PTSD to a nuanced, individualised and context dependant use:

PTSD as a diagnosis maybe varies for people, it's a category that we can use and it will be helpful for people.

PTSD, it's a category that will help you to predict what he wants, to predict what he will do, and to understand what he has gone through.

Many health professionals refer to a PTSD diagnosis as an instrument: useful in certain contexts, for certain purposes, for a certain audience. For some, it's a useful clinical tool which serves to further their own understanding of a patient's experience, guiding treatment pathways. It provides a common language of understanding for themselves and other health professionals. For others, the clinical use lies in helping the patient themselves make sense of this experience. In **chapter eleven**, for example, I explore how both refugees and professionals use it for the asylum tribunal.

A smaller percentage of health professionals, 11 out of the 43 interviewed, appear openly critical of the diagnosis:

I am very critical of PTSD

It's difficult to define [trauma] in, um, such a rigid, uh, diagnostic configuration. There's the, the category of PTSD and there's each individual patient or different ways to express them.

PTSD is a social control construction which has a certain history in medical anthropology field - there were a lot of critique.

Looking at the elements which organize these positions, several factors seem to play one role. Firstly, this type of professional training is followed by a factor influencing the acceptance or not of the PTSD On the one hand, we have pure a biomedical model with some medical doctors and psychiatrists, and on the other, a model that is rather psychoanalytic, which takes into account a subjective and individual perspective. Secondly, professionals having more work experience with refugee populations seem, for the most part, more conscious of the cultural influencing factors with which these individuals express their distress or suffering and face them. The scientific literature reveals that, when facing culturally foreign contexts, health professionals oscillate between "normalization" processes (based on the dominant western medical models, by imposing symptomatically and explanatory norms related to the PTSD, for instance), and the "customization" (taking into account the singularity of each individual, including their socio-cultural context, for instance) (Bourassa-Dansereau, 2013; Leanza, 2011).

Health professionals are constantly juggling these two positions. The majority of those interviewed seem to have representations of trauma in refugee populations which serves as an attempt to reconcile the "normalised" with the "customised" position:

> The individual is never just a trauma.
>
> Someone may have PTSD, but that doesn't define them.
>
> There is no one size fits all.

Above all else, what is highlighted is the need to see the individual beyond the trauma. It is not about accepting the diagnosis or not, but about being conscious of the limitations and concrete social, political, and legal implications of using it, as well as the need to recognize the unique complexities of individual experiences of trauma. We need to go beyond PTSD.

References

Adame, A. L., & Knudson, R. M. (2007). Beyond the counter-narrative: Exploring alternative narratives of recovery from the psychiatric survivor movement. *Narrative Inquiry, 17*(2), 157–178.

Afana, A.-H., Pedersen, D., Rønsbo, H., & Kirmayer, L. J. (2010). Endurance is to be shown at the first blow: Social representations and reactions to traumatic experiences in the Gaza Strip. *Traumatology: An International Journal, 16*(4), 73–84.

Andreasen, N. C. (2010). Posttraumatic stress disorder: A history and a critique. *Annals of the New York Academy of Sciences, 1208*(1), 67–71.

American Psychiatric Association. (1980). *Diagnostic and statistical manual of mental disorders* (3rd ed.). Arlington, VA: American Psychiatric Association.

American Psychiatric Association. (2013). *Diagnostic and statistical manual of mental disorders* (5th ed.). Arlington, VA: American Psychiatric Association.

Aroche, J., & Coello, M. J. (2004). Ethnocultural considerations in the treatment of refugees and asylum seekers. In J. Wilson & B. Drožđek (Eds.), *Broken spirits: The treatment of traumatized asylum seekers, refugees, war and torture victims* (pp. 53–80). New York, NY: Brunner-Routledge.

Becker, D. (1995). The deficiency of the concept of posttraumatic stress disorder when dealing with victims of human rights violations. In R. J. Kleber, C. R. Figley, & B. P. R. Gersons (Eds.), *Beyond trauma: Cultural and societal dynamics* (pp. 99–110). New York, NY: Plenum Press.

Becker, D. (2004). Dealing with the consequences of organised violence in trauma work. *Transforming ethnopolitical conflict* (pp. 403–420). New York: Springer.

Becker, D., Lira, E., Castillo, M. I., Gómez, E., & Kovalskys, J. (1990). Therapy with victims of political repression in Chile: The challenge of social reparation. *Journal of Social Issues, 46*(3), 133–149.

Bourassa-Dansereau, C. (2013). Exercer la pédiatrie en contexte multiculturel: une approche complémentariste du rapport institutionnalisé à l'Autre. *Alterstice-Revue Internationale de la Recherche Interculturelle, 3*(1), 103–108.

Bracken, P. (2001). Post-modernity and post-traumatic stress disorder. *Social Science and Medicine, 53*(6), 733–743.

Bracken, P. (2002). *Trauma: Culture, meaning and philosophy*. London, U.K.: Whurr Publishers.

Bracken, P., Giller, J., & Summerfield, D. (2016). Primum non nocere. The case for a critical approach to global mental health. *Epidemiology and Psychiatric Sciences, 25*(6), 506–510.

Brewin, C. R., Lanius, R. A., Novac, A., Schnyder, U., & Galea, S. (2009). Reformulating PTSD for DSM-V: Life after criterion A. *Journal of Traumatic Stress, 22*(5), 366–373.

Brinkmann, 2017.Brinkmann, S. (2017). Perspectives on diagnosed suffering. In *Nordic psychology*. Taylor & Francis.

Brown, P. (1995). Naming and framing: the social construction of diagnosis and illness. *Journal of Health and Social Behavior, 35*, 34–52.

Burgess, A. W., & Holmstrom, L. L. (1974). Rape trauma syndrome. *American Journal of Psychiatry, 131*(9), 981–986.

Calhoun, L. G., & Tedeschi, R. G. (2014). *Handbook of posttraumatic growth: Research and practice*. London: Routledge.

Campbell, C., & Cornish, F. (2014). Reimagining community health psychology: Maps, journeys and new terrains. *Journal of Health Psychology, 19*(1), 3–15.

Cloitre, M., Stolbach, B. C., Herman, J. L., Kolk, B. V. D., Pynoos, R., Wang, J., & Petkova, E. (2009). A developmental approach to complex PTSD: Childhood and adult cumulative trauma as predictors of symptom complexity. *Journal of Traumatic Stress, 22*(5), 399–408.

Cloitre, M., Courtois, C. A., Ford, J. D., Green, B. L., Alexander, P., Briere, J., Herman, J. L., Lanius, R., Stolbach, B. C., Spinazzola, J., Van der Kolk, B. A., & Van der Hart, O. (2012). The ISTSS expert consensus treatment guidelines for complex PTSD in adults. Retrieved from https://www.traumacenter.org/products/pdf_files/ISTSS_Complex_Trauma_Treatment_Guidelines_2012_Cloitre,Courtois,Ford,Green,Alexander,Briere,Herman,Lanius,Stolbach,Spinazzola,van%20der%20Kolk,van%20der%20Hart.pdf. On 11 February, 2020.

Copping, A., Shakespeare-Finch, J., & Paton, D. (2010). Towards a culturally appropriate mental health system: Sudanese-Australians' experiences with trauma. *Journal of Pacific Rim Psychology, 4*(01), 53–60.

d'Halluin, E. (2009). La santé mentale des demandeurs d'asile. *Hommes et migrations. Revue française de référence sur les dynamiques migratoires, 1282*, 66–75.

d'Halluin, E., Latté, S., Fassin, D., & Rechtman, R. (2004). La deuxième vie du traumatisme psychique. *Revue française des affaires sociales, 1*, 57–75.

Devereux, G. (1967). *Essais d'ethnopsychiatrie générale*. Barcelona: Barral Editores.

Drožđek, B., & Wilson, J. P. (2007). *Voices of trauma: Treating psychological trauma across cultures*. New York, N. Y.: Springer.

Drožđek, B., Noor, A. K., Lutt, M., & Foy, D. W. (2003). Chronic PTSD and medical services utilization by asylum seekers. *Journal of Refugee Studies, 16*(2), 202–211.

Drožđek, B., Rodenburg, J., & Moyene-Jansen, A. (2020). "Hidden" and diverse long-term impacts of exposure to war and violence. *Frontiers in Psychiatry, 10:975*, 1–12.

Eagle, G. (2014). From evolution to discourse: Key conceptual debates in the history and study of traumatic stress. *Psychology in Society, 47*, 1–20.

Eagle, G., & Kaminer, D. (2013). Continuous traumatic stress: Expanding the lexicon of traumatic stress. *Peace and Conflict: Journal of Peace Psychology, 19*(2), 85.

Fassin, D. (2000). Les politiques de l'ethnopsychiatrie: La psyché africaine, des colonies africaines aux banlieues parisiennes. *L'Homme, 153,* 231–250.

Fassin, D., & d'Halluin, E. (2005). The truth from the body: Medical certificates as ultimate evidence for asylum seekers. *American Anthropologist, 107*(4), 597–608.

Fassin, D., & Rechtman, R. (2009). *The Empire of trauma: An inquiry into the condition of victimhood*. Princeton, N.J.: Princeton University Press.

Fisher, M. P. (2014). PTSD in the U.S. military, and the politics of prevalence. *Social Science and Medicine, 115,* 1–9.

Foa, E. B., & Kozak, M. J. (1986). Emotional processing of fear: Exposure to corrective information. *Psychological Bulletin, 99*(1), 20–35.

Foucault, M. (1988). *Madness and civilization: A history of insanity in the age of reason*. New York, NY: Vintage.

Friedman, M. J., & Marsella, A. J. (1996). Posttraumatic stress disorder: An overview of the concept. In A. J. Marsella, M. J. Friedman, E. Gerrity, & R. Scurfield (Eds.), *Ethnocultural aspects of posttraumatic stress disorder: Issues, research, and clinical applications* (pp. 11–32). Washington, DC: American Psychological Association.

Goguikian Ratcliff, B. G., & Rossi, I. (2015). Santé mentale et sociétés plurielles. *Alterstice-Revue Internationale De La Recherche Interculturelle, 4*(2), 3–12.

Gold, S. D., Marx, B. P., Soler-Baillo, J. M., & Sloan, D. M. (2005). Is life stress more traumatic than traumatic stress? *Journal of Anxiety Disorders, 19*(6), 687–698.

Haans, T., Lansen, J., & ten Brummelhuis, H. (2007). Clinical supervision and culture: A challenge in the treatment of persons traumatised by persecution and violence. In B. Drožđek & J. P. Wilson (Eds.), *Voices of trauma: Treating psychological trauma across cultures* (pp. 339–366). New York, N.Y: Springer.

Herman, J. (1992). Complex PTSD: A syndrome in survivors of prolonged and repeated trauma. *Journal of Traumatic Stress, 5*(3), 377–391.

Herman, J. (1997). Trauma and recovery. 1992. Basic.

Hinton, D. E., & Lewis-Fernández, R. (2010). Idioms of distress among trauma survivors: Subtypes and clinical utility. *Culture, Medicine, and Psychiatry, 34*(2), 209–218.

Hinton, D. E., & Lewis-Fernández, R. (2011). The cross-cultural validity of posttraumatic stress disorder: Implications for DSM-5. *Depression and Anxiety, 28*(9), 783–801.

Hynie, M. (2018). The social determinants of refugee mental health in the post-migration context: A critical review. *The Canadian Journal of Psychiatry, 63*(5), 297–303.

Janoff-Bulman, R. (1985). The aftermath of victimization: Rebuilding shattered assumptions. *Trauma and Its Wake, 1,* 15–35.

Jenkins, J. H. (1996). Culture, emotion, and PTSD In A. J. Marsella, M. J. Friedman, E. T. Gerrity, & R. M. Scurfield (Eds.), *Ethnocultural aspects of posttraumatic stress disorder: Issues, research, and clinical applications* (pp. 165–182). American Psychological Association.

Khan, M. M. R. (1977). *Selbsterfahrung in der Therapie: Theorie und praxis [Self-experience in therapy: Theory and practice]*. Munich: Kindler Verlag.

Kirmayer, L. J. (2001). Cultural variations in the clinical presentation of depression and anxiety: Implications for diagnosis and treatment. *Journal of Clinical Psychiatry, 62,* 22–30.

Kirmayer, L. J., Kienzler, H., Afana, A. H., & Pedersen, D. (2010). Trauma and disasters in social and cultural context. *Principles of Social Psychiatry, 2,* 155–177.

Kleinman, A. (1978). Concepts and a model for the comparison of medical systems as cultural systems. *Social Science and Medicine Part B: Medical Anthropology, 12,* 85–93.

Knaevelsrud, C., Liedl, A., & Maercker, A. (2010). Posttraumatic growth, optimism and openness as outcomes of a cognitive-behavioural intervention for posttraumatic stress reactions. *Journal of Health Psychology, 15*(7), 1030–1038.

Koss, M. P., & Harvey, M. R. (1991). *The rape victim: Clinical and community interventions*. Sage Publications, Inc.

Laqueur, T. (2010). We are all victims now. *London Review of Books, 8,* 19–23.

Larrabee, M. J., Weine, S., & Woolcott, P. (2003). The wordless nothing: Narratives of trauma and extremity. *Human Studies, 26*(3), 353–382.
Leanza, Y. R. (2011). *Exercer la pédiatrie en contexte multiculturel: une approche complémentariste du rapport institutionnalisé à l'autre*. Georg éditeur.
Lewis-Fernández, R., & Aggarwal, N. K. (2013). Culture and psychiatric diagnosis. In R. D. Alarcón (Ed.), *Cultural psychiatry* (Vol. 33, pp. 15–30). Rochester, MN: Karger Publishers.
Lindy, D. C., Morales, R., & Lindy, J. D. (2007). Latino new yorkers and the crash of flight 587: Effects of trauma on the bicultural self. In B. Drožđek & J. P. Wilson (Eds.), *Voices of trauma: Treating psychological trauma across cultures* (pp. 321–338). New York, NY: Springer.
Linton, R. (2015). A presumption of disclosure: Towards greater transparency in asylum proceedings. *Seattle UL Rev, 38,* 1069–1139.
Losi, N. (2002). Some assumptions on psychological trauma interventions in post-conflict communities. In R. Papadopoulos (Ed.), *Therapeutic care for refugees: No place like home* (pp. 103–120). London: Karnac.
Maercker, A., & Hecker, T. (2016). *Broadening Perspectives on Trauma and Recovery: A Socio-Interpersonal View of PTSD European Journal of Psychotraumatology, 7,* 29303.
Maercker, A., Brewin, C. R., Bryant, R. A., Cloitre, M., Reed, G. M., van Ommeren, M., et al. (2013). Proposals for mental disorders specifically associated with stress in the international classification of diseases-11. *the Lancet, 381*(9878), 1683–1685.
Maier, T., & Straub, M. (2011). My head is like a bag full of rubbish: Concepts of illness and treatment expectations in traumatized migrants. *Qualitative Health Research, 21*(2), 233–248.
Maqueda, F. (2005). L'accès aux soins psychiques pour les demandeurs d'asile: Position soignante, position citoyenne. *L'Autre, 6*(1), 111–123.
Marlowe, J. M. (2010). Beyond the discourse of trauma: Shifting the focus on Sudanese refugees. *Journal of Refugee Studies, 23*(2), 183–198.
Marsella, A. J. (2010). Ethnocultural aspects of PTSD: An overview of concepts, issues, and treatments. *Traumatology, 16*(4), 17.
Marsella, A. J., Friedman, M. J., & Spain, E. H. (1996). *Ethnocultural aspects of posttraumatic stress disorder: Issues, research, and clinical applications*. American Psychological Association.
Mattar, S. (2011). Educating and training the next generations of traumatologists: Development of cultural competencies. *Psychological Trauma: Theory, Research, Practice, and Policy, 3*(3), 258–265.
Mollica, R., Caspi-Yavin, Y., Bollini, P., Truong, T., Tor, S., & Lavelle, J. (1992). The Harvard trauma questionnaire: Validating a cross-cultural instrument for measuring torture, trauma, and posttraumatic stress disorder in Indochinese refugees. *The Journal of Nervous and Mental Disease, 180*(2), 111–116.
Mollica, R., McInnes, K., Poole, C., & Tor, S. (1998). Dose-effect relationships of trauma to symptoms of depression and post-traumatic stress disorder among Cambodian survivors of mass violence. *The British Journal of Psychiatry, 173*(6), 482–488.
Momartin, S., Silove, D., Manicavasagar, V., & Steel, Z. (2003). Dimensions of trauma associated with posttraumatic stress disorder (PTSD) caseness, severity and functional impairment: A study of Bosnian refugees resettled in Australia. *Social Science & Medicine, 57*(5), 775.
Moro, M. R. (1992). Principes théoriques et méthodologiques de l'ethnopsychiatrie. *Santé Mentale Au Québec, 17,* 71–98.
Moro, M. R., & Baubet, T. (2013). *Psychopathologie Transculturelle*. Issy-les-Moulineaux: Elsevier Masson.
Nathan, T. (1986). Trauma et mémoire. *Nouvelle revue d'ethnopsychiatrie, 6,* 7–18.
Neace, R. T., Thaier, C., & Nasir, S. (2020). Understanding refugees: A complex discussion. In J. Kottler, S. Banu, & S. Jani (Eds.), *Handbook of refugee experience: Trauma, resilience, and recovery* (pp. 9–20). California Cognella Academic Publishing: San Diego.
Nickerson, A., Bryant, R. A., Brooks, R., Steel, Z., Silove, D., & Chen, J. (2011). The familial influence of loss and trauma on refugee mental health: A multilevel path analysis. *Journal of Traumatic Stress, 24*(1), 25–33.

Nickerson, A., Cloitre, M., Bryant, R. A., Schnyder, U., Morina, N., & Schick, M. (2016). The factor structure of complex posttraumatic stress disorder in traumatized refugees. *European Journal of Psychotraumatology, 7,* 33253.

Nicolas, G., Wheatley, A., & Guillaume, C. (2015). Does one trauma fit all? Exploring the relevance of PTSD across cultures. *International Journal of Culture and Mental Health, 8*(1), 34–45.

Papadopoulos, R. (2002b). *Therapeutic care for refugees: No place like home.* Karnac Books.

Pupavac, V. (2002). Pathologizing populations and colonizing minds: International psychosocial programs in Kosovo. *Alternatives, 27*(4), 489–511.

Roberto, S., & Moleiro, C. (2016). Looking (also) at the Other side of the story. Resilience processes in Migrants. *Journal of International Migration and Integration, 17*(3), 929–946.

Schore, A. N. (2003). *Affect dysregulation and disorders of the self (norton series on interpersonal neurobiology)* (Vol. 1). New York, NY: WW Norton & Company.

Schweitzer, R., Melville, F., Steel, Z., & Lacherez, P. (2006). Trauma, post-migration living difficulties, and social support as predictors of psychological adjustment in resettled Sudanese refugees. *Australian and New Zealand Journal of Psychiatry, 2*(40), 179–187.

Selye, H. (1950). *The physiology and pathology of exposure to stress.* Montréal: Acta Endocrinologia.

Selye, H. (1956). *The stress of life.* New York, NY: McGraw-Hill.

Silove, D. (1999). The psychosocial effects of torture, mass human rights violations, and refugee trauma: Toward an integrated conceptual framework. *The Journal of Nervous and Mental Disease, 187*(4), 200–207.

Silove, D., Steel, Z., McGorry, P., & Mohan, P. (1998). Trauma exposure, postmigration stressors, and symptoms of anxiety, depression and post-traumatic stress in Tamil asylum-seekers: Comparison with refugees and immigrants. *Acta Psychiatrica Scandinavica, 97*(3), 175–181.

Silove, D., Ventevogel, P., & Rees, S. (2017). The contemporary refugee crisis: An overview of mental health challenges. *World Psychiatry, 16*(2), 130–139.

Sironi, F. (1999). *Bourreaux et victimes: Psychologie de la torture.* Odile Jacob.

Staeuble, I. (2004). De-centering Western perspectives: Psychology and the disciplinary order in the First and Third World. In A. C. Brock, J. Louw, & W. van Hoorn (Eds.), *Rediscovering the history of psychology: Essays inspired by the work of Kurt Danziger* (pp. 183–205). New York, NY: Kluwer.

Steel, Z. (2001). Beyond PTSD: Towards a more adequate understanding of the multiple effects of complex trauma. In C. Moser & D. Nyfeler (Eds.), *Traumatiserungen von Flüchtlingen und Asyl Schenden: Einflus des politischen, sozialen und medizinischen Kontextes* (pp. 66–84). Zurich: Seismo.

Steel, Z., Chey, T., Silove, D., Marnane, C., Bryant, R. A., & Ommeren, M. V. (2009). Association of torture and other potentially traumatic events with mental health outcomes among populations exposed to mass conflict and displacement: A systematic review and meta-analysis. *JAMA, 302*(5), 537–549.

Struwe, G. (1994). Training health and medical professionals to care for refugees: Issues and methods. In A. J. Marsella, T. Bornemann, S. Ekblad, & J. Orley (Eds.), *Amidst peril and pain: The mental health and well-being of the world's refugees* (pp. 311–324). Washington DC: American Psychological Association.

Sturm, G., Baubet, T., & Moro, M. R. (2010). Culture, trauma, and subjectivity: The French ethnopsychoanalytic approach. *Traumatology, 16*(4), 27–38.

Summerfield, D. (1996). *L'impact de la Guerre et des Atrocités sur les Populations Civiles: Principes Fondamentaux pour les Interventions des ONG et une Analyse Critique des Projets sur le Traumatisme Psychosocial.* London: Overseas Development Institute.

Summerfield, D. (1999). A critique of seven assumptions behind psychological trauma programmes in war-affected areas. *Social Science and Medicine, 48*(10), 1449–1462.

Summerfield, D. (2001). The invention of post-traumatic stress disorder and the social usefulness of a psychiatric category. *British Medical Journal, 322*(7278), 95–98.

Tang, C.S.-K. (2007). Culturally relevant meanings and their implications on therapy for traumatic grief: Lessons learned from a Chinese female client and her fortune-teller. In B. Drožđek & J. P. Wilson (Eds.), *Voices of trauma: Treating psychological trauma across cultures* (pp. 127–150). New York: Springer.

Tankink, M., & Richters, A. (2007). Silence as a coping strategy: The case of refugee women in the Netherlands from South-Sudan who experienced sexual violence in the context of war. In B. Drožđek & J. Wilson (Eds.), *Voices of trauma: Treating psychological trauma across cultures* (pp. 191–210). New York: Springer.

Tedeschi, R. G., & Calhoun, L. G. (2004). Posttraumatic growth: Conceptual foundations and empirical evidence. *Psychological Inquiry, 15*(1), 1–18.

ter Heide, F. J. J., Mooren, T. M., & Kleber, R. J. (2016). Complex PTSD and phased treatment in refugees: A debate piece. *European Journal of Psychotraumatology, 7*(1), 28687.

Tummala-Narra, P. (2007). Conceptualizing trauma and resilience across diverse contexts. *Journal of Aggression, Maltreatment and Trauma, 14*(1–2), 33–53.

Turner, B. (1992). *Regulating bodies: Essays in medical sociology*. London: Routledge.

Van Der Kolk, B. (2015). *The body keeps the score: Brain, mind, and body in the healing of trauma*. Penguin Books.

Van Ommeren, M., de Jong, J. M., Sharma, B., Komproe, I., Thapa, S. B., & Cardeña, E. (2001). Psychiatric disorders among tortured bhutanese refugees in nepal. *Archives of General Psychiatry, 58*(5), 475–482. https://doi.org/10.1001/archpsyc.58.5.475.

Ventevogel, P., & Faiz, H. (2018). Mental disorder or emotional distress? How psychiatric surveys in Afghanistan ignore the role of gender, culture and context. *Intervention, 16*(3), 207.

Viñar, M. N. (2005). The specificity of torture as trauma: The human wilderness when words fail. *The International Journal of Psychoanalysis, 86*(2), 311–333.

Wagner, B., Knaevelsrud, C., & Maercker, A. (2007). Post-traumatic growth and optimism as outcomes of an internet-based intervention for complicated grief. *Cognitive Behaviour Therapy, 36*(3), 156–161.

Wang, S. (2016). Aidez-nous à comprendre vos Chinois! *Genèses, 4*, 141–156.

Wasco, S. M. (2003). Conceptualizing the harm done by rape applications of trauma theory to experiences of sexual assault. *Trauma, Violence, & Abuse, 4*(4), 309–322.

Watters, C. (2001). Emerging paradigms in the mental health care of refugees. *Social Science and Medicine, 52*(11), 1709–1718.

Weine, S., Danieli, Y., Silove, D., Ommeren, M. V., Fairbank, J. A., & Saul, J. (2002). Guidelines for international training in mental health and psychosocial interventions for trauma exposed populations in clinical and community settings. *Psychiatry, 65*(2), 156–164.

Wilson, J. P., & Drožđek, B. (2004). *Broken spirits: The treatment of traumatized asylum seekers, refugees and war and torture victims*. London: Routledge.

Wilson, J. P., & Drožđek, B. (2007). Are we lost in translations?: Unanswered questions on trauma, culture and posttraumatic syndromes and recommendations for future research. In B. Drožđek & J. P. Wilson (Eds.), *Voices of trauma: Treating psychological trauma across cultures* (pp. 367–386). New York: Springer.

Young, A. (1995). *The harmony of illusions*. Princeton: Princeton University Press.

Chapter 5
Culturally Informed Manifestations of Trauma

Human beings have an inherent need to make sense of their experiences. This may be particularly true of traumatic experiences which have the potential to shake the bedrock on which one's belief systems are based (Droždek & Wilson, 2007; Herman, 1992). Globally, the literature attests to substantial variations in how people worldwide respond to traumatic events. These culturally-determined variations are seen in how experiences of trauma are described and labelled, beliefs about the causes of psychological distress, ways in which people heal from trauma (including both formal and informal mental health interventions), and how people experiencing trauma are treated within their communities (Weissbecker et al., 2018). Furthermore, recent research has provided evidence that post-traumatic responses "involve bodily and social processes that are based on cultural models, social scripts and scenarios; much of this knowledge is tacit or implicit and emerges in response to specific cultural affordances that depend on social context." (Kirmayer et al., 2018, p. 173). Simply put, "culture matters when it comes to understanding and treating psychological sequelae of traumatic events" (Chentsova Dutton & Maercker, 2019, p. 1).

This chapter provides an overview of the literature exploring the pertinent question raised by Droždek and Wilson (2007):

> Does culture (i.e. cognitive-affect belief systems) act as a perceptual filter to the cognitive appraisal and interpretation of psychic trauma? If so, how do internalized belief systems and culturally shaped patterns of coping and adaptation, govern the posttraumatic processing of traumatic experience? (p. 372).

Early approaches to the study of psychological phenomena from a cultural perspective was concerned with the application of biomedical psychiatric categories in non-Western settings. Since the mid-twentieth century, however, a variety of new fields have developed. These contemporary approaches (such as transcultural, ethno—and ecosocial psychiatry as well as new cross-cultural psychology) have shifted away from treating culture purely as a confounding factor to be taken

G. Theisen-Womersley, *Trauma and Resilience Among Displaced Populations*,
https://doi.org/10.1007/978-3-030-67712-1_5

into consideration towards recognizing culture as constitutive of different worldviews with an inherently complex impact on experiences of trauma (Kaiser & Jo Weaver, 2019). Many are based on the seminal works of medical anthropologist and cross-cultural psychiatrist, Arthur Kleinman, who was among the first to highlight cross-cultural differences in "causal models" or narratives of traumatic experiences (Kleinman, 1977, 1978; Kleinman & Good, 2004). The approaches have particularly highlighted the importance of paying attention to the ways in which culture shapes expressions of distress and help- and health-seeking (Kienzler et al., 2019). Importantly, this also includes an acknowledgement of the broader political, social, and economic processes affecting mental health—such as the powerful effects of structural violence and social inequality (Kienzler et al., 2019; Kirmayer, 2019, 2018; Kirmayer et al., 2010; Kleinman, 1977, 1978; Petit & Wang, 2018). This chapter offers an exploration of these approaches. It aims in particular to examine the complex interplay between culture and trauma as it relates to refugee populations.

Defining Culture from a Sociocultural Perspective

Firstly, in order to enter into this debate, the word "culture" itself needs to be deconstructed and examined– as it is neither a static, reified, nor tangible concept. Culture is the ever-changing result of negotiated "compromises between the already established and the imaginatively possibly" (Amsterdam & Bruner, 2000, p. 231). According to Drožđek & Wilson (2007):

> The concept of culture is about the process of being and becoming a social creature, about the rules of a society and about the ways in which these are enacted, experienced, and transmitted ... Culture regulates the impact and expression of emotions and shapes individual expressions and perceptions of how to suffer under stress and these modes are taught sometimes openly, sometimes indirectly (p. 6)

From the specific perspective of sociocultural psychology, Sharapova and Goguikian Ratcliff (2018) define it thus:

> Culture here is considered as a set of practices executed in a tangible and observable way by a social group, as well as internal patterns and belief systems, each level mutually reinforcing the other. Furthermore, culture is not a static characteristic of an individual who continually adapts to ever-changing environments. Human development is thus embedded in social networks, interpersonal relations, and local environment. Therefore, culture plays an important role in shaping our identity, and constructs our reality via a process of cultural representations within a specific historical and cultural context (p. 2).

Such sociocultural approaches to understanding experiences of trauma therefore consider it to be a process that exists both in the intrapsychic realm of the individual as well as within sociocultural realm of relations and interactions—that is "embedded, situated, distributed, and co-constructed within contexts while also being intrinsically interwoven into these contexts" (Stetsenko, 2008, p. 7).

According to Marsella (2010), culture is:

> Shared learned behavior and meanings acquired in life activity contexts that are passed on from generation to another for purposes of promoting survival, adaptation, and adjustment. These behaviours and meanings are dynamic, and are responsive to change and modification in response to individual, societal, and environmental demands and pressures. Culture is represented externally in artefacts, roles, settings, and institutions. Culture is represented internally in values, beliefs, expectations, consciousness, epistemology (i.e., ways of knowing), ontology, and praxeology, personhood, and worldviews. Cultures can be situational, temporary, or enduring (p. 19).

Culture here is thus considered both as a set of practices physically executed in a tangible and observable sense by the group, as well as integral to belief systems located internally within individual members, each level mutual reinforcing the other. Furthermore, culture is not static but continually adapts to ever-changing environments.

Culturally-Informed Narratives of Trauma: Perspectives of Diverse Theoretical Traditions

Tankink and Richters (2007) note that culture is created, maintained and sustained among groups through dominant narratives or discourses:

> Every cultural group creates its own cultural discourse which is built up from cultural assumptions, the tracks of its collective past, cultural notions of femininity, sexuality, gender identity and roles, discursive and symbolic formations and practices, and ideas of how to deal with order and chaos. Equally important are ideas of the values of personal responsibility, of how to control the environment, of how daily life should be arranged, and of an orientation toward the future. Those narrative constructions, often called cultural master narratives, inform a person about what gives life meaning and what is inspiring, and also what is dangerous, risky or worth taking a risk for. Such a cultural discourse has the function of a "cultural script, a kind of social character," directing individual narratives, behaviour and the making of meaning…It is important to realize that a cultural master narrative is not a fixed, static entity but the result of creative activity in which ideas and notions are developed and shared. Its production takes place in a continuous process of dialogue between individuals and the group they belong to; it is linked with specific contexts, and it is always culturally based (p. 198–199).

The importance of such culturally-informed narratives of trauma or collective representations of psychological distress has similarly been explored by, among others, those following in the French tradition of ethnopsychiatry founded by Georges Devereux (Baubet & Moro, 2003; Devereux, 1967, 1980; Moro, 1992; Nathan, 1986; Petit & Wang, 2018; Sturm et al., 2007, 2010). In order to examine the role of collective representations in healing from trauma, authors from within this French tradition have drawn on Foucauldian notions that language, political systems and religion are structures of culture. They argue that collective representations of trauma provide a frame for the construction of narrations. This frame informs the processing of traumatic experiences and the way in which the individual may be able to convey their distress in socially understandable and acceptable ways. Collective representations of trauma enable coherent narratives to be constructed through establishing connections between the present and the past and by providing a meaning behind painful or frightening experiences—thereby bridging gaps between different aspects of an individual's life experiences which may have become shattered or disconnected as a result of the trauma. This includes, for example, theories about the origins of pain and the possibilities of healing, conceptions of family and social bounds, religious or metaphysical conceptions of the world, ideologies or positions in a field of political conflicts (Sturm et al., 2010). In other words, these theories assist in the construction of narratives as a fundamental part of the healing process. Despite the significant impact of collective representations and symbols in the processing of trauma, individuals necessary reproduce them with transformations in personal ways. They may be commented, questioned, or re-interpreted, or reorganised in a *bricolage* using different symbolic universes (Sturm et al., 2007).

Collective representations or cultural scripts of trauma have alternatively been conceptualised as narrative "master scripts" by the transcultural psychiatrist Laurence Kirmayer and colleagues (Kirmayer, 2019; Kirmayer & Jarvis, 2019; Kirmayer et al., 2018). He notes that "we are narrative beings, fashioning ourselves from the stuff of stories, locating our biographies and life projects in discursive webs of shared meaning" (Kirmayer, 2019, p. 31). He argues that culturally determined linguistic structures provide the context and rules for interactional processes that underlie complex emotions and provides a lexical base in which emotional experience is embedded (Kirmayer et al., 2010; Kirmayer, 2001). It are these narrative master scripts, or culturally determined linguistic structures which form the "landscape of memory" (Kirmayer, 1996). This emerging field of transcultural psychiatry (alternatively ecosocial psychiatry), spearheaded by Kirmayer among others, has provided some striking examples of how cultural variations in ways of life and social contexts shape embodied experience, and how experiences of trauma (including behavioral expressions of distress) vary with cultural knowledge, beliefs, and interpretations. He and others within this tradition (Greene et al., 2017; Kirmayer, 2019; Kirmayer et al., 2010; Kirmayer & Ramstead, 2016; Kirmayer & Minas, 2000) have demonstrated that, while evolutionary history reaches all the way up from brain circuitry to cultural forms of life, culture reaches all the way down to neuroplastic circuitry and epigenetic regulation. Cultural psychiatry, therefore, considers that

> human biology is fundamentally cultural biology and human environments are social environments, constituted by relationships with others and with cooperatively constructed institutions and practices… experience is always preceded by and embedded in cultural systems of meanings and practices, which influence modes of attention and interpretive frames or models. (Kirmayer & Ramstead, 2016, p. 3).

As illustrated in the above figure (Kirmayer & Ramstead, 2016, p. 48, Fig. 5.1)—cultural psychiatry explores how embodied experiences of trauma give rise to metaphors, which structure and shape individual experience, and to narratives, which are amplified, stabilized, and extended through collective enactments. In turn, discursive practices give rise to new metaphors and modes of embodiment.

Other approaches conceptualising mental health from a sociocultural perspective include "medical sociology"—which examines the interplay between social and

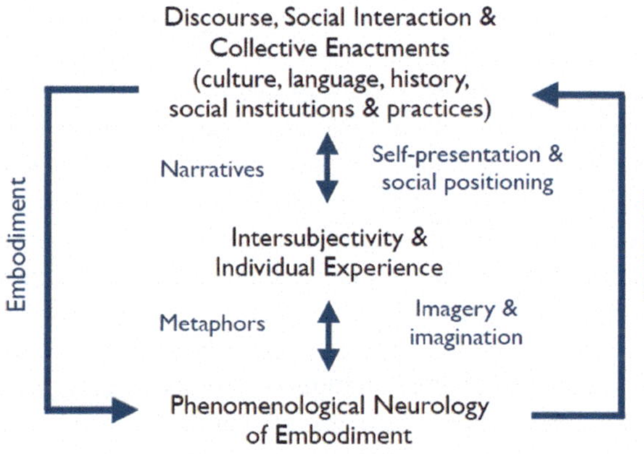

Fig. 5.1 Embodiment and enactment in experience

medical conditions, with the premise that mental health challenges are mediated and modified by social activities and the cultural environment (Nicolas et al., 2015), "social psychiatry" (Di Nicola, 2019), "transcultural psychiatry" (Schouler-Ocak et al., 2019)—which is particular concerned with mental health care for refugee populations—as well as "cultural-clinical psychology." The latter argues for an integrative approach to understanding clinical disorders in psychology with a consideration of the contextual embedding of these disorders within culturally-determined networks of local meanings, norms, institutions, and cultural products (Ryder et al., 2011). Within cultural-clinical psychology, master narratives of trauma have been referred to as "cultural scripts" (Ryder et al., 2011). Originally described by cognitive psychologists in the 1980s, these cultural scripts are defined in cultural-clinical psychology as "specific behavioural and experiential sequences of elements such as thoughts, memories, attention patterns, bodily sensations, sleep abnormalities, emotions and affective expressions, motivation, coping attempts, and ritualized behaviours that are relevant to posttraumatic adjustment" (Chentsova Dutton & Maercker, 2019, p. 1). They are partly culturally shared and intersubjective in nature. They are understood as sequences that are not only familiar to oneself, but also to others, serving to ground interactions between people. They are guides for understanding and interpreting behaviour as well as rules for behaving. Moreover, they need not be personally experienced to be understood and described by informants in a given cultural context.

Outside of these trans—or socio—cultural traditions, cultural narratives have equally been referred to in the cognitive sciences as "multirepresentational cognitive theorizing in psychopathology" (Brewin et al., 1996; Dalgleish, 2004). Dalgleish (2004, for example, refers to the role of various mental representational constructs (e.g., schemas, propositional representations, pictorial or image representations, distributed networks etc.) in the cognitive modelling of psychopathological states of trauma. The models originate in broader cognitive psychology work on schema and artificial intelligence and draws on the literature on the effects of schema on processing information (Chentsova Dutton & Maercker, 2019). Indeed, "cultural neuroscience" is another tradition exploring the culture-trauma nexus—attesting to the influence of culture on the underlying neural mechanisms involved in the development and maintenance of PTSD Research within this field increasingly supports the view that mental processes are intrinsically social. It explores how the circuits of the mind extend out into the world, through our tools, discourse, practices, and institutions that enable cooperation. This social view of the brain has now received new recognition and precision thanks to advances in computational neuroscience (Kirmayer, 2019). In relation to culturally-informed narratives of trauma specifically, cultural neuroscience argues that those with PTSD have difficulty in updating these trauma narratives—which are shaped by culturally derived self-representations that manifest at both the collective and individual level. Such variations in trauma narratives, they argue, may strengthen specific neural processes that diverge by culture, consolidating particular culturally-informed responses to traumatic events (Liddell & Jobson, 2016; Liddell et al., 2017).

These diverse approaches seem to agree on the notion that the individual's processing of traumatic events is informed by internalized representational constructs, which is both influenced by and reflected through culture, which is in itself in turn influenced by and reflected through language. The process is inevitably socially situated. Culture thus constructs our reality via a process of socialization within a specific historical and cultural context (Marsella, 2010). It fundamentally affects how people understand and express psychological distress related to trauma. As summarized by Van Maanen (1995):

> Language is auditioning for an a priori role in the social and material world. Moreover, it is a role that carries constitutional force, bringing facts into consciousness and therefore being. No longer then is something like an organization or, for that matter, an atom or quark thought to come first while our understandings, models or representations of an organization, atom or quark come second. Rather, our representations may well come first, allowing us to see selectively what we have described. (p. 134).

The Impact of Trauma

From a sociocultural perspective, ruptures created by trauma are embedded within an intersubjective context wherein severe emotional pain cannot find a relational home in which to be held and integrated (Atwood et al., 2002; Stolorow, 2011). Trauma creates ruptures at the intersection of the individual and their social context and related to safety, trust, independence, power, esteem, intimacy as well as spiritual and existential beliefs. *S*hould this prove to be the case, the lack of connection of past and present can also be understood as preventing the emergence of possible futures. Viewed through the lens of a dialogic systems sensibility, the traumatic world's slipping away from the categories of meaning can be seen as a severe disruption of those relational processes in which meaning is formed (Sucharov et al., 2007). More recently, this rupture in core schemas has been theorised as representing a threat not only to one's core sense of self, but furthermore a violation of self-understanding and worldviews to the extent that it disrupts attachment and interpersonal processing systems necessary for meaning making in the social world (Liddell & Jobson, 2016;

Maercker & Hecker, 2016). From within this sociocultural paradigm, this lack of connection to the future is intrinsically linked to a severe disruption of the relational processes by which meaning is dialogically created—the bedrock of which is social recognition. Indeed, research attests to the importance of social recognition in protecting against the development of post-traumatic symptomatology—defined as "positive individual or societal reactions that recognize and acknowledge victims' traumatic experiences and difficulties" (van der Velden et al., 2019, p. 287).

Trauma begets trauma. Exposure to trauma, itself connected to a breakdown in social connection and exacerbated by the process of migration, risks the individual being caught up in a vicious cycle where no addressee may be found, no language exists to form a coherent narrative whereby the event may itself be collectively represented and made sense of. Indeed, many authors highlight that trauma remains simply inaccessible to verbal recollection (Brewin, 2001; Brewin et al. 1996; Brewin et al., 2009), paradoxically the very recollection itself necessary for healing. Returning to the specific context of migration in particular, itself characterized by a rupture in connection to "home" (and all the social, cultural, professional and linguistic connections that this implies)—the physical, social and political isolation so typically experienced by asylum seekers upon arrival to host countries and often imposed by the state through legal requirements, serves only to feed monstrous feelings of invisibility and disconnectedness (Bhimji, 2015). In such a state, there is no coherently constituted Self: no memory, no clear defining of the Self and of the world in the safe confines of time—only psychological rumination and speaking in embodied signs. Disaffiliation, de-culturation and de-linking both in terms of family and social ties similarly affects the internal capacity to make links between different events and moments in life. Without the container of home-as-it-was, there is little membrane to hold the symbolic (Goguikian Ratcliff, 2012).

According to Kirmayer (1996):

> Traumatic experience is not a story but a cascade of experiences, eruptions, crevasses, a sliding of tectonic plates that undergird the self. These disruptions then give rise to an effort to interpret and so to smooth, stabilize and recalibrate. The effect of these processes is to create a specific narrative landscape. This landscape must fit with (and so is governed by) folk models of memory (p. 14)

Narratives of trauma, then, may be understood then as cultural constructions of personal and historical memory: What is registered is highly selective and thoroughly transformed by interpretation and semantic encoding at the moment of experience (Kirmayer, 1996). Particularly in cases where trauma has been prolonged, "the survivor may be left with large chunks of endured experience with no meaning, creating disquieting gaps and discontinuities in the experience of one's life history" (Sucharov et al., 2007, p. 2).

For those whose landscapes have been ruptured by trauma, "their problem is not the limits of memory but of language—the inadequacy of ordinary words to express all they have witnessed" (p.4). When words fail, when "the temporality of linguistic convention, considered as ritual, exceeds the instances of its utterance, and that excess is not fully capturable or identifiable (the past and future of the utterance cannot be narrated with any certainty)" (Butler, 1997, p. 1), it is naturally falls upon the body to become the site of (re-constructive) action. Métraux (1999a,1999b) explains this phenomenon as "memory-pain" sticking to the body with an intensity of experience untranslatable by words. Kirmayer (1996) further posits that when the image or content of a traumatic memory is unavailable, it is the bodily aspects of memory which persist. In the absence of narrative, the body holds what the mind cannot.

The Interplay of Factors

Given the complexity of the interrelation between culture and experiences of trauma, an examination of the interplay of factors regarding the impact of culture on trauma and trauma on culture requires consideration on several levels:

(1) The pre-existing cultural context

⇩

(2) The nature of the event

⇩

(3) What meaning is attributed to the event (individually and collectively)
Why did the event occur? What is considered "traumatic" or abnormal versus what is considered "normal?" Arguably, evaluating the 'toxicity' of an experience will depend in part on pre-existing cultural norms and "master narratives," belief structures and group experiences (including exposure to previous potentially traumatizing events) and the meaning attributed to that event on both an individual as well as a group level.

⇩

(4) How this sense making determines symptomatic responses
E.g. Guilt due to a belief that bad behaviour caused the rape; fear due to a belief that the tsunami was caused by angry gods who could strike again, acceptance due to a belief in fate…

⇩

(5) What meaning is attributed to the symptomatic responses
E.g. I'm experiencing flashbacks because I've been possessed by an evil spirit; I am a weak person because I cannot stop crying; my nightmares are messages from the ancestors…

Once again, the meaning attributed to the event is both individual and collective.

(6) Healing: How the meaning made of symptomatic response informs health seeking behaviour and treatment outcomes

For a more in-depth exploration of these mechanisms, Marsella (2010, p. 21) has developed an interaction model from within an ethno-cultural perspective of how culture influences the clinical parameters of the diagnostic criteria for PTSD and related stress disorders that may occur in response to "traumatic" events. These multi-layered factors may go some way in explaining the interesting cultural variations in response to trauma which have been noted in the literature, not only among individuals but also among different cultural groups (Bracken, 2002; Hinton & Lewis-Fernández, 2011; Lewis-Fernández & Kirmayer, 2019; Marsella et al., 1996; Perilla, Norris, & Lavizzo, 2002; Rousseau et al., 1997; Summerfield, 2001). (Fig. 5.2).

This model speaks to a larger theoretical debate over the meaning of medical diagnoses in transcultural settings in general. This debate has been well defined by Kleinman (1977, 1978; Kleinman & Good, 2004) who examines concepts of disease, sickness and illness. He defines the concept of "disease" as describing and categorizing disorders firmly within a Western medical model. "Illness," however, refers to the subjective experience of this disease, and "sickness" is the social phenomenon which defines the role of the patient and societal expectations around this (Goguikian Ratcliff & Rossi, 2015). As Maier and Straub (2011) note, illness according to Kleinman's definition is therefore based on conceptual models used by individuals, communities or cultures which provide an explanatory model for the illness. This explanatory model includes more than just ideas about the cause of an illness; they also incorporate ideas about estimating the severity of illness, appropriate treatment, and the meaning of the illness. In other words, explanatory models are based on a.

> "belief system about illness including which symptoms the ill subjectively experience, beliefs about etiology of the illness, assumptions of the time line or course that the illness will take, perceived consequences (e.g., social consequences) that occur as a result of the illness, and beliefs about what constitutes acceptable treatment options" (Benish et al., 2011, p. 281).

In relation to PTSD in particular, Maercker and colleagues (Maercker & Hecker, 2016; Maercker & Horn, 2013) have noted that it is one of the rare psychiatric diagnoses that requires an environmental context by its very definition. Not only does it require an exposure to a particular event—the event itself needs to have been interpreted by the individual as being traumatic. They have recently developed a framework model which situates the experience of trauma within socio-interpersonal context. The model describes three layers: (1) social affects comprising shame, guilt, anger, revenge, etc.; (2) close relationships including trauma disclosure, social support or negative exchange, empathy, etc.; and (3) culture and society, comprising aspects like the collective experience of trauma, social acknowledgment as victim or survivor, cultural value orientation, etc.

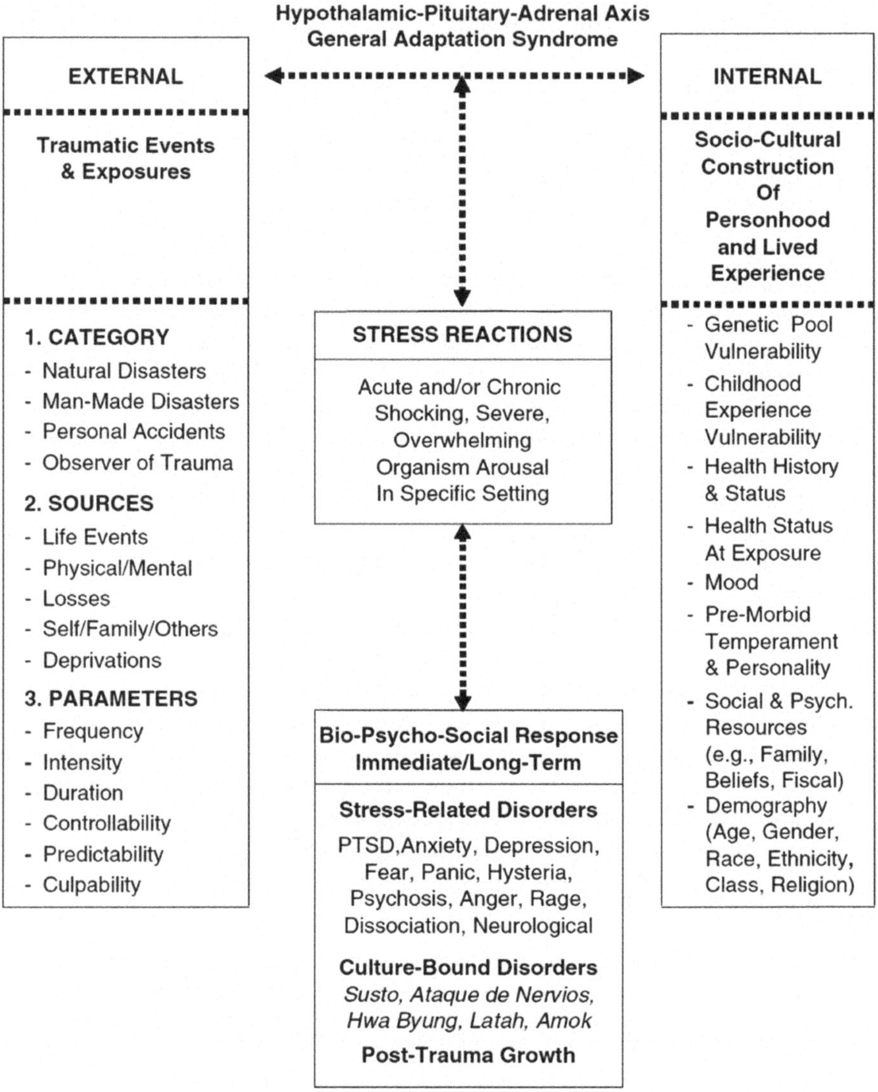

Fig. 5.2 The complex trauma and PTSD ecology: An interactional model

Culturally-Informed Responses to Trauma: Attributing Meaning to the Experience

Given the significance of the sociocultural environment on experiences of trauma, it is therefore no surprise that while symptoms of PTSD have been found among trauma survivors of both genders, all ages, and diverse racial, ethnic, and cultural groups, it is also true that particular events (such as incest, rape, or spousal abuse) and symptoms (such as dissociation, somatic complaints, *ataques nervios*) may have quite different meanings across different cultural contexts (Harvey, 2007). Drožđek and Wilson (2007), highlight some of these differences: Among Cambodian refugees who had suffered multiple life-threatening trauma during the Khmer Rouge regime, many who suffered from PTSD and depression understood their symptoms in light of their Buddhist beliefs in karma as a station in life, an incarnate level of being and fate where personal suffering is considered from a particular religious-cosmological perspective on the meaning of life. Among the Native American people, illness is thought to result from imbalance, loss of harmony and being dispirited with oneself due to a loss of vital connectedness. A common explanation for the 1988 Yuannan earthquake in China was that a "great dragon" was moving below the earth because he was angry with the people…

Other examples from the literature include Sao Tomean explanations of trauma among migrants in Portugal—where idioms of mental distress typically involved supernatural phenomena rooted in a Christian religious discourse, mixed with indigenous beliefs around withcraft, "unsatisfied spirits" and the evil eye (Trovão, Ramalho, & David, 2017). A study exploring causal attributions of mental health challenges among Somali refugees in Finland (Kuittinen, Mölsä, Punamäki, Tiilikainen, & Honkasalo, 2017) found that the most commonly endorsed causal attributions were jinn, jealousy related to polygamous relationships, and various life problems. The authors identified five attribution categories which they argue play a crucial role in shaping experiences of trauma: (a) somatic, (b) interpersonal, (c) psychological, (d) life experiences, and (e) religious causes. Similarly, in a recent investigation of lay beliefs among asylum seekers of African descent in Germany, asylum seekers attributed symptoms of post-traumatic stress less strongly to traumatic experiences, but more strongly to religious and supernatural causes such as sorcery, spiritual possession, and being cursed or bewitched (Grupp et al., 2018).

Many researchers and practitioners have made more concerted efforts to engage with these local "idioms of distress,"[1] and to use this knowledge to re-frame or re-orient interventions to fit with local understandings and lived experience (Kidron & Kirmayer, 2018; Lewis-Fernández & Kirmayer, 2019). A plethora of examples, in response to trauma in particular, have been documented in the literature (Afana et al., 2010; Hinton & Lewis-Fernández, 2010; Jayawickreme et al., 2012; Lewis-Fernández & Kirmayer, 2019; Summerfield, 1996). Afana et al. (2010), for example, highlight how Palestinian communities have processed continual exposure to war through particular linguistic constructs of trauma: *Sadma* (trauma as a sudden blow with immediate impact), *Faji'ah* (tragedy), and *Musiba* (calamity). *Sadma* is used metaphorically to refer to painful events that happen suddenly, *Faji'ah* is used to describe the reaction to an extraordinary event (mainly the loss of a loved one) and *Musiba* is used when traumatic events are persistent and have long-term consequences. They use these examples to show how such distinctive, historically-bound idioms illustrate communal reflections on the meaning behind experiences of

---

[1] Defined by Nichter (Nichter, 2010) as "socially and culturally resonant means of experiencing and expressing distress in local worlds" (p. 405).

violence, forced displacement, social exclusion, and humiliation. Behind all of the various idioms of distress found across the world lie the social representations of trauma and ways in which it is defined and processed on a socio-cultural level:

> The idioms we have described borrow from everyday language to make sense of the impact of violence in a situation of protracted conflict. They do not represent discrete syndromes or sharply delimited categories. Rather, they are familiar ways of speaking about traumatic events that invoke specific networks of meaning. They serve to communicate to others within the community about the dimensions of suffering through language that references collective experience and that conveys assumptions about the expected bounds of behaviour, the likely course of distress, and outcome of clinical or social intervention. Generally, these cultural idioms of trauma are not diagnostic entities that require treatment but a vocabulary through which distress is expressed and social support mobilized (Afana et al., 2010, p. 82).

In research conducted among the Adivasis indigenous people in tribal communities in Pune, India, the most prevalent metaphorical concepts of trauma were found to be related to shock and wound. The most predominant expression, which was used by all of the participants of the study, was "this should not have happened" (asa nahi vhayala pahije hota) (Rechsteiner et al., 2019).

If the meaning attributed to the event is significantly determined by cultural factors, so too are the responses. In a meta-review of 917 patients with symptoms of possessive trance disorders from 14 low—and middle-income countries, Hecker et al. (2015) found that spirit possession following trauma exposure is a phenomenon occurring worldwide which can be understood as a global idiom of distress. Indeed, Mozambique, a country that experienced almost three decades of war and devastation, exhibits a possession prevalence rate of more than 18% of the population. They similarly conclude that social and cultural factors also seem to play an important role in the reported disease models and healing rituals related to PTSD and other forms of pathological spirit possession.

A variety of "cultural concepts of distress" (CCDs) have been explored in recent decades throughout the literature. Hassan et al. (2005) note that many Syrian refugees attribute obsessive rumination to satanic temptations, using the Arabic word wisswas (وسواس) meaning both the devil and unpleasant recurrent thoughts. Among Albanian migrants in Switzerland, this has been referred to as a "point in the heart" or "Brenge": the beginning of rumination triggered by different causes (Shala et al., 2020). Drožđek and Wilson (2007) highlight some more examples from the literature: In the experience of many Salvadoran refugees who report "attaques nervios," a somatic response involving feelings of anxiety, fear, and anger, and calor, an experience of intense heat that extends through one's body. Such high rates of somatic responses have equally been found among tortured Bhutanese refugees in Nepal (Van Ommeren et al., 2001), American prisoners of war and holocaust survivors (Herman, 1992), refugees seeking treatment for PTSD in Switzerland (Morina et al., 2017), as well as South African victims of torture during the apartheid period (Eagle & Kaminer, 2013).

Bowles and Mehraby (2007) write about a particular young male client in Australia from Afghanistan, had symptoms which were "consistent with symptoms of grief, anxiety (PTSD) and depression, although he described them as 'burning in his heart' and understood them as part of God's will. If it was God's will, he would recover and find his family again" (p. 316). Weissbecker et al. (2018) classify these various idioms of distress noted in the literature according to:

- Idioms related to thoughts, e.g. kufungisisa meaning 'thinking too much' in Shona in Zimbabwe and yeyeesi meaning 'many thoughts' in Kakwa in South Sudan
- Idioms related to the heart, e.g. poil-heart meaning 'heavy hearted' in Krio in Sierra Leone, qalbi-jab meaning 'broken heart' in Somalia, qalb maaboud meaning 'squeezed heart' in Arabic (referring to dysphoria and sadness) and houbout el qalb meaning 'falling or crumbling of the heart' (referring to the somatic reaction of sudden fear)
- Idioms related to the head, e.g. amutwe alluhire meaning 'my head is tired' in Nande in the Democratic Republic of Congo
- Idioms related to the general body, e.g. jiu sukera gayo meaning 'drying of the body' used by Bhutanese refugee in Nepal to indicate a situation of loss and desperation or lashe mn grana meaning 'my body is heavy' in the Kirmanji Kurdish dialect

The list of differences in cultural responses to trauma is vast. The above examples are just the tip of the iceberg. A comprehensive review of various anecdotal evidence is beyond the scope of this chapter. What is noteworthy is the multitude of differences being noted across all layers of processing, from the meaning attributed to the event to the symptomatic responses to the meaning attributed to the symptomatic response. Furthermore, ethnographic research suggests that such "idioms of distress take on their communicative meaning in specific social contexts, and therefore require a broad understanding of complex and fluid cultural conceptions of wellness and distress and a detailed exploration of their actual use in a particular instance." (Kidron & Kirmayer, 2018, p. 3).

Pathways to Healing

A central concern of addressing trauma among refugee populations is the efficacy and cross-cultural applicability of methods of coping and treatment intervention (Kirmayer, 2018). Just as the meaning attributed to traumatic events and responses to them vary significantly among cultures, so to do healing practices and health-seeking behavior:

> Each culture develops specific forms and mechanisms… based on 'cultural wisdoms' ... for posttraumatic recovery, stabilization and healing… Considered from an evolutionary and adaptational perspective, cultures develop rituals, helper roles, ceremonies and other modalities to facilitate recovery from distressing psychological conditions including those produced by trauma. The viability of culture in the face of collective trauma illustrates … that there can be no experience of psychological trauma without a cultural history, grounding or continuity of background. (Boris Drožđek & Wilson, 2007) p. 381–382)

Culturally-determined metaphorical idioms for overcoming trauma—notably related to post-traumatic growth and resilience—have been aptly described by Meili et al. (2018). Elsewhere in the literature, in their study on trauma among a population of refugees in Switzerland, Maier and Straub (2011) identified 4 categories regarding their psychiatric patients' 'concept of illness' and healing regarding the diagnosis of PTSD: They termed the first concept drawn upon by patients a "scientific/technical" model. This fits most comfortably into the medical model paradigm on an individual level and medical care consequently is deemed the most appropriate treatment method. The second concept was a chronological, time-bound model implying that patients believed that the current psychological difficulties will naturally improve over time. A third concept was a model of "sociocultural depravity"—a model wherein suffering is linked to the current socio-economic and political context and in which healing can only occur once these material conditions have improved. The fourth and least common concept drawn upon by their patients was based on "personal guilt" and implies a more internalized, depressive state of psychological suffering.

Rousseau and Bagalishya (2007) refer to the African family council, a traditional way of resolving trauma or healing among families which may not be available to migrant communities in "Western" host countries:

> In many African societies, God is thought to be responsible for various social conditions, for the unequal distribution of good luck and bad, for the birth defects and for accidents of every kind. Ruin, illness, loss, premature death and accidents may all be punishments of an offended God, but more often than not they are attributed either to the anger of ancestors or to the witchcraft of living people (p. 262).

Bigfoot and Schmidt (2010) have emphasised the significant role that indigenous knowledge plays in cultural adaptation in the aftermath of trauma, demonstrating how native American communities intuitively rely on behavioral principles that they practiced for many generations before learning theory came into the literature. Eagle (2014) gives the example of "African cosmology" wherein falling victim to a traumatic event may be interpreted as an indication that one's ancestors have withdrawn their favour and protective function, and that the likely origins of their displeasure need to be identified and remedied. She similarly remarks that highly religious people of different faiths are likely to draw upon explanatory frameworks concerning suffering, victimization, aggression, violence and loss, located within the particular creeds of their belief systems. Among the Kubandwa cult across the African Great Lakes Area, people afflicted by trauma enter into a peaceful and accepting relationship with a possessing spirit in order to be healed. Part of this ritual includes a technique known as Gucekera, whereby unknown spirits are aggressively driven out of the individual in a form of exorcism (Ventevogel et al., 2018).

Tankink and Richters (2007) highlight the role of religion in healing in particular, which they argue allows people to convey an internal feeling to something outside them, to God, which can help to reduce their pain. They cite Geertz (1993) who notes that religion offers

> the formulation, by means of symbols, of an image of such a genuine order of the world which will account for, and even celebrate, the perceived ambiguities, puzzles, and paradoxes in human experiences. The effort is not to deny the undeniable—that there are unexplained events, that life hurts, or that rain falls upon the just—but to deny that there are inexplicable events, that life is unendurable, and that justice is a mirage (Geertz, 1993, p. 108 as cited in Tankink & Richters, 2007).

The importance of religiously- or spiritually-informed meaning making to inform healing from traumatic events has similarly been highlighted among Sudanese refugees in Australia (Copping et al., 2010), Filipino, Sao Tomean and Indo-Mozambican migrant mothers settled in Portugal (Trovão et al., 2017), and sub-Saharan refugees in Canada—where nearly half of participants privileged prayer as the best treatment for mental health challenges (Langevin et al., 2017). These studies highlight the role of religion in providing cultural resources aimed at transforming the trauma narrative—as well as the importance of religious networks as generating "social capital" (Tortelli et al., 2017) and opportunities for social mobility and activism.

In a study exploring resilience among Mexican refugees in Texas, the authors demonstrate how culture was a key mediating factor in healing from trauma. Culture assigned meaning to the traumatic events to which participants in the study had been exposed through the construction of narratives. The following cultural resources emerged as essential components in—family support, the ability to talk to others about their own experiences, the idea that there is no personal control over the circumstances (fatalism) and religious faith (Lusk & Baray, 2017a). In a study on the Cambodian idiom of distress known as *baksbat,* (Kidron & Kirmayer, 2018), ethnographic research among a population of trauma survivors suggests that the idiom itself may signify resolution and self-healing rather than continued distress. This highlights an inherent relationship, within the concept of *baksbat* itself, between the context of distressing events, responses to these events, and pathways to healing. The authors of the study note that in daily family life and in Cambodian communities, the idiom indeed referenced a far richer and dynamic network of meanings than for which the "static" concepts of trauma operating at the health clinics may account.

Within the "dynamic narrative" approach of Colette Daiute (Daiute, 2016, 2017; Daiute & Lightfoot, 2004; Daiute et al., 2015; Tarchi et al., 2019), she refers to the process of "narrative sense making" defined as a dynamic meaning of accounts of specific events and different perspectives towards these events which change over time. She uses the example of refugee communities involved in conflict and displacement during and after the 1990s wars of the former Yugoslavia to demonstrate how the changes afforded by narrative sense making allow for new perceptions and interpretations of potentially traumatic events experienced. She and colleagues argue that culturally-informed narratives are not only an important means of communication, but that they represent a "sophisticated decontextualized form of reflection and meaning-making" (Tarchi et al., 2019) p. 80). This quality of connecting with others and the world through narratives, of assessing and developing meaning in relational contexts, is defined as "dynamic storytelling." From within this perspective, Daiute explains, we use storytelling as a complex process for connecting with others for a wide range of purposes:

> We use storytelling to do things in the world—to figure out what is going on, to connect with others, and sometimes to imagine how life could be. Language genres like narrative are thus human resources for making sense of extremely challenging circumstances, gaining symbolic control over them and possibly creating a path for action... In this way, the **narrative becomes a possible world** (Daiute, 2017, p. 9).

The act of narrating is thus understood to be a major relational and developmental tool, especially with positive engagement in collectives addressing bad situations in challenging and rapidly changing environments (Daiute, 2016). In this way, narratives can be resources for engaging critically and creatively with environments and their social structures.

(Daiute et al., 2015), a "potential process of possibility—imagining and enacting social change with narrative—a lifelike yet creative symbolic system" (Daiute, 2015, p. 157). Daiute similarly highlights the power dynamics inherent to narrative practice, including the flexible uses of narrating as a mechanism of socio-political engagement and change: "as mediators of human interaction, symbolic discourses, like narrative language, are created in cultures allowing for a range of dynamic relations, not only oppressive functions of master narratives but also counter narratives and complex interactions in daily life" (Daiute et al., 2015, p. 46). Further research in the field of narrative psychology has found that redemption—a narrative sequence in which people recount emotionally negative experiences as having positive endings—is a useful mechanism for coping with adversity; in other words, redemption may serve as a cultural master narrative providing individuals with a socially valued script for narrating challenging life experiences (Blackie et al., 2020).

This chapter has explored some key concepts of cultural psychiatry (transcultural psychiatry, cross-cultural psychiatry, or ethnopsychiatry): the interdisciplinary field of research and clinical practice concerned with the impact of culture on mental health and illness (Kirmayer, 2018). These different terms for the field reflect particular intellectual and research traditions as well as changing configurations of the social world, but all address questions of enduring importance concerning variations in the causes, experience, expression, and course of mental health problems and the efficacy of specific modes of individual or collective coping, social response, and healing practices.

As recently noted by Kirmayer et al. (2018),

> Exploring cultural meanings requires attention to over-arching discourse, embodied practices, and everyday engagements with an ecosocial environment. Restitution, treatment and recovery can then be guided by knowledge of cultural meanings, dynamics, and strategies for coping with catastrophic threats, injury, humiliation, helplessness and loss. (p. 84).

According to Kirmayer, then, any consideration of experiences of trauma among refugee populations therefore needs to include "biological processes of learning and memory; embodied experiences of injury, pain, and fear; narratives of personal biography; the knowledge and practices of cultural and social systems; and the power and positioning of political struggles enacted on individual, family, and community and national levels" (Kirmayer et al., 2010, p. 170). Elsewhere, he notes that.

> In research, an ecosocial perspective urges us to move an exclusive focus on the brain to consider the developmental trajectories and situations that shape its architecture and function. We may function well in a range of contexts but expect certain resources to be ready-to-hand and find some kinds of situations, especially challenging. Understanding the mechanisms of mental disorders thus requires attention to the world beyond the individual, including families, communities, and networks, both local and global. (Kirmayer, 2019, p. 32).

Such ecosocial approaches to understanding trauma from a cultural perspective go beyond a reductionist focus on "cultural differences" wherein "culture" is perceived to be a reified, crystallised concept and viewed as a potential barrier to be overcome in a process of psychiatric classification (Watters, 2001). In other words, it is a move away from conceptual models dominated by implicit colonial hierarchies or reified notions of culture as a homeostatic variable to be taken into consideration. The aim is not to rely on overly-crude or misleading cultural stereotypes (Kirmayer et al., 2018). Instead, the focus is on ever-changing cultural and social systems which determine the various forms of an individual subjective experience of illness, an experience inevitably in constant flux (Goguikian Ratcliff & Rossi, 2015). This framework similarly recognises that healing from trauma is not an individual project, but a communal process which necessarily recognises the social, economic, and political context affecting the mental health of refugee populations (Sousa & Marshall, 2017).

These developments in theories of culture, and traumatology have enriched cross-cultural understanding of mental health dynamics and case conceptualization, informing the development of intervention models which aim to go beyond a single-trauma focus to address cumulative trauma dynamics as well collective identity and culture-specific traumas (Groen et al., 2017; Kira, 2010). The implications for both mental health interventions and for research is a focus on the dynamic inter-relationship of past traumatic experiences, ongoing daily stressors and the fundamental ruptures to core psychosocial systems extending beyond the individual to their sociocultural environment (Silove et al., 2017). I explore this by drawing on clinical examples from my work in the field—notably the case of 8 women from the Murle tribe affected by conflict in South Sudan who experienced an episode of mass fainting spells, as well as the case in Greece of a refugee victim of torture from Guinea confronted with a different cultural belief system of trauma between herself and her psychologist in Athens. These cases are used to highlight the important role of belief systems around trauma, the meaning given to the traumatic event, culturally determined idioms of distress and symptom manifestations, as well as implications for health seeking behaviour and explanatory models of healing.

Case Study 1: Mass Fainting Spells Among the Murle Tribe of South Sudan

Introduction to the Context

Gumuruk is a rural village in war-torn Jonglei state, South Sudan. It is populated by a tribe of people known as the Murle—predominantly nomadic cattle herders who have been heavily affected by conflict between themselves and the rival tribes of Dinke and Nuer. This is a conflict that dates back generations. It has been particularly intense over the past couple of years following the birth of South Sudan, the youngest country in the world. In the second half of 2011, relations between the Murle and Lou Nuer became increasingly strained. A number of clashes broke out with cattle raiding, looting and destruction of property, killing of civilians including women and children, in a dramatic escalation from the inter-communal conflicts of the previous years. In June 2011 the Lou Nuer perpetrated a violent attack on Pibor county (Gumuruk and Lekongole), with an estimated 430 deaths and 7000–10,000 people displaced. On 18 August 2011 the Murle counterattacked in Pieri (Uror county), with an estimated 340 deaths and 26,800 people displaced. Between 23 December 2011 and 3 January 2012, 6000–8000 armed youth, militarily organized and primarily of the Lou Nuer ethnic group, calling themselves the "White Army," launched a series of systematic attacks on areas inhabited by the Murle. Pibor was also attacked and parts of the town looted. According to the UNMISS, there were an estimated 612 deaths (including 88 women and 88 children) and 140,000 people were affected. As a result of this conflict, the majority of Murle men from this village were killed and nearly all of the cattle stolen during a violent clash. This has left the women of the village to take care of the children without any access to a food supply. Especially during the dry season, it's nearly impossible for vegetables or other sources of food to grow.

In August 2013, following interethnic clashes between Murle and Lou Nuer in July 2013, *Médecins Sans Frontières* (MSF) arrived in Pibor to run mobile clinics. I was part of the team as a clinical psychologist. We set up a hospital in Gumuruk, ready to receive victims of violence, but relatively few victims arrived to the clinic to seek medical care. This was possibly related to fears of being attacked by the Lou Nuer in coming to the clinic. Therefore, in an effort to reach those still hiding in the bush, MSF set up mobile clinics at the same time as the World Food Programme (WFP) organised food distributions. On these days, people would flock from neighbouring villages or, in some cases, come out from hiding in the bush. Many of them were women with young children. Many had to walk for two or three days to arrive. The WFP would mark all of their fingers with black ink—much like voting in certain countries of the world—to track who had received their bag of rice. On these days, our clinic would also experience a significant influx of patients. A lot took the opportunity to seek medical care in the same village. Otherwise, it was seen as too long a distance and too unsafe a risk to come to the clinic.

A Case of "Mass Hysteria"?

During one particular "food distribution" day, a group of community members arrived at our clinic carrying two women on a stretcher. The women had collapsed waiting in line to receive food. Both of their fingers were stained with a black ink that the WFP used to mark people who were in line to receive food. Neither of them were able to walk. They lay limply, occasionally jerking their entire bodies as though in a trance or experiencing a seizure. The two women were not related. The community was furious. Some of the other women were howling and crying hysterically and men were shouting angrily in Murle. We discovered that one of the women's three-month-old baby had just died while waiting in line to receive the food. The death was possibly linked to dehydration—her mother having had to walk for three days with her in the scorching heat in order to come to the food distribution. The baby's little finger had also just been stained with the same black ink. Rumours spread that the black ink was poisoned. It was the black ink itself that had killed the baby. It now also had poisoned the women. The community was blaming the neighbouring Lou Nuer tribe. The Nuer had allegedly cursed the ink using traditional African witchcraft. After that, we immediately heard cases of seven more women who had collapsed after having ink put on their fingers. Most experienced generalised pain all over their bodies followed by seizures and collapsing on the ground. Most couldn't open their eyes. All were too weak to walk. In my time in the clinic, I had already started to see such cases of what might be considered in psychoanalytic terms as "hysterical conversion." Nearly every evening in the clinic, the community would bring in women to the emergency room with the same presentation and same physical complaints. This became so common that as a psychologist, I was also 'on call' in the emergency room in the evenings. I became the "go-to" woman for doctors who understandably felt frustrated and lacked the time, patience, or expertise to attend to such cases.

The doctor explained to the community the likelihood that the child had died of starvation and dehydration, after having had to stand in line in 40° heat. This was not accepted by the community. The doctors' explanations were met with indignation, panic, and accusations that he didn't know what he was talking about. He and I went with some of our local staff and had ink put on our own fingers to prove to the people waiting in line that it wasn't poisoned. They answered that it was because we were both "Khawaja" (white people) that it had a different effect. Our translators (also from the Murle tribe) did the same. The community remained unconvinced. All seven women were brought for observation at the clinic, had a medical check-up and stayed overnight. They all slept soundly through the night. When I met with them the following day, they presented as calm, healthy and were able to walk easily. There didn't seem to be a sense of shame or distress. Four complained of headaches and three continued to experience generalised bodily pain but they all asked to be discharged. Feelings of sadness or anger were denied. Affect remained neutral or blunted. The main feeling was that they had indeed been poisoned but that the poison had been weak and was now metabolised.

Reflections

In the span of one month, I saw 30 cases of patients presenting at the clinic in Gumuruk with symptoms of psychosomatic complaints/conversion disorder. The vast majority were women (93%). There was a broad age range including children, teenagers, as well as adults. Just over half the cases (53%) were admitted to the emergency room at night. Typical presentation included collapsing, "convulsing," shaking, eyes forced close, arched back, intermittent hiccups or vocalisations of pain, extreme and exaggerated slowness of movement and generalized body pain. No other medical complications were found. The number of cases rose steadily over in this period.

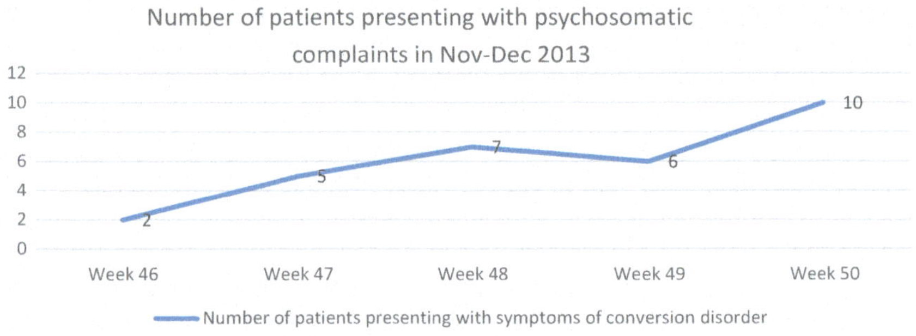

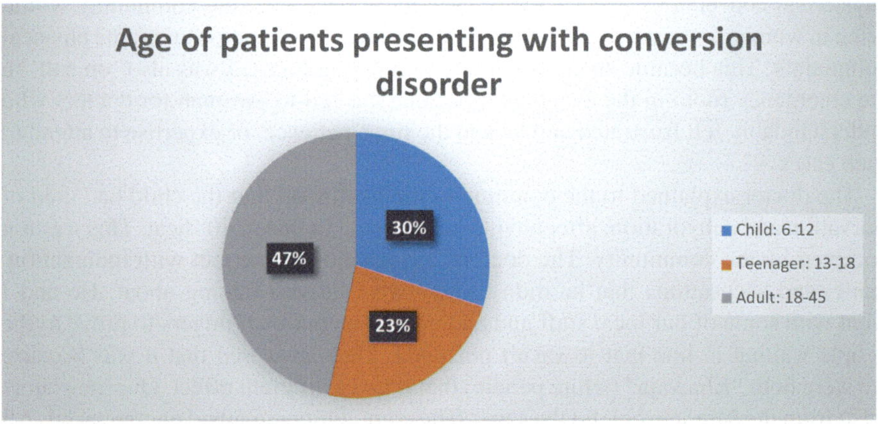

The steady increase in cases could possibly be in response to increased tension in Gumuruk regarding potential conflict with the arrival of the dry season. Dry season in Gumuruk means that armed men are able to move more easily across the land. Conflict typically erupts during this period.

There are a few different ways in which we can make sense of this. From a psychoanalytic perspective, psychically painful memories or feelings are repressed and converted into physical symptoms. For Murle, this repression may be a necessary means of psychic survival. Repression protects people from experiencing unbearable emotional pain. From the perspective of evolutionary psychology, non-combatants during or after times of attack unconsciously use these symptoms as nonverbal signal of not being a dangerous combatant/not carrying infectious disease. This explains group effect and gender difference in prevalence. From a sociological perspective, many studies have found prevalence to be higher in rural, lower socio-economic groups due to poorer understanding of medical/psychological concepts. From a neurophysiological perspective, symptoms are genuine and result from the physiological stress in the body (patient suffering trauma under continuous "flight or fright" response mode—leading to changes in hormonal levels, significant muscle tension etc.). Symptoms therefore result from an over-activation of the fear circuit/adrenaline response in the body. Research suggests that conversion disorder is associated with alterations in regional cerebral blood flow as well as greater functional connectivity between the right amygdala and the right supplementary motor area (Stone et al., 2005; Voon et al., 2010; Yazici & Kostakoglu, 1998).

None of these perspectives is necessarily at odds with the other. All offer relevant insights into the case. From a sociocultural perspective in particular, we need to ask ourselves the following questions:

- What systemic factors may be contributing to this group presentation of hysterical conversion?
- Is there a role for a more classically western psychoanalytic understanding or intervention?
- What ethical concerns might arise out of implementing a psychological intervention from a western/clinical perspective in this context?
- How would one work with such cases given the nature of short-term "humanitarian" interventions in such under-resourced settings?

Case Study 2: Psychotherapy with a Guinean Refugee Victim of Torture in Athens

Brigitte is a Guinean refugee victim of torture aged 40, diagnosed with the PTSD I met her in the course of my research among refugee victims of torture in Athens, Greece. She was referred to the clinic after presenting with symptoms of trauma. Nightmares were particularly troubling for her. In the course of the year that we spent together, she described her experiences of sessions with a psychologist:

> B: The psychologist told me that the nightmares are linked to the past, because I told him that I'm being chased. He told me that it's linked to the past, that's it.
>
> Interviewer: And what do you think?
>
> B: Me, I told him that it's spiritual, but afterwards, when he spoke, I told myself that "I don't know" but it's also possible that it's linked to what I'm thinking in my head. It's also that. Because I leave what's in my head. If I remove what's in my head, it can sort itself out. Apparently, when you have dreams where people are chasing you, we, we say that it's witchcraft. Among the Africans, we say that it's witchcraft. But he, he explained to

me that … for example, I had a dream the night before last. I remember two dreams. Where they chained me up, he said that it's linked to my past and that it's me myself who is chaining myelf up. Because of, maybe, what I refuse to think, I chain myself. So it's me myself who has to cut the chains. Nobody is chasing me. I need to liberate myself. Even though it's not easy, I need to liberate myself, scientifically.

Interviewer: He said that?

B: Yes, he said, scientifically … me, I told him about the spirituality but he said that scientifically, dreams are expressing what we're feeling […] I think it's witchcraft, it's the ancestors […] Yes, it's someone who wants to … but he said that scientifically it's our thoughts, in my head, my thoughts because I have children at home [in Guinea] that I had with different fathers, not with the same man. And because I'm Christian, sometimes I feel guilty and I tell myself that it's not a good image as a Christian. He told me that that's what I think […] I told myself that it's also probable that it's the truth. Because maybe, in my head, I am guilty, it's true. Even though I listen to the word of God, one could say that I did something that I couldn't pardon myself for. But Christ has already forgiven me. That's also the problem […] spiritually, it's complex. What I see, I explain spiritually with the hand of witchcraft. It means that the family isn't leaving me in peace. Spiritually, they are following me, they followed me two nights ago until I was scared. I don't know, there are two explanations […] Apparently there is an explanation that's different to what I think myself. So I don't know which to leave or take. I don't know…but I told myself that maybe that one's right as well.

In this extract, Brigitte is confronted with a different explanatory model to that of her own ("apparently there is an explanation that's different to what I think myself"). Her understanding of the nightmares is framed as being a "spiritual" one—linked to the ideology of African witchcraft. According to this model, the nightmares are as a result of someone else chasing her and putting a spell on her. It is the family who will not leave her in peace. She is bewitched, and the nightmares are a cause of an external individual or group of individuals deliberately trying to harm her. She is then confronted with the psychologist who "explains" a "scientific" model to her. The use of the words "explain" and "scientific" hint at the asymmetry inherent to the therapeutic relationship mentioned above. They imply that the knowledge of the psychologist is to be taken as undisputed scientific fact (hierarchically superior to other forms of knowledge falling outside of the western scientific paradigm). The represented situation of the psychologist who is "explaining" this science to her places him in the position of knowledgeable teacher and her in the position of the hither-to ignorant learner.

The temporal challenges play a role in these two different conceptions: the scientific "model" represented by the psychologist is rather based on the past—and consequently, it is more static and unchangeable, it is a model in which the individual is the passive victim of what is happening to him or her. On the other hand, with the "spiritual" model there is a more active, dynamic and changing conception, based on the current and external, instead of the internalized past. Throughout her speech, her own position in relation to the "scientific" model appears ambivalent. It is a dynamic and constantly shifting one, where the psychologist's explanation is both contested and accepted. When confronted with the explanatory model of her psychologist, she begins by saying: "I need to liberate myself. Even though it's not easy, I need to liberate myself, scientifically." Implied in these words is an acceptance of his model, based on an individualised and westernised understanding of trauma, where distress is solely located at the level of the individual and the individual has the power and obligation to heal themselves. The contradictions between this explanatory model and that of hers is highlighted in the words "me, I told him about the spirituality *but* [my emphasis] he said that scientifically, dreams are expressing what we're feeling." It is as though, metaphorically, she holds up the two models to examine them; it is the spiritual versus the scientific; her model *but* his. She then continues to directly contradict the model offered by the psychologist in saying "I think it's witchcraft".

Despite these contradictions, she continues by saying "he told me that's what I think". Let's consider the inherent imbalance of power implicit to these words: one individual telling another individual what they think. When faced with this interpretation, Brigitte grapples with the truth of what the psychologist is saying. She repositions herself once more. Faced with this interpretation, she continues: "I told myself that it's also probable that it's the truth." By telling herself this, she engages in an internal monologue where she grapples with the truth of the psychologist's words in light of the apparent dissonance between his explanation and hers. She appears to resolve this conflict, to some extent, by taking an "also" approach. His explanation is "also" correct, as is hers. The *"also"* instead of a *"but"* would therefore seem to suggest that she would like to incorporate this newfound understanding into her own explanatory model, thus accepting both points of view as valid. The conclusion of this is illustrated in her words "I don't know…but I told myself that maybe that one's right as well." The case of Brigitte offers an example of the fact that working with refugee populations in the field of mental health requires a knitting together a variety of worldviews brought together in the meeting between health professionals and the refugees themselves. Brigitte and her psychologist are both French-speakers, yet despite sharing a common language, the meeting of both worlds during a consultation necessitates constant mediation. Despite this challenge, she draws on the words of her psychologist as a resource to enhance her resilience. Weaving together the "spiritual" and "medical" explanations for the nightmares is a significant part of the process by which she comes to term with the traumatic experiences she's faced, and by which she constructs a new, more hopeful future for herself.

Conclusion: Introducing a Collective, Sociocultural Approach to Understanding Trauma and Recovery

In order to address some of the needs for more research on trauma among refugee populations, I draw on a socio-cultural framework that focuses on the intersubjective, mediational space between the individual and culture-society-interaction to account for the experience of humans in time and in particular social and cultural environments (O'Connor, 2015). Such an approach presupposes human beings inhabit shared forms of life, and utilize semiotic resources with reference to social structures and institutions. Meaning is continually negotiated within the social sphere and "cultural products, like language and other symbolic systems, mediate thought and place their stamp on our representations of reality" (Bruner, 1991, p. 3). In other words, the sociocultural context informs symbolic realities—products of human beings embodying different histories—which objectify themselves in language, discursive practices, social representations, myths, normative systems, religions, and other cultural products. Within these symbolic networks of cultural facts, individuals, institutions, and groups develop their complex and singular subjective organisations. As noted by Dafermos et al. (2015), "the approach differs radically from theories based on the psychologisation and pathologisation of human development, primarily because it clearly posits that there are inexorable links between social and individual development" (p. 74). It focuses on the exploration of complex, multidimensional, dynamic phenomena (Dafermos, 2018).

Within this framework, the individual constructs the social and at the same time is constructed by the social (Zepke & Leach, 2002). Similarly, the meaning attributed to an event (for example, whether or not the experience of being forced to marry at 14 years old is experienced by a young woman as traumatic or not) is both a reflection of the individual and their sociocultural environment. Attributing meaning to events is itself a co-constructed activity—with human beings conceived of as communicational agents that are constantly responding to situations within their sociocultural environment, in dialogue with others (Gonçalves & Ribeiro, 2012).

As argued by González Rey (2008),

> social and individual subjectivities are configured recursively through the interactions of active subject's in the functioning of groups and social institutions. The dialogue between individuals is only a moment within these subjective social dynamic systems that integrate social practices and relations; systems within which the individual is an author rather than a recipient in the dialogical processes. These dynamics represent particular configurations within the broader scenario of social subjectivity. (p. 187)

To summarize a few fundamental tenants of the theoretical framework of sociocultural psychology:

- The focus is on the way in which individuals, within their sociocultural environment, render reality significant
- Individuals are inevitably situated within a specific sociocultural and historic time and place, and are actively engaged in the construction of the meaning of reality with others
- Thoughts, feelings and actions of individuals are formed within a sociocultural milieu, mediated by cultural resources (considered as a collective accumulation of experiences of past generations). This relates to Vygotsky's "first law of development" which states that every acquisition is first social, before being reconstructed on an individual, psychological plane through the process of mediation
- Consequently, social and psychological phenomena are processes that exist in the realm of relations and interactions—that is, as embedded, situated, distributed, and co-constructed within contexts while also being intrinsically interwoven into these contexts

This perspective therefore involves a focus on the thread of language and related underlying semiotic systems. It is inherently dialogical (Marková, 2006, 2016). It understands dialogue to be the fundamental dimension of language as well as of human experience (Greco, 2016; Salazar-Orvig & Grossen, 2008). It likewise includes a recognition that all languages are composed of different social languages (Bakhtin, 1981; Gee, 2014). It emphasizes the contextual and unfinished nature of meaning (Gillespie & Cornish, 2014), inevitably situated within a specific sociocultural, historical and political context. As such, this theoretical framework highlights the heterogeneous, fluid and dynamic nature of individual subjectivities (Gee, 2014; González Rey, 2016; Squire, 2008).

Within this framework, an individual's experience of a potentially traumatic event, for example, necessarily is influenced by and reflected through language and culture. Culture (as explored in a previous chapter) is considered both as a set of practices physically executed in a tangible and observable sense by the group, as well as integral to belief systems lying internally within individual members (Brewin et al., 1996; Droždek & Wilson, 2007; Sturm et al., 2007, 2010). In other words, the approach highlights the ways in which life experience (in this case, experiences of trauma linked to migration) are mediated through language and culture.

Such an approach would include an acknowledgement that current concepts of mental health, notably a diagnosis of PTSD, are to some extent socially constructed objects produced within a specific historical period (Goguikian Ratcliff & Rossi, 2015). The perception of the potentially traumatic event, then, is mediated, among others, through collective memory and the inter-generationally transmitted historic experiences, myths or stories from the past shaping worldviews (Droždek & Wilson, 2007). Here, elements of temporality are considered, as is the continual interaction of the person with their environment in a given social and historical context. It would therefore follow that not only do reactions to potentially traumatic events differ according to cultural norms, but the very making sense of what is or what is not considered to be "traumatic" may similarly be informed by socio-cultural context (Daiute, 2017; Zittoun, 2014; Zittoun, & Sato 2018). Simply put, "culture shapes and gives meaning to the whole of human experience, including potentially traumatic experiences. Both cultural idioms of distress and narratives influence the nature of a pathological experience" (Rechtman, 2000, pg 404). These socioculturally determined idioms of distress have been defined in the D.S.M.-V as "ways of expressing distress that may not involve specific symptoms or syndromes, but that provide shared ways of experiencing and talking about personal or social concerns" (APA, 2003; Lewis-Fernández & Aggarwal, 2013).

Manifestations of trauma from within this socio-cultural framework are seen as unfolding within the context of systems of relationships which form the ever-changing environment. As Harvey (2007) notes, this ecological perspective is needed to guide inquiries into the understanding of trauma resilience. This is because it incorporates a "resource perspective" which assumes that human communities, like other living environments, evolve adaptively and are deeply embedded in complex and dynamic social contexts in which resources are exchanged. Individuals within this system are capable of negotiating and influencing, as well as being influenced by, this system. Equally, symptom severity is viewed as not static but fluid and changing according to a continuum of pathological reactions (Drožđek, 2015). For people whose lives are characterized by ongoing hardship, often shaped by discrimination, poverty and other current and future dangers, traumatic events may fall within a continuum of suffering and may not be singled out or experienced with the same precision as the definition of PTSD appears to demand (Eagle, 2014). This is a particularly relevant consideration for the mental health of refugees in light of the multiple and arguably ongoing environmental stressors and potentially traumatic experiences with which they are faced.

As noted by Daiute (2016), "trauma is *real, [my emphasis]* and many scholars are studying and treating trauma as a social as well as an individual phenomenon" (p. 130). Trauma experienced by displaced populations cannot be conceived of as a process having an inherent value occurring outside the network of sociocultural and historic experience. This is because it cannot be disconnected from its consequences for the *concrete* life of the individual. Trauma is related to individuals, as well as social histories and resources (Goulart, 2017; Goulart & González Rey, 2016; González Rey, 2008). It cannot be divorced from *daily-lived reality*. We cannot study the development of trauma trajectories among displaced populations without considering the concrete: concrete individuals and the concrete reality of their environment. Firstly, an understanding of the sociocultural resources drawn upon by various communities in the face of exposure to traumatic events should fundamentally inform mental health interventions for migrant populations. The under-utilization and mistrust of mainstream mental health services by migrants—and ethnic minorities in general—has been well documented (Bigfoot & Schmidt, 2010; Mattar, 2011; Watters, 2001) and may be in part due to the variations in healing practices determined by culture as noted above.

As recently highlighted in a study among mental health services for refugees in Greece, Karageorge et al. (2016) note the absence of knowledge regarding the acceptability and validity of current mental health interventions for this population. Their research highlights how both refugees and mental health professionals expressed challenges related to understanding and respecting respective cultures—a significant barrier to accessing such services. They identify the following barriers to the acceptability and validity of mental health services: (1) mistrust or uncertainty of intentions/expectations (2) having more immediate (practical) concerns than talk, (3) difficulty discussing trauma and (4) the inadequate cultural competence of health professionals. A recent desk review released by the World Health Organization (WHO) and UNHCR, the United Nations Refugee Agency, has argued that the development of effective mental health and psychosocial support programs requires knowledge of existing health systems and socio-cultural context, and that familiarizing international humanitarian practitioners with local culture and contextualizing programs is essential to minimize risk of harm, maximize benefit, and optimize efficient use of resources (Greene et al., 2017). Another key report recently released by the *International Society for Traumatic Stress Studies* (Nickerson et al., 2018) exploring trauma among refugee populations similarly highlights that the majority of current refugee crises of the twenty-first century are situated well outside the cultural contexts in which DSM-5 and ICD-10 nosologies have been organized. The report highlights key cultural barriers to accessing adequate and culturally relevant mental health services include "differential symptom expressions across cultures, the potential for limited construct validity of disorders in different groups, and unclear cultural validity of clinical interventions" (p. 15).

Some concrete implications for interventions—as noted by Nicolas et al. (2015)—include an integrated, multi-disciplinary approach which recognises the importance of a social response. This might include, for example, addressing issues aligned with social role and social support disruption; including a focus on current material concerns around living conditions, family reunification, legal and social justice, employment, establishing sociocultural-informed systems of meaning etc. He and his colleagues (2015), for example, have argued for a "social ecology of trauma risk and recovery" wherein interventions addressing trauma take into account structures of family, community and wider social institutions—and a focus on the social positioning of the individual within these structures. They argue that such interventions must be based on the following premises: (a) a recognition that culturally shaped narratives of distress play a role in subjective experiences of trauma across cultures and (b) a degree of ethnocentricity is inherent in Western understandings of trauma. The field of community psychology, more specifically the "ecological analogy" of community psychology as defined by Harvey (2007) similarly argues for an understanding healing traumatic wounds within a collective, social context. What is required for healing within this "ecological analogy," she argues, is a deeper understanding of life trajectories, dynamic processes, interactions and the continual development and change in psychological symptoms. The past decade indeed has seen a rise in interventions considering trauma interventions from a cultural perspective which have expanded to include services designed and delivered by paraprofessionals who are refugees themselves working in a collaborative team approach with mental health providers (Mitschke et al., 2017).

It is with this perspective that the following two sections of the book address trauma among displaced populations: firstly through exploring collective experiences of trauma and recovery affecting entire communities of displaced populations (as well as aspects of resilience and aspirations for a better future), and secondly through exploring some practical applications for professionals working with this population.

References

Afana, A.-H., Pedersen, D., Rønsbo, H., & Kirmayer, L. J. (2010). Endurance is to be shown at the first blow: Social representations and reactions to traumatic experiences in the Gaza Strip. *Traumatology: An International Journal 16*(4), 73–84.

American Psychiatric Association. (2013). Diagnostic and statistical manual of mental disorders (5th ed.). Arlington, VA: American Psychiatric Association

Amsterdam, A. G., & Bruner, J. (2000). *Minding the law*. Cambridge, MA: Harvard University Press.

Atwood, G. E., Orange, D. M., & Stolorow, R. D. (2002). Shattered worlds/psychotic states: A post-Cartesian view of the experience of personal annihilation. *Psychoanalytic Psychology, 19*(2), 281.

Bakhtin, M. (1981). *The dialogic imagination (translated by Caryl Emerson and Michael Holquist).* Austin, TX: University of Texas Press.

Baubet, T., & Moro, M. R. (2003). *Psychiatrie et migrations.* Paris: Masson.

Benish, S. G., Quintana, S., & Wampold, B. E. (2011). Culturally adapted psychotherapy and the legitimacy of myth: A direct-comparison meta-analysis. *Journal of Counseling Psychology, 58*(3), 279–289.

Bhimji, F. (2015). Collaborations and performative agency in refugee theater in Germany. *Journal of Immigrant and Refugee Studies, 1,* 1–23.

Bigfoot, D. S., & Schmidt, S. R. (2010). Honoring children, mending the circle: Cultural adaptation of trauma-focused cognitive-behavioral therapy for American Indian and Alaska Native children. *Journal of Clinical Psychology, 66*(8), 847–856.

Blackie, L. E. R., Mcdonald, S., Mclean, K. C., & Colgan, J. E. V. (2020). *A qualitative investigation into the cultural master narrative for overcoming trauma and adversity in the United Kingdom.* Qualitative Psychology: Advance online publication.

Bowles, R., & Mehraby, N. (2007). Lost in limbo: cultural dimensions in psychotherapy and supervision with temporary protection visa holder from Afghanistan. In B. Drožđek & J. P. Wilson (Eds.), *Voices of trauma: Treating psychological trauma across cultures* (pp. 295–320). New York, NY: Springer.

Bracken, P. (2002). *Trauma: Culture, meaning and philosophy.* London, U.K.: Whurr Publishers.

Brewin, C. R. (2001). A cognitive neuroscience account of posttraumatic stress disorder and its treatment. *Behaviour Research and Therapy, 39*(4), 373–393.

Brewin, C. R., Dalgleish, T., & Joseph, S. (1996). A dual representation theory of posttraumatic stress disorder. *Psychological Review, 103*(4), 670–686.

Brewin, C. R., Lanius, R. A., Novac, A., Schnyder, U., & Galea, S. (2009). Reformulating PTSD for DSM-V: Life after criterion A. *Journal of Traumatic Stress, 22*(5), 366–373.

Bruner, J. (1991). The narrative construction of reality. *Critical Inquiry, 18*(1), 1–21.

Butler, J. (1997). *Excitable speech: A politics of the performative.* London: Routledge.

Chentsova Dutton, Y., & Maercker, A. (2019). Cultural scripts of traumatic stress: Outline illustrations and research opportunities. *Frontiers in Psychology, 10,* 2528.

Copping, A., Shakespeare-Finch, J., & Paton, D. (2010). Towards a culturally appropriate mental health system: Sudanese-Australians' experiences with trauma. *Journal of Pacific Rim Psychology, 4*(01), 53–60.

Dafermos, M. (2015). Reflection on the relationship between cultural-historical theory and dialectics. *J Психологическая наука и образование, 20*(3), 16-24.

Dafermos, M. (2018). Developing creativity in science: The case of vygotsky. In M. Dafermos (Ed.), *Rethinking cultural-historical theory* (pp. 215–242). Singapore: Springer.

Daiute, C. (2015). Narrating possibility. In G. Marsico (Ed.), *Jerome S. Bruner beyond 100* (pp. 157–172). London: Springer.

Daiute, C. (2016). A relational approach to human development research and practice in 21st century violence and displacement. *Journal of Human Development, 59*(2–3), 128–151.

Daiute, C. (2017). Narrating refuge. *Europe's Journal of Psychology, 13*(1), 1–15.

Daiute, C., & Lightfoot, C. (2004). Narrative analysis: Studying the development of individuals in society. London: Sage.

Daiute, C., Todorova, R. S., & Kovács-Cerović, T. (2015). Narrating participation and power relations in a social inclusion program. *Language Communication, 45,* 46–58.

Dalgleish, T. (2004). Cognitive approaches to posttraumatic stress disorder: The evolution of multirepresentational theorizing. *Psychological Bulletin, 130*(2), 228.

Devereux, G. (1967). *Essais d'ethnopsychiatrie générale.* Barcelona: Barral Editores.

Devereux, G. (1980). The works of george devereux. In G. D. Spindler (Ed.), *The making of psychological anthropology* (pp. 364–406). Los Angeles: University of California Press.

Di Nicola, V. (2019). A person is a person through other persons: A social psychiatry manifesto for the 21st century. *World Social Psychiatry, 1*(1), 8–21.

Droždek, B. (2015). Challenges in treatment of posttraumatic stress disorder in refugees: Towards integration of evidence-based treatments with contextual and culture-sensitive perspectives. *European Journal of Psychotraumatology, 6,* 24750.

Droždek, B., & Wilson, J. P. (2007). *Voices of Trauma: Treating psychological trauma across cultures.* New York, N.Y.: Springer.

Eagle, G. (2014). From evolution to discourse: Key conceptual debates in the history and study of traumatic stress. *Psychology in Society, 47,* 1–20.

Eagle, G., & Kaminer, D. (2013). Continuous traumatic stress: Expanding the lexicon of traumatic stress. *Peace and Conflict: Journal of Peace Psychology, 19*(2), 85.

Gee, J. P. (2014). *An introduction to discourse analysis: Theory and method.* London: Routledge.

Gillespie, A., & Cornish, F. (2014). Sensitizing questions: A method to facilitate analyzing the meaning of an utterance. *Integrative Psychological and Behavioral Science, 48*(4), 435–452.

Goguikian Ratcliff, B. (2012). Repenser les liens entre migration, exil et traumatisme. *(Re)penser l'Exil, 1,* 1–8.

Goguikian Ratcliff, B. G., & Rossi, I. (2015). Santé mentale et sociétés plurielles. *Alterstice-Revue Internationale De La Recherche Interculturelle, 4*(2), 3–12.

Gonçalves, M. M., & Ribeiro, A. P. (2012). Therapeutic change, innovative moments and the reconceptualization of the self: A dialogical account. *International Journal of Dialogical Science, 6*(1), 81–98.

González Rey, F. (2008). Subject, subjectivity, and development in cultural-historical psychology. In B. van Oers, W. Wardekker, E. Elbers, & R. Van der Veer (Eds.), *The transformation of learning: Advances in cultural-historical activity theory* (pp. 137–156). Cambridge: Cambridge University Press.

González Rey, F. (2016). Advancing the topics of social reality, culture, and subjectivity from a cultural–historical standpoint: Moments, paths, and contradictions. *Journal of Theoretical and Philosophical Psychology, 36*(3), 175.

Goulart, D. M. (2017). The psychiatrization of human practices worldwide: Discussing new chains and cages. *Pedagogy, Culture and Society, 25*(1), 151–156.

Goulart, D. M., & González Rey, F. (2016). Mental health care and educational actions: From institutional exclusion to subjective development. *European Journal of Psychotherapy and Counselling, 18*(4), 367–383.

Greco, S. (2016). Analysing multiple addressivity in research interviews: A methodological suggestion from argumentation theory. *Learning, Culture and Social Interaction, 8,* 61–74.

Greene, M. C., Jordans, M. J., Kohrt, B. A., Ventevogel, P., Kirmayer, L. J., Hassan, G., et al. (2017). Addressing culture and context in humanitarian response: Preparing desk reviews to inform mental health and psychosocial support. *Conflict and Health, 11*(1), 21.

Groen, S. P., Richters, A., Laban, C. J., & Devillé, W. L. (2017). Cultural identity among Afghan and Iraqi traumatized refugees: Towards a conceptual framework for mental health care professionals. *Culture Medicine and Psychiatry, 42*(1), 69–91.

Grupp, F., Moro, M. R., Nater, U. M., Skandrani, S. M., & Mewes, R. (2018). "It's that route that makes us sick": Exploring lay beliefs about causes of post-traumatic stress disorder among sub-saharan african asylum seekers in Germany. *Frontiers in Psychiatry, 9,* 628.

Geertz, C. (1993). The Interpretation of Culture. London: Fontana Press.

Harvey, M. R. (2007). Towards an ecological understanding of resilience in trauma survivors: Implications for theory research and practice. *Journal of Aggression Maltreatment and Trauma, 14*(1–2), 9–32.

Hassan, G., Kirmayer, L. J., Mekki-Berrada, A., Quosh, C., El Chammay, R., Deville-Stoetzel, J., . . . Coutts, A. (2015). Culture, context and the mental health and psychosocial wellbeing of Syrians: a review for mental health and psychosocial support staff working with Syrians affected by armed conflict, (pp. 14–15). Geneva: UNHCR

Hecker, T., Braitmayer, L., & van Duijl, M. (2015). Global mental health and trauma exposure: The current evidence for the relationship between traumatic experiences and spirit possession. *European Journal of Psychotraumatology, 6*(1), 29126.
Herman, J. (1992). Complex PTSD: A syndrome in survivors of prolonged and repeated trauma. *Journal of Traumatic Stress, 5*(3), 377–391.
Hinton, D. E., & Lewis-Fernández, R. (2010). Idioms of distress among trauma survivors: Subtypes and clinical utility. *Culture Medicine and Psychiatry, 34*(2), 209–218.
Hinton, D. E., & Lewis-Fernández, R. (2011). The cross-cultural validity of posttraumatic stress disorder: Implications for DSM-5. *Depression and Anxiety, 28*(9), 783–801.
Jayawickreme, N., Jayawickreme, E., Atanasov, P., Goonasekera, M. A., & Foa, E. B. (2012). Are culturally specific measures of trauma-related anxiety and depression needed? The case of Sri Lanka. *Psychological Assessment, 24*(4), 791.
Kaiser, B. N., & Jo Weaver, L. (2019). Culture-bound syndromes, idioms of distress, and cultural concepts of distress: New directions for an old concept in psychological anthropology. *Transcultural Psychiatry, 56*(4), 589–598.
Karageorge, A., Rhodes, P., Gray, R., & Papadopoulos, R. (2016). Refugee and staff experiences of psychotherapeutic services: A qualitative systematic review. *Intervention, 15(1)*, 51-69
Kidron, C. A., & Kirmayer, L. J. (2018). Global mental health and idioms of distress: The paradox of culture-sensitive pathologization of distress in Cambodia. *Culture Medicine and Psychiatry, 43*(2), 1–25.
Kienzler, H., Spence, C., & Wenzel, T. (2019). A culture-sensitive and person-centred approach: Understanding and evaluating cultural factors social background and history when working with refugees. In T. Wenzel & B. Droždek (Eds.), *An uncertain safety: Integrative health care for the 21st century refugees* (pp. 101–116). New York, NY: Springer.
Kira, I. A. (2010). Etiology and treatment of post-cumulative traumatic stress disorders in different cultures. *Traumatology, 16*(4), 128.
Kirmayer, L. J. (1996). Landscapes of memory: Trauma, narrative and dissociation. In P. Antze & M. Lambek (Eds.), *Tense past: Cultural essays on memory and Trauma* (pp. 173–198). London: Routledge.
Kirmayer, L. J. (2001). Cultural variations in the clinical presentation of depression and anxiety: Implications for diagnosis and treatment. *Journal of Clinical Psychiatry, 62,* 22–30.
Kirmayer, L. J. (2018). Ethno-and cultural psychiatry. In H. Callan (Ed.), *The international encyclopedia of anthropology* (pp. 1–11). Hoboken, NJ: Wiley.
Kirmayer, L. J. (2019). Toward an ecosocial psychiatry. *World Social Psychiatry, 1*(1), 30.
Kirmayer, L. J., & Jarvis, G. J. H. (2019). Culturally responsive services as a path to equity in mental healthcare. *Healthcare Papers, 18*(2), 11–23.
Kirmayer, L. J., & Minas, H. (2000). The future of cultural psychiatry: An international perspective. *Canadian Journal of Psychiatry Revue Canadienne De Psychiatrie, 45,* 438–446.
Kirmayer, L. J., & Ramstead, M. J. (2016). Embodiment and enactment in cultural psychiatry. In C. Durt, T. Fuchs, & C. Tewes (Eds.), *Embodiment enaction and culture: Investigating the constitution of the shared World* (pp. 397–422). Cambridge, MA: MIT Press.
Kirmayer, L. J., Kienzler, H., Afana, A. H., & Pedersen, D. (2010). Trauma and disasters in social and cultural context. *Principles of Social Psychiatry, 2,* 155–177.
Kirmayer, L. J., Ban, L., & Jaranson, J. (2018). Cultural logics of emotion: Implications for understanding torture and its sequelae. *Torture Journal, 28*(1), 84–100.
Kleinman, A. (1977). Depression somatization and the new cross-cultural psychiatry. *Social Science and Medicine, 11*(1), 3–9.
Kleinman, A. (1978). Concepts and a model for the comparison of medical systems as cultural systems. *Social Science and Medicine Part B: Medical Anthropology, 12,* 85–93.
Kleinman, A., & Good, B. (2004). Culture and depression. *New England Journal of Medicine, 351,* 951–952.

Kuittinen, S., Mölsä, M., Punamäki, R.-L., Tiilikainen, M., & Honkasalo, M.-L. (2017). Causal attributions of mental health problems and depressive symptoms among older somali refugees in finland. *Transcultural Psychiatry, 54*(2), 211–238.
Langevin, R., Lavoie, É., & Laurent, A. (2017). Les croyances culturelles sur la santé mentale: Points de vue de parents francophones migrants de l'Afrique subsaharienne. *Neuropsychiatrie De l'Enfance Et De l'Adolescence, 66*(2), 81–89.
Lewis-Fernández, R., & Aggarwal, N. K. (2013). Culture and psychiatric diagnosis. In R. D. Alarcón (Ed.), *Cultural psychiatry* (Vol. 33, pp. 15–30). Rochester, MN: Karger Publishers.
Lewis-Fernández, R., & Kirmayer, L. J. (2019). Cultural concepts of distress and psychiatric disorders: Understanding symptom experience and expression in context. *Transcultural Psychiatry, 56*(4), 786–803.
Liddell, B. J., & Jobson, L. (2016). The impact of cultural differences in self-representation on the neural substrates of posttraumatic stress disorder. *European Journal of Psychotraumatology, 7,* 30464.
Liddell, B. J., Nickerson, A., & Bryant, R. A. (2017). Clinical science and torture survivors' rights to rehabilitation. *The Lancet Psychiatry, 5*(2), 101–103.
Lusk, M., & Baray, S. C. (2017). Mental health and the role of culture and resilience in refugees fleeing violence. *Environment and Social Psychology, 2*(1), 1–13.
Maercker, A., & Hecker, T. (2016). Broadening perspectives on trauma and recovery: A socio-interpersonal view of PTSD. *European Journal of Psychotraumatology, 7,* 29303.
Maercker, A., & Horn, A. B. (2013). A socio-interpersonal perspective on PTSD: The case for environments and interpersonal processes. *Clinical Psychology and Psychotherapy, 20*(6), 465–481.
Maier, T., & Straub, M. (2011). My head is like a bag full of rubbish: Concepts of illness and treatment expectations in traumatized migrants. *Qualitative Health Research, 21*(2), 233–248.
Marková, I. (2006). On 'the inner alter'in dialogue. *International Journal for Dialogical Science, 1*(1), 125–147.
Marková, I. (2016). *The dialogical mind: Common sense and ethics.* Cambridge: Cambridge University Press.
Marsella, A. J. (2010). Ethnocultural aspects of PTSD: An overview of concepts issues and treatments. *Traumatology, 16*(4), 17.
Marsella, A. J., Friedman, M. J., & Spain, E. H. (1996). *Ethnocultural aspects of posttraumatic stress disorder: Issues research and clinical applications*: American Psychological Association.
Mattar, S. (2011). Educating and training the next generations of traumatologists: Development of cultural competencies. *Psychological Trauma: Theory Research Practice and Policy, 3*(3), 258–265.
Meili, I., Heim, E., & Maercker, A. (2018). Culturally shared metaphors expand contemporary concepts of resilience and post-traumatic growth: Contrasting an indigenous Brazilian community and a Swiss rural community. *Medical Humanities, 45*(4), 335-345.
Métraux, J.-C. (1999b). Dons de mémoire: Lecture anthropologique et sociale d'une psychothérapie interculturelle. *Psychothérapies, 19*(4), 225–234.
Métraux, J.-C. (1999a). Au temps du silence, la nosographie reste muette. Le syndrome post traumatique en question. In F. Maqueda (Ed.), *Traumatisme de guerre. Actualités cliniques et humanitaires.* (pp. 41–66). Paris Hommes et Perspectives
Mitschke, D. B., Praetorius, R. T., Kelly, D. R., Small, E., & Kim, Y. K. (2017). Listening to refugees: How traditional mental health interventions may miss the mark. *International Social Work, 60*(3), 588–600.
Morina, N., Kuenburg, A., Schnyder, U., Bryant, R. A., Nickerson, A., & Schick, M. (2017). The association of post-traumatic and postmigration stress with pain and other somatic symptoms: An explorative analysis in traumatized refugees and asylum seekers. *Pain Medicine, 19*(1), 50–59.
Moro, M. R. (1992). Principes théoriques et méthodologiques de l'ethnopsychiatrie. *Santé Mentale Au Québec, 17,* 71–98.
Nathan, T. (1986). Trauma et mémoire. *Nouvelle revue d'ethnopsychiatrie*(6), 7–18.

Nichter, M. (2010). Idioms of distress revisited. *Culture Medicine and Psychiatry, 34*(2), 401–416.
Nickerson, A., Liddell, B., Asnaani, A., Carlsson, J., Fazel, M., Knaevelsrud, C., Morina, N., Neuner, F. Newnham, E., & Rasmussen, A. (2018). Trauma and mental health in forcibly displaced populations: An international society for traumatic stress studies briefing paper. ISTSS, Chicago. Retrieved from https://istss.org/getattachment/Education-Research/Briefing-Papers/Trauma-and-Mental-Health-in-Forcibly-Displaced-Pop/Displaced-Populations-Briefing-Paper_Final.pdf.aspx on the 12th of Febrauary 2020.
Nicolas, G., Wheatley, A., & Guillaume, C. (2015). Does one trauma fit all? Exploring the relevance of PTSD across cultures. *International Journal of Culture and Mental Health, 8*(1), 34–45.
O'Connor, K. (2015). Activity theory. In K. Tracy (Ed.), *International encyclopedia of language and social interaction* (Vol. 1, pp. 27–34). Hoboken, NJ: Wiley.
Perilla, J. L., Norris, F. H., & Lavizzo, E. A. (2002). Ethnicity, culture, and disaster response: Identifying and explaining ethnic differences in PTSD six months after Hurricane Andrew. *Journal of Social and Clinical Psychology, 21*(1), 20–45.
Petit, V., & Wang, S. (2018). Éditorial: La santé mentale en migrations internationales. *Revue Européenne Des Migrations Internationales, 34*(2/3), 7–20.
Rechsteiner, K., Tol, V., & Maercker, A. (2019). It should not have happened: Metaphorical expressions idioms, and narrative descriptions related to trauma in an indigenous community in India. *International Journal of Qualitative Studies on Health Well-Being, 14*(1), 1667134.
Rechtman, R. (2000). Stories of trauma and idioms of distress: From cultural narratives to clinical assessment. *Transcultural Psychiatry, 37*(3), 403–415.
Rousseau, C., & Bagilishya, D. (2007). Survival as subversion: When youth resistance strategies challenge tradition, religion, and political correctness. In B. Drožđek & J. Wilson (Eds.), *Voices of trauma: Treating psychological trauma across cultures* (pp. 257–269). New York, NY: Springer.
Rousseau, C., Drapeau, A., & Corin, E. (1997). The influence of culture and context on the pre- and post-migration experience of school-aged refugees from central America and Southeast Asia in Canada. *Social Science and Medicine, 44*(8), 1115–1127.
Ryder, A. G., Ban, L. M., & Chentsova-Dutton, Y. E. (2011). Towards a cultural–clinical psychology. *Social and Personality Psychology Compass, 5*(12), 960–975.
Salazar-Orvig, A., & Grossen, M. (2008). Le dialogisme dans l'entretien clinique. *Langage Et Société, 1,* 37–52.
Schouler-Ocak, M., Laban, C. J., Bäärnhielm, S., Kastrup, M. C., Dein, S., & Wintrob, R. (2019). Transcultural psychiatry: refugee, asylum seeker and immigrant patients over the globe. In J. A. & F. K. (Eds.), *Advances in psychiatry* (pp. 637–655). Cham: Springer.
Shala, M., Morina, N., Gross, C. S., Maercker, A., & Heim, E. (2020). A point in the heart: concepts of emotional distress among albanian-speaking immigrants in Switzerland. *Culture Medicine Psychiatry, 44,* 1–34.
Sharapova, A., & Goguikian Ratcliff, B. (2018). Psychosocial and sociocultural factors influencing antenatal anxiety and depression in non-precarious migrant women. *Frontiers in Psychology, 9,* 1200.
Silove, D., Ventevogel, P., & Rees, S. (2017). The contemporary refugee crisis: An overview of mental health challenges. *World Psychiatry, 16*(2), 130–139.
Sousa, C., & Marshall, D. J. (2017). Political violence and mental health: Effects of neoliberalism and the role of international social work practice. *International Social Work, 60*(4), 787–799.
Squire, C. (2008). Experience-centred and culturally-oriented approaches to narrative. In M. Andrews, C. Squire, & M. Tamboukou (Eds.), *Doing narrative research* (pp. 42–63). London: Sage.
Stetsenko, A. (2008). From relational ontology to transformative activist stance on development and learning: Expanding Vygotsky's (CHAT) project. *Cultural Studies of Science Education, 3*(2), 471–491.
Stolorow, R. D. (2011). *World affectivity Trauma.* New York: Routledge.
Stone, J., Carson, A., & Sharpe, M. (2005). Functional symptoms and signs in neurology: assessment and diagnosis.*Neurosurgery and Psychiatry, 76*(suppl 1), i2-i12.

Sturm, G., Baubet, T., & Moro, M. R. (2007). Mobilising social and symbolic resources in transcultural therapies with refugees and asylum seekers: The story of Mister Diallo. In B. Drožđek & J. Wilson (Eds.), *Voices of trauma: Treating psychological trauma across cultures* (pp. 211–231). New York: Springer.

Sturm, G., Baubet, T., & Moro, M. R. (2010). Culture trauma and subjectivity: The French ethnopsychoanalytic approach. *Traumatology, 16*(4), 27–38.

Sucharov, M. S., Buirski, P., & Kottler, A. (2007). Kafka's window and Kohut's mirror: A dialogic journey to the center of traumatic worlds. In P. Buirski & A. Kottler (Eds.), *New developments in self psychology practice* (pp. 193–206). Lanham: Jason Aranson.

Summerfield, D. (1996). *L'impact de la Guerre et des Atrocités sur les Populations Civiles: Principes Fondamentaux pour les Interventions des ONG et une Analyse Critique des Projets sur le Traumatisme Psychosocial.* London: Overseas Development Institute.

Summerfield, D. (2001). The invention of post-traumatic stress disorder and the social usefulness of a psychiatric category. *British Medical Journal, 322*(7278), 95–98.

Tankink, M., & Richters, A. (2007). Silence as a coping strategy: The case of refugee women in the Netherlands from South-Sudan who experienced sexual violence in the context of war. In B. Drožđek & J. Wilson (Eds.), *Voices of trauma: Treating psychological trauma across cultures* (pp. 191–210). New York: Springer.

Tarchi, C., Surian, A., & Daiute, C. (2019). Assessing study abroad students' intercultural sensitivity with narratives. *European Journal of Psychology of Education, 34*(4), 1–22.

Tortelli, A., Sauzé, D., & Skurnik, N. (2017). Capital social, santé mentale et immigration. *Annales Médico-Psychologiques Revue Psychiatrique, 175*(6), 573–576.

Trovão, S., Ramalho, S., & David, I. (2017). Mental health among Asian and African migrant working mothers: New vulnerabilities old religious coping resources. *Mental Health Religion and Culture, 20*(2), 1–13.

van der Velden, P. G., Oudejans, M., Das, M., Bosmans, M. W., & Maercker, A. (2019). The longitudinal effect of social recognition on PTSD symptomatology and vice versa: Evidence from a population-based study. *Psychiatry Research, 279,* 287–294.

Van Maanen, J. (1995). Crossroads style as theory. *Organization Science, 6*(1), 133–143.

Van Ommeren, M., de Jong, J. M., Sharma, B., Komproe, I., Thapa, S. B., & Cardeña, E. (2001). Psychiatric disorders among tortured bhutanese refugees in nepal. *Archives of General Psychiatry, 58*(5), 475–482. https://doi.org/10.1001/archpsyc.58.5.475.

Ventevogel, P., Niyonkuru, J., Ndayisaba, A., Reis, R., & de Jong, J. T. (2018). Change and continuity in Burundian divinatory healing. *Journal of Eastern African Studies, 12*(1), 22–43.

Voon, V., Brezing, C., Gallea, C., Ameli, R., Roelofs, K., LaFrance, W. C., Jr., & Hallett, M. (2010). Emotional stimuli and motor conversion disorder. *Brain, 133*(5), 1526–1536.

Watters, C. (2001). Emerging paradigms in the mental health care of refugees. *Social Science and Medicine, 52*(11), 1709–1718.

Weissbecker, I., Hanna, F., El Shazly, M., Gao, J., & Ventevogel, P. (2018). Integrative mental health and psychosocial support interventions for refugees in humanitarian crisis settings. In T. Wenzel & B. Drožđek (Eds.), *An uncertain safety: Integrative health care for the 21st century refugees* (pp. 117–153). New York: Springer.

Yazici, K. M., Kostakoglu, L. J. P. R. N. (1998). Cerebral blood flow changes in patients with conversion disorder. *83*(3), 163-168

Zepke, N., & Leach, L. (2002). Contextualised meaning making: One way of rethinking experiential learning and self-directed learning? *Studies in Continuing Education, 24*(2), 205–217.

Zittoun, T. (2014). Three dimensions of dialogical movement. *New Ideas in Psychology, 32,* 99–106.

Zittoun, T., & Sato, T. (2018). Imagination in adults and the aged person. In T. Zittoun & V. P. Glăveanu (Eds.), *Handbook of imagination and culture* (pp. 187–208). New York, NY: Oxford University Press.

Chapter 6
Collective Trauma, Collective Healing

Trauma associated with forced displacement has a psychosocial impact not only on the individual, but also families, communities and larger society. At the family level, this includes the dynamics of single parent families, lack of trust among members, and changes in significant relationships and child-rearing practice. Communities tend to be more dependent, passive, silent, without leadership, mistrustful and suspicious. Additional adverse effects noted in the literature include the breakdown of traditional structures, institutions and familiar ways of life, and deterioration in social norms, ethics and loss of social capital (Somasundaram, 2014). Saul's (2013) landmark definition of collective trauma highlights its larger social impact, occurring at multiple levels, with "shared injuries to a population's social, cultural, and physical ecologies" (p. 1). In another seminal work on collective trauma, Erikson (1976) defines it as "a blow to the basic tissues of social life that damages the bonds attaching people together and impairs the prevailing sense of communality." (p. 154).

Considering experiences of trauma solely on an individual level, and solely related to an isolated event, is not enough. One needs to consider the impact of collective trauma—and recovery—among refugee populations from a sociocultural and historic perspective. Entire communities may have undergone traumatic experiences, and at various moments across history, disrupting core attachments to families, friends and cultural systems (Lindert et al., 2016). The literature suggests that the consequences of trauma exposure in a population of refugees may go beyond individual suffering to impacting family members and entire communities due to impaired psycho-social functioning in everyday life (Ainamani et al., 2017; Womersley & Arikut-Treece, 2019).

Over the past few decades, a plethora of research has highlighted the importance of the sociocultural environment for the way in which individuals, and indeed entire communities, experience trauma (Bracken et al., 1997; Eagle & Kaminer, 2013; Nickerson et al., 2016; Wilson & Drožđek, 2007). As stated by Jenkins (1996)

G. Theisen-Womersley, *Trauma and Resilience Among Displaced Populations*,
https://doi.org/10.1007/978-3-030-67712-1_6

> Because traumatic experience can also be conceptualized collectively, person-centred accounts alone are insufficient to an understanding of traumatic reactions. In addition to the social and psycho-cultural dynamics surrounding any traumatic response, the collective nature of trauma may be related to ... the political ethos characterizing an entire society (p. 177).

Eagle (2014) refers to notions of collective or historical traumatizations whereby whole groups of people carry a sense of common persecution or victimization:

> The idea of historical trauma is associated most strongly with the history of first nation people in America and the genocidal violence to which they were subjected. Collective trauma is the term that tends to be used about the response of groups of South Africans subject to a brutal apartheid and colonial history, as well as about the response of groups of Jewish people to the Holocaust. Such trauma may be understood to be transmitted intergenerationally via both conscious and unconscious mechanisms, such that those of generations post those directly victimized nevertheless carry the experience of trauma within themselves. In some respect identity and collective trauma come to be intertwined. Such conceptualizations of trauma may encompass a somewhat broader definition of traumatic stressors including not only relations of oppression that threaten actual survival of the group, but also more ideological forces that threaten the eradication of cultural or group identity. In this framework racism, xenophobia or fundamentalisms based on oppression may be understood to produce collective traumatisation. (p. 13)

She suggests that people may be traumatized at multiple levels. This includes collective/social, personal/physical and role identity levels. This point is no more pertinent to bear in mind than in the case of refugee populations often faced with a plethora of traumatic events on a collective level. Becker's (1995, 2004; Becker et al., 1990) concept of extreme trauma further encapsulates the extremity of such collective and historic trauma, defined as the following:

> Extreme traumatisation is an individual and collective process that refers to and is dependent on a given social context; a process that is marked by its intensity, its extremely long duration and the interdependency between the social and the psychological dimensions. It exceeds the capacity of the individual and of social structures to respond adequately to this process. Its aim is the destruction of the individual, of his sense of belonging to society and of his social activities. Extreme traumatisation is characterized by a structure of power within the society that is based on the elimination of some of its members by other members of the same society. The process of extreme traumatisation is not limited in time and develops sequentially. (Becker, 2004, p. 5).

Considering trauma thus as a process, elements of temporality are highlighted, as is the continual interaction of the person with their environment in a given social and historical context. What is particularly interesting in this definition is the highlighting of the socio-political context and power dynamics at play in influencing the mental health of whole populations. Considering the "elimination of some of its members by other members of the same society" referred to in the definition is pertinent both to situations of conflict as well as to societal dynamics at play for refugee communities attempting to integrate into host societies and facing possible discrimination. Following prolonged or repetitive traumatisation, entire communities may thus develop a complex constellation of shared feelings, attitudes and behavioural patterns deeply informed by post-traumatic responses and which may force groups into the role of victim—passive, unskilled, unable and unsure (Makhashvili & Tsiskarishvili, 2007).

Loss of "Home" as Container

Among a sample of Iraqi asylum seekers in the Netherlands, 87.6% reported experiencing the loss of a loved one, with traumatic and multiple losses independently predicting psychopathology (Hengst et al., 2018). Yet, even among those refugees who have not directly experienced the loss of a loved one, loss is an inevitable component of the migration experience. As noted by Du and Witmer (2020), loss associated with the refugee experience is not only that of loved ones as well as the geographical home (often representing a loss of decades, if not centuries, of investment), but also of the familiar sociocultural context (which they refer to as the "psychosocial milieu") as well as a disruption of the life biography (which they define as "a unique web of situated life episodes" [p. 38]) at the level of the individual, the community, and the generations that lived in a certain place at a certain time.

Volkram (2004) argues that "since moving from one country to another involves loss—loss of country, friends and of previous identity—all dislocation experiences can be examined in terms of the immigrant's ability to mourn and/or resist the mourning process." (p. 8). The seemingly paradoxical nuance referred to within this literature is that not all refugees suffer from PTSD on an individual level, yet that pre-migration experiences necessarily involve loss at the communal level which in itself is potentially traumatic. In other words, in order to reflect on the traumatic experiences of refugees, one cannot neglect to examine what has been necessarily been lost to entire communities before embarking on the journey of migration. Rousseau et al. (2014) note the impact of the cumulative effects of a grieving process for communal losses and separations related to forced migration, referring to what Eisenbruch (1991) terms "cultural bereavement." A multi-level path analysis conducted by Nickerson and colleagues (Nickerson et al., 2011) similarly demonstrates how loss and trauma significantly impacted on psychological outcomes among refugee families as a whole in a way that extends beyond individual mental health.

Papadopoulos (2002a, 2002b, 2007) draws on the notion of "nostalgic disorientation" to refer to the uniqueness of this bewildering predicament:

> The loss is not only about a concrete object or condition but it encapsulates the totality of all dimensions of home.... Refugees sense the impact of this multidimensional, deep and pervasive loss and they feel disorientated because it is difficult to pinpoint the clear source and precise nature of this loss...Whenever the home is lost, all the organizing and containing functions break wide open, and there is the possibility of disintegration at all of these three levels: at the individual-personal level; at the family-marital; and at the socio-economic/cultural-political level (Papadopoulos, 2002a, p. 15, p.24).

His main argument is that the loss of home is not just about the conscious loss of the family home with all its material, sentimental and psychological values, but it is a loss of a much more fundamental and symbolic kind which necessarily creates a psychological disturbance.

An important characteristic of home, which inevitably is lost to some extend in the process of migration, is that it grounds and provides coherence to the stories of families. Each family has a story which, its own story which does not necessarily coincide with an external historical account of it. Like all stories, it consists of many more smaller stories of specific facets of the family. As such, "family stories express the interconnection between the personal, family and wider parameters within the context of a sense of home that enables the holding and containing of all opposite and contradictory elements that threaten to disrupt the sense of continuity and predictability" (Papadopoulos, 2002a, p. 25). As Masade (2007) notes 'home embodied objects, languages, practices (which evolved into traditions), histories, myths and faiths [are] all bound to a specific location' (p. 94) which is lost in the process of migration. This loss necessarily contributes towards a sense of empowerment, identity and meaning in life being compromised on a community level (Drožđek & Wilson, 2007; Schweitzer et al., 2006). Falicov (2002) similarly reflects on the loss and resilience inherent to the family migration experience, noting that what refugees have in common is the painful loss of home and separations from loved ones and the inevitable mixed emotion of sadness for what they have lost as well as the elation for what they could gain, the ambivalence of wanting to stay and wanting to go.

Collective Responses to Trauma

Not only may traumatic events be experienced collectively, the psychological impact and manifestation of such trauma is similarly thought to be informed by the sociocultural context. The burgeoning field of cultural psychiatry highlights how cultural variations in ways of life and social contexts shape the embodied experience of trauma and recovery (Kirmayer & Ramstead, 2016). This research demonstrates how particular symptoms or behavioural expressions of distress vary with cultural knowledge, beliefs and interpretations (Kleinman, 1978) and that individuals interpret and respond to their own symptoms with culturally varied coping strategies that may influence the experience of trauma and recovery (Ryder et al., 2011). The work of Kirmayer and colleagues (Kirmayer, 2019; Kirmayer & Jarvis, 2019; Kirmayer & Minas, 2000) for example, demonstrates how the experience of trauma is always preceded by and embedded in cultural systems of meanings and practices, which influence modes of attention and interpretive frames or models. Cultural models may be organised in many ways, including collective symbols, images or representations and forms of cooperative activity. In other words, experience of trauma is an intersubjective, temporal, dynamic process shaped by culture. This approach goes beyond a reductionist focus on "cultural differences," wherein "culture" is perceived a reified, crystallised concept and viewed as a potential barrier to be overcome in a process of psychiatric classification (Watters, 2001). Instead, it focuses on ever-changing cultural and social systems, which determine the various forms in which trauma manifests on a collective level.

Collective, Culturally-Based Interventions

The under-utilisation and mistrust of mainstream mental health services by ethnic minorities in general—and displaced populations in particular—has been well documented (Bigfoot & Schmidt, 2010; Mattar, 2011; Watters, 2001). In the literature, this mistrust been attributed in part due to the variations in culturally informed healing practices and perceptions of mental health services. Indeed, contemporary health related approaches have a western medical illness model perspective that is primarily individualistic in orientation, in contrast to more collectivist ways of understanding relationships between self, society, mind, and body (Somasundaram, 2014). Research conducted among displaced populations by Karageorge et al. (2016) identified the following barriers to the acceptability and validity of mental health services among displaced populations in Greece:

(1) Mistrust or uncertainty of intentions/expectations,
(2) Having more immediate (practical) concerns than talk,
(3) Difficulty discussing trauma and
(4) The inadequate cultural competence of health professionals.

A recent desk review released by the World Health Organization (WHO) and the United Nations High Commissioner for Refugees (UNHCR), the United Nations Refugee Agency, has argued that the development of effective MHPSS programmes requires knowledge of existing health systems and sociocultural context, and that familiarising international humanitarian practitioners with local culture and contextualising programmes is essential to minimise risk of harm, maximise benefit and optimise efficient use of resources (Greene et al., 2017). Developments in theories of identity, culture and traumatology have enriched cross-cultural understanding of mental health dynamics and case conceptualisation, informing the development of intervention models which aim to address cumulative trauma dynamics as well collective identity and culture-specific traumas (Groen et al., 2017; Kira, 2010). As noted by Wind & Komproe (2018), researchers and practitioners have called for interventions which incorporate the socioecological perspective into their design. Their research reveals the links between the individual process that determines disaster mental health and the social community one lives in—highlighting the necessity of interventions to consider the shared context on mental health outcomes.

For communities affected by genocide in particular, literature from Rwanda (Pearlman, 2013; Kanyangar et al., 2007; King, 2011; Staub et al., 2005), Guatemala (Marín Beristain et al., 2000) and Bosnia (Ba & LeFrangois, 2011; Clark, 2008; Denborough, 2011) all highlight the profound impact of public rituals of mourning and remembrance in healing from collective and historic trauma. In Rwanda, this involved engaging in Gacaga tribunals (Kanyangara et al., 2007; King, 2011), and in Guatemala, this involved collective sharing, commemorative activities and funeral rites for the Mayas—including symbolically identifying and punishing those responsible (Marín Beristain et al., 2000). In Bosnia, collective healing was shown to revolve around the principles of the "three Rs"—retributive justice, restorative justice and reconciliation, as mediated for example by the International Criminal Tribunal for the former Yugoslavia (Clark, 2008).

One striking example of collective healing may be drawn from my experience of working with the displaced Yezidi population of Northern Iraq: when the highly traumatised girls and women returned from Islamic State (ISIS) captivity, the spiritual leader of the community welcomed them back. The symbolic gesture was intended to lift the shame, which so often accompanies survivors of trauma (Maercker & Horn, 2013). This precious act seems to have enabled the women to be accepted back within the community. Some of the released hostages performed a purifying ceremony at Lalish, considered the holiest temple of the Yezidi faith. These healing interventions were enacted on a collective level—drawing on cultural and symbolic resources known to the community. One could argue that without these interventions, the released hostages would risk further traumatisation because of subsequent guilt, shame and social stigma: the rupture with the community is in itself traumatic. Within this context, individual trauma-focused therapy as typically prescribed within a Western model would be simply insufficient at best, harmful at worst.

To explore the collective impact of trauma on entire displaced communities, this chapter will draw on two case studies from my work in Iraq and the Philippines, first introduced in chap. 3: the forcibly displaced Yezidi community of Kurdistan Northern Iraq, (200 women whom I interviewed in the context of a project evaluation—where PTSD prevalence was an estimated 82%), and displaced communities affected by the recent conflict in Marawi, Philippines (factors of collective trauma and recovery explored by myself and colleagues among 80 participants in the context of a mental health needs assessment, where PTSD prevalence was an estimated 78%).

Case Study One: The Displaced Yezidi Community of Northern Iraq

This case is first introduced in chap. 3—where the staggering estimate of PTSD prevalence among the Yezidi community is shown to be 82%. In this chapter, I explore the impact of this collective trauma at multiple levels: collective/social, personal/physical and role identity. I also explore the substantial impact of the political, legal, and socio-cultural environment on these experiences of collective trauma and recovery. The case study also appears in an article published in *Intervention* entitled "Collective trauma among displaced populations in Northern Iraq: A case study evaluating the therapeutic interventions of the Free Yezidi Foundation" (Womersley & Arikut-Treece, 2019).

According to Mohammadi (2016), the Yezidi community in particular is facing "not just the individual recent trauma related to the 2014 attacks, but a historical trauma too—they faced genocide 73 times during the Ottoman Empire" (p. 410). This research highlights both the historic and collective nature of the trauma to which the Yezidi population has been exposed, related to historic and ongoing oppression and exposure to violence, as well as identity-related trauma among displaced populations attempting to integrate into host communities (Gerdau et al., 2017; Groen et al., 2017). It is not only individuals facing traumatic events but entire communities.

Among the Yezidi community, Ceri et al., (2016) note a variety of culturally informed idioms of distress drawn on by Yezidis to express their emotional distress:

> The term "Ferman" is an expression for destruction and holocaust and reminds them of massacres against Yazidis; it means at once genocide and trauma. Every Yazidi knows the word "Ferman" because the term passes on from one generation to the next. In the context of the terror attacks by ISIS, the term "Ferman" regained a massive impact for Yazidis. It evokes feelings of mourning and fright. Two further idioms of distress are "nefsî" (arab. psyche), which is used synonymously for all mental disorders and traumas, and "liver burned" (cigera min shewiti), which means emotional suffering (p.146).

The trauma is transmitted inter-generationally. It is experienced collectively, within a particular cultural context. If we're not localising trauma on an individual but rather a community level, what are the practical implications for mental health interventions? What is being done efficiently and what needs to change? How can interventions consider the underlying sources of collective trauma in a way which reflects "local histories and systemic issues of politics, identity and community" (Kirmayer et al., 2010, p. 14)? How can we facilitate collective healing? To explore this question, I conducted 16 focus group discussions (FGDs) with Yezidi women attending the Free Yezidi Foundation, and six in-depth interviews with members of the project team.

Direct quotes from transcripts of these interviews and FGD are presented under the following identified themes:

- Impact of events
- Manifestations of trauma
- Collective trauma
- Culturally informed idioms of distress
- Perceptions of mental health services

The Impact of Events

The Yezidi community's experiences are characterised by a context of complex trauma. Trauma was related to not only exposure to human rights violations and other atrocities in 2014, but compounded variables related to.

- Multiple losses (home, family members, possessions, socioeconomic status)
- Fear of ongoing attacks
- Breakdown of the family unit (due to loss, separation and family members seeking refuge abroad)
- Poverty
- Gender roles being threatened due to men losing employment opportunities
- Poor living conditions in the camps (including cramped living quarters)
- Feeling "trapped" in the camps
- Uncertain futures
- Ethnic discrimination

The following quotes highlight some ways in which members of the Yezidi community described their current situation:

> Years are lost from our lives
>
> In general, we are still, we're just as scared about the future and what will happen, so it's all in our mind. They're saying that the same thing will happen again because they say 'you are a minority' and usually there is no one, for example, to protect you.
>
> The trauma is bigger than the time with ISIS, because, maybe you are not—you just want to be at home, not going alone, you just don't want to see a friend. It's like from social person to person who is avoiding everything. In each way. Like the day is one trauma, during ISIS it's trauma, after ISIS also it's trauma and it's been like four years, we've been here in the tents, it's a big trauma here, obviously.

For the Yezidi community, the trauma is "bigger than the time with ISIS." In other words, the trauma is not related to a specific single, isolated (or isolatable) event. It extends beyond the news headlines. It extends beyond the borders of time. It is both related to the past, to generations of oppression, conflict, and violence; as much as it is related to the future, a future which makes them "just as scared." It impacts social relationships within the community ("you don't want to see a friend"). It's exacerbated by appalling current living conditions in the camp. The trauma of displacement pervades the community—leading to a generation who have "lost years" of their lives. As one woman noted,

> We are thinking about the past and the future at the same time

Manifestations of Trauma

Nightmares and insomnia were the most common symptoms reported in the FGD. Many reported feeling scared, jumpy or alert—particularly at night. Increased aggression was also noted—with augmented propensity towards conflict in the family (e.g. fighting with husbands, or shouting at the children). Trauma also manifested physically (psychosomatic symptoms). In every single FGD, mention was made of family members with heart problems or "fainting spells" starting after the attacks and displacement. Other physical difficulties reported included celiac disease, asthma and constant headaches.

These manifestations are illustrated in the following quotes:

> Even in dreams, we just want to see our homes in dreams.
>
> I'm always thinking about another genocide.
>
> I get really angry when someone says something that's not the right thing, it makes me really upset.
>
> When it becomes dark I feel like we're going to have to run another time, to escape.
>
> All these come to me, for example seeing dead people—all of these all things come to my mind, when I just want to go to bed or shower. I am very nervous all the time.

Collective Trauma

Throughout the FGD and interviews, trauma was commonly referred to on a collective level. In other words, when describing the psychological impact of events on themselves as individuals, many would refer to the impact of events on "us" as a Yezidi community. Many referred to the Yezidi community as close-knit community from which it was difficult to exit or enter (we are a circle, you can't go out and find someone or bring someone inside). The suffering of one member of the community was expressed as suffering from all, with many referring to a collective "we" as opposed to individual "I." Notably, even those not directly exposed to the conflict reported experiencing symptoms of trauma.

The collective trauma, as indicated by the pronoun "we," is illustrated in the following quotes:

> We're forced to be thinking too much about relatives—not only thinking about ourselves… Yezidi are kidnapped every day.
>
> We think about relatives, so it's very difficult because of this, so it's always very new, that's why it's very difficult.
>
> When every single [kidnapped hostage] comes back, we can feel better.
>
> From my family, nobody's kidnapped but, I feel like all the whole community—when they're kidnapped I feel as if they're part of me.

The above-mentioned quotes are testament to the powerful impact of trauma on a collective level. Healing from this collective trauma is seen to be possible only "when every single" Yezidi returns unharmed. Many of the women who participated in these FGDS have directly experienced unspeakable violence and abuse at the hands of ISIS. Many have not. All are affected. As noted by Erikson (1976), in the case of collective trauma,

> 'I' continue to exist, though damaged and maybe even permanently changed. 'You' continue to exist, though distant and hard to relate to. But 'we' no longer exist as a connected pair or as linked cells in a larger communal body (p. 154).

Culturally Informed Idioms of Distress

Yezidi women drew on a variety of culturally informed idioms of distress to describe the ways in which they experience trauma, as illustrated in the following direct quotes:

> We are scared, they are always in our hearts and minds these things.
>
> Our mind is not comfortable.
>
> It's still in our all minds what they did.
>
> My very spirit changes. I have difficulty sleeping at night, I'm thinking and thinking and thinking
>
> I'm an old person because of these things that happened to me.
>
> I'm thinking a lot.
>
> It's like it's not stopping. It's always there.

Note again the use of the collective nouns—even metaphors of the mind and heart are considered in the plural ("our hearts," "our minds"). The vast majority of the idioms of distress were centred on the notion of 'thinking too much'. As noted in the literature on transcultural psychiatry, such idioms of distress include more than just ideas about the cause of an illness; they also incorporate ideas about estimating the severity of illness, appropriate treatment and the meaning of the illness. In other words, it reflects a process of sense making situated within a specific sociocultural context (Harvey, 2007; Kleinman, 1978; Maier & Straub, 2011), which should be taken into consideration by the programme design of any intervention. It is important to note that many of the women taking part in these FGD have been diagnosed with PTSD However, none referred to the diagnosis—or any related medical terminology—to describe their experiences of trauma.

Perceptions of Mental Health Services

In general, a significant shift in perceptions of mental health services among the Yezidi community appears to have occurred. Whereas before the attacks of 2014, mental health services were seen as being only for people who are "crazy" (with a significant social stigma attached)—this has now changed. Paradoxically, this shift may possibly be related to the alarmingly high levels of trauma in the community, which have led to an easier and more obvious recognition of the need for mental health support. In other words, one reason for this acceptance could possibly be due to the significant efforts the project undertook to sensitize the community about the importance of taking care of their mental health, for example by implementing psycho-education sessions. It could also be simply due to the overwhelming impact of collective trauma on this community: an impact too significant, too evident, and too debilitating to be ignored.

This shift towards a more positive perception of mental health services is illustrated in the following quotes:

> Before people were thinking it's shame, for example, if you see a doctor or a psychologist but for now for Yezidi community, it's become something very general since all of them are affected, it's something very normal and general for every Yezidi.

> They know what is trauma. They know that for example if the kids are traumatized then they have to be treated. It is something psychological; we shouldn't consider them as crazy or mad.

> I have right now, like, about 28 people, 26 waiting list [to see the psychologist], and I think that's why because right now they understand.

Case Study Two: Displaced Populations Affected by ISIS in Marawi, Philippines

Following the recent crises of extreme violence in Marawi (the country's largest Muslim-majority city) and natural disaster in two Lanao provinces, 450,000 citizens find themselves in IDP camps or 'homestays' with no own home to return to. In addition, some 1,500 families are grieving for the loss of loved ones—many under horrifying circumstances.

In response to these events, a five-member team of the Global Initiative for Stress and Trauma Treatment (GIST-T), in consultation with EMDR Philippines, Philippines Psychiatric Association, Nonviolent Peaceforce (NP) and World Bank Manila, conducted a needs assessment to understand the psychosocial impact of the recent crises in Marawi on the affected population—individuals, families, and local communities. The aim was to gather first-hand information from IDPs, review the state of current psychological services available, identify unmet mental health needs, and propose immediate and medium-term ways to strengthen capacity of mental health professionals and paraprofessionals to provide appropriate treatment. All team members participated in the data collection and information gathering, and contributed to the development of this final report. Data and thematic analysis was undertaken by Dr. Derek Farrell.

Apart from psychometric testing, the results of which are presented in chap. 3, the following semi-structured interview questionnaire was used to interview 80 respondents from the community:

> Question 1: What happened to you?
> Question 2: Of all these things that happened to you, which one is currently bothering you the most? Which one causes you the most distress/ worst?
> Question 3: Are you able to say who your perpetrator/ assailant was?
> Question 4: Did you sustain any physical injuries?
> Question 5: What impact do you think your experiences of adverse events have had on you?
> Question 6: What impact do you think your experiences have had on those close to you?
> Question 7: Have you been feeling guilty about the trauma or your response to it? Shamed? Angry? How much have these feelings been present for you?
> Question 8: How has your mood been since the trauma?
> Question 9: What behavioural changes did you notice in yourself after the trauma experience?
> Question 10: What behavioural changes did you notice in significant others?
> Question 11: Since the trauma, have you ever thought that life is not worth living, or thought of suicide? If yes, how often?
> Question 12; What strategies/ interventions have you used in managing your trauma symptoms?

Origins and Layers of Trauma

The findings from this mission attest to the alarmingly high rates of trauma among the population. Furthermore, they highlight the substantial impact of the political, legal, and sociocultural environment on both the prevalence of trauma, as well as processes of psychosocial rehabilitation. Indeed, trauma among this population was also shown to be experienced on a complex, collective level, related to:

- Historic trauma
- Intra-familial trauma
- Religious conflict
- Violent extremism
- Sexual and gender-based violence (SGBV)
- Natural disasters
- History of forced evacuations and displacements

Intergenerational Transmission

The cycle of trauma and violence appears to have continued for generations, as indicated by the high level of adverse childhood experiences to which this adult population has been exposed. Given the significant concern raised by parents and teachers over the impact of trauma on the mental health of children in the community, the perpetuation of this cycle of trauma and violence is a significant cause for concern. The scientific literature reports that children exposed to violence and exhibiting with higher levels of trauma, have an increased vulnerability towards appetitive aggression (i.e. aggressive behaviour related to actively searching violence) and engaging in acts of extremism.

Effect on Adults and Children

Serious symptoms of depression, anxiety, and trauma were clinically observed by the consultant psychologists—confirming the results of the psychometric screening. Among the most disturbing observations was the increase in physical violence and aggression reported—particularly among the youth. Children, for example, were seen to play "Isis-Isis"—dressing up as fighters and "re-enacting" the traumatic events to which they had been exposed. Others were too afraid to attend school—jumping at the slightest sound of a motorcycle or a helicopter, as the noise would trigger memories of traumatic events. The emotional distress among adults was similarly observed to affect their ability to function productively.

Self-awareness of Trauma

The majority of actors with whom the team engaged, including the military, teachers and humanitarian workers, spontaneously referred to themselves needing psychological assistance for their own trauma—with some becoming visibly emotionally distressed/in tears when speaking about their experiences. Despite the stigma surrounding mental health in general, many spoke directly and openly about their psychological distress and need for assistance.

Thematic Analysis of Qualitative Data

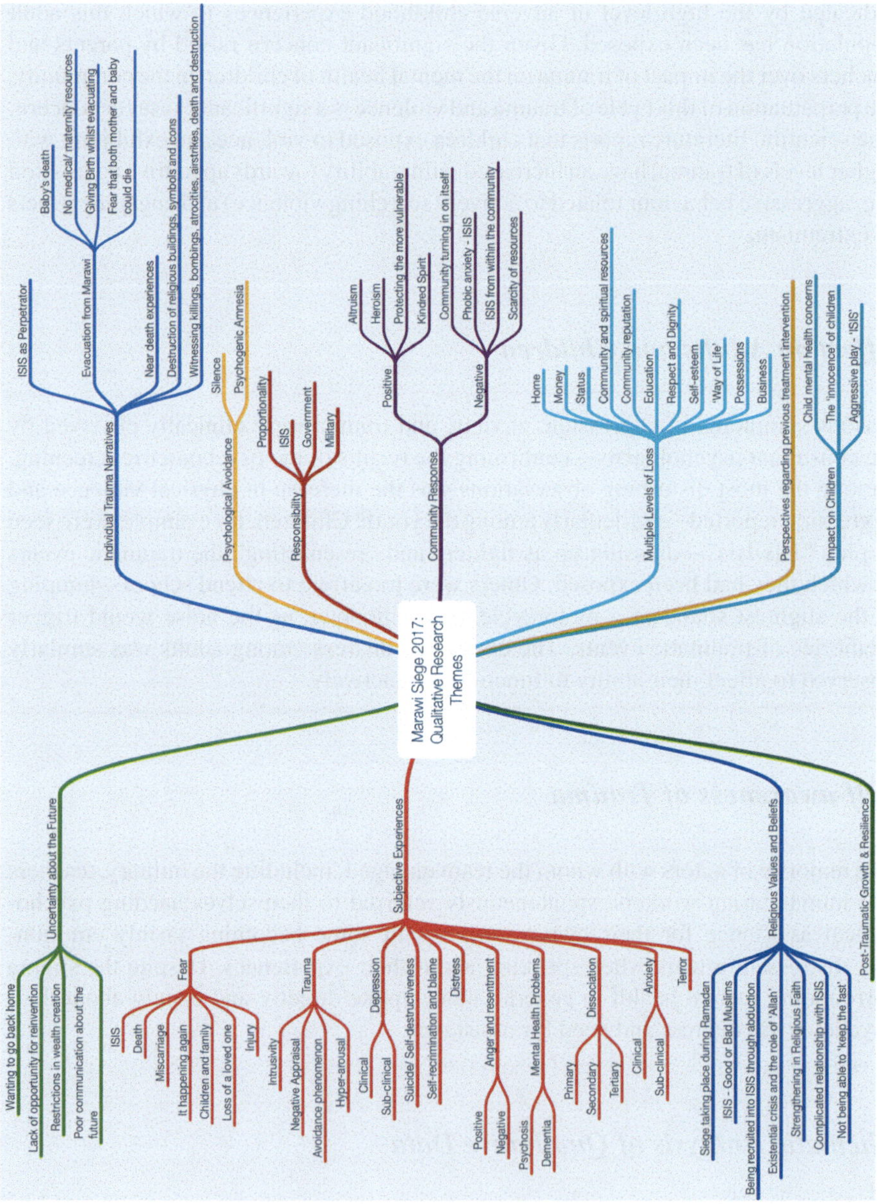
Marawi Siege 2017: Qualitative Research Themes
Individual Trauma Narratives
ISIS as Perpetrator
Evacuation from Marawi
Baby's death
No medical/ maternity resources
Giving Birth whilst evacuating
Fear that both mother and baby could die
Near death experiences
Destruction of religious buildings, symbols and icons
Witnessing killings, bombings, atrocities, airstrikes, death and destruction
Psychological Avoidance
Silence
Psychogenic Amnesia
Responsibility
Proportionality
ISIS
Government
Military
Community Response
Positive
Altruism
Heroism
Protecting the more vulnerable
Kindred Spirit
Negative
Community turning in on itself
Phobic anxiety - ISIS
ISIS from within the community
Scarcity of resources
Multiple Levels of Loss
Home
Money
Status
Community and spiritual resources
Community reputation
Education
Respect and Dignity
Self-esteem
'Way of Life'
Possessions
Business
Perspectives regarding previous treatment intervention
Impact on Children
Child mental health concerns
The 'innocence' of children
Aggressive play - 'ISIS'
Uncertainty about the Future
Wanting to go back home
Lack of opportunity for reinvention
Restrictions in wealth creation
Poor communication about the future
Subjective Experiences
Fear
ISIS
Death
Miscarriage
It happening again
Children and family
Loss of a loved one
Injury
Trauma
Intrusivity
Negative Appraisal
Avoidance phenomenon
Hyper-arousal
Depression
Clinical
Sub-clinical
Suicide/ Self-destructiveness
Self-recrimination and blame
Distress
Anger and resentment
Positive
Negative
Mental Health Problems
Psychosis
Dementia
Dissociation
Primary
Secondary
Tertiary
Anxiety
Clinical
Sub-clinical
Terror
Religious Values and Beliefs
Siege taking place during Ramadan
ISIS - Good or Bad Muslims
Being recruited into ISIS through abduction
Existential crisis and the role of 'Allah'
Strengthening in Religious Faith
Complicated relationship with ISIS
Not being able to 'keep the fast'
Post-Traumatic Growth & Resilience

Subjective Experiences of the Marawi Siege

Within the Trauma Interview Schedule, the first question—What happened to you?—implies no negativity, blame, proportionality or indication of responsibility or prejudice. Rather, the intention is to capture a series of subjective narratives.

Question 1: What happened to you?—brings out traumatic experiences at a subjective level. Supporting narratives are given below.

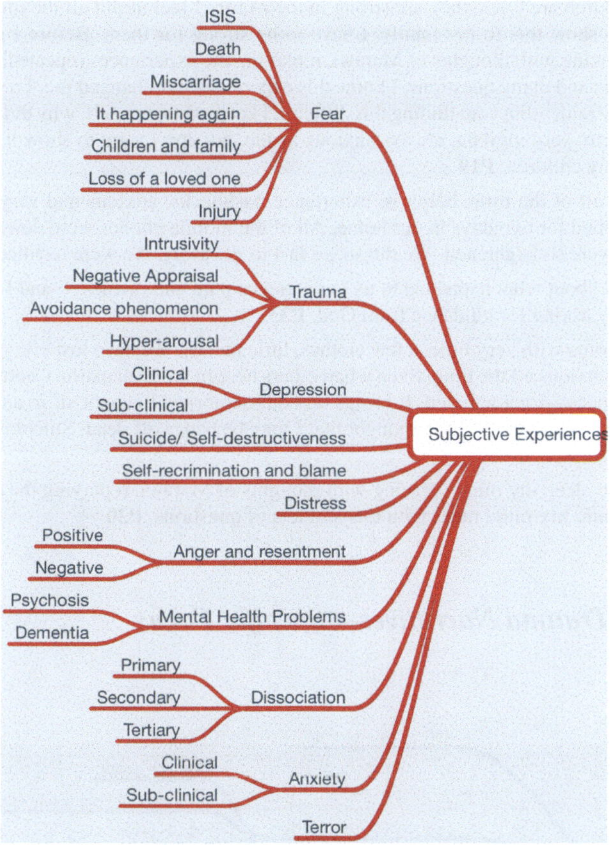

Sub-theme of subjective experience

Many of the following narratives capture subordinate themes of:

- Trauma
- Terror
- Fear
- Depression
- Suicide/ Self-destructiveness

- Self-recrimination
- Distress
- Anger and resentment
- Mental health problems
- Anxiety

> What we experienced in Marawi was terrifying. On the day we evacuated we were very frightened, we had guns pointed at us, and they threatened to fire—ISIS fighters threatened to kill us. We all thought we were going to die. It is so sad to see what has happened to Marawi. We are still troubled, but we put our faith in Allah and ask for his forgiveness. My wife and children are OK—they are strong in their faith. I feel afraid all the time, but I am frightened to show this to my family. I have to be strong for them. Before I go to sleep, my mind is racing with thoughts of Marawi, replaying the experiences repeatedly. My mind races with lots and many questions. I know this experience has changed me. I try to connect more with my faith—but I am finding this difficult. I keep asking myself, why did this happen to us. Now I am very vigilant, always anxious inside, but don't want to show it. I just want the best for my children. **P19**

> I feel scared all of the time, helpless, experience flashbacks, anxious and very depressed. We were trapped for two days in our home. All of the mobile phones were down. When we escaped we were so frightened. We ran so, so fast to get away. We were terrified. **P38**

> When I think about what happened to us I experience pain and rawness—and I am angry. I am constantly asking for guidance from God. **P33**

> We left our home with very little, a few clothes, little money. We have lost everything. I feel stressed and anxious all the time. Even when others here in the Evacuation Centre talk about their experiences—I get agitated. It brings on bad memories. I cannot sit in any one place for any period. Sometimes I have thought that I may be better off dead. Suicide has crossed my mind. **P29**

> Before I go to sleep my mind is racing with thoughts of Marawi, replaying the experiences again and again. My mind races with lots and lots of questions. **P20**

Individual Trauma Narratives—Specific Focus

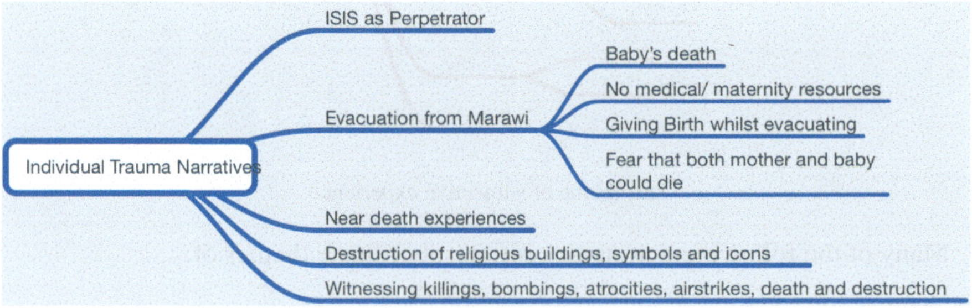

Sub-theme of individual narratives of note

Subordinate themes:

- ISIS as perpetrator
- Evacuation from Marawi
- Near death experiences
- Destruction of buildings, symbols and icons
- Witnessing killings, bombings, atrocities, death and destruction

I was three months pregnant when we had to escape. I was afraid for me, my husband, and my unborn child. I was petrified of losing my baby during the siege. ISIS threatened me. The worst part of the evacuation was that my father died as we were trying to escape. We could not grieve properly for the loss of our father. My baby was born here in the centre. This is no place to bring up a new baby. **P9**

At first I didn't want to leave our home. I was very scared and frightened. We had to travel on foot in order to escape. We left in a hurry which meant that we could take very little—only what we could carry. I witnessed somebody being killed right in front of me. He was killed by ISIS. It was a boy, maybe nine or ten. He had stolen some food from a local market. So, they killed him, in front of everyone. **P2**

I was born in Marawi. When the siege started, I was trapped for three days. I thought it would stop. I remember bullets hit our house. We had vehicles that we could use for escape, but none of us could drive. Eventually, when we did escape, it was on foot—ISIS fighters stopped us. They focussed on me, as they said my hair was too long. They reprimanded my father for allowing his son's hair to be too long. He ordered my father to cut it—and then they let us go. We were terrified that they were going to hurt us. There are times when I cry when I think of the happiness we had before. **P55**

I have very painful memories of the war and the siege. I have very vivid memories of the activities of ISIS fighters. We thought we were going to die. When we were evacuating we took off our shoes so that we would not be heard. We ended up with lots of cuts and injuries to our feet. I'm very concerned about my father—he is angry all the time. I just feel lonely and sad. **P46**

We were trapped in Marawi for three days during the siege (23–26 May 2017). Our house was burned and then we witnessed it being bombed. Thankfully, we were not in our house at the time. Our house was in an elevated position; we had moved to stay lower down the city. I was frightened being in Marawi as I am a Christian and this felt more scary and unsafe. We left with very little, no money—we are uncertain about the future. **P50**

During the conflict, I was nine months pregnant at the time. As we were fleeing I had to give birth to my child. It didn't go OK. I was rushed to hospital where I was operated on. I survived, but my baby died. Now I'm overwhelmingly sad and fearful all of the time. **P12**

We know that our home and business was destroyed by the siege. Loud noises are very distressing. We thought we would be separated from our family. Any loud noise makes my body shake and tremble, I have bad dreams and feel like I cannot control my emotions. We are afraid for our children that in the future they may join ISIS. We know of children who attended the Madrasa and were never seen again. As a parent, it is terrifying to lose one's children in this way. Why is this happening to us—have I not been a good Muslim, is Allah disappointed in us, in me? **P24**

The most terrifying part was that people thought we were part of ISIS, and there was a point when people turned on us, but we were able to reassure them that we were not ISIS. We were very afraid. The bombings and airstrikes were very frightening. We also came across ISIS fighters and they started to follow us. We were terrified. As we were fleeing, we all started reciting words from the Quran—like in unison, and eventually ISIS left us alone. **P18**

23rd May 2017. I initially thought that it was a family skirmish or conflict and thought that things would settle down. Then we got the message 'ISIS' is here. I was very distressed. We started to hear gunshots, but this is not unusual for here. Then we got text messages to say that ISIS was in the Cathedral. We initially thought it would be over in a few days, but it took five months. We were very afraid. The military cordoned off the whole area. They were afraid that ISIS fighters would try to escape. We could hear the airstrikes. We could not leave as my husband was an electrician and he was told that he needed to keep the lights on for the military. Whenever the airstrikes occurred, the ground would shake. We could often see the planes as they were flying very low. Most people left –but we had to stay. We had to feed many dogs from our Catholic community for those that fled. We were afraid that our chapel would be destroyed. We feared for our children, how would we get food, we felt unsafe. It is God's will. **P42**

I'm ashamed at having to give birth on the road as we were trying to evacuate. **P6**

We escaped the day after the burning of the church, school and jail. We transferred from place to place along with our neighbours. **P13**

Psychological Avoidance

Subordinate themes:

- Silence
- Psychogenic amnesia

The whole thing is too distressing. I don't want to talk about. An ISIS fighter put a gun to my head—I don't want to talk about it. **P5**

I had a near death experience—but I don't want to talk about it. I thought I was going to die. The bombings were terrible. I just want to go home. **P10**

I can't remember anything about the crisis—it is all just a blank. It is all a bad memory. I struggle to remember what happened. What happened in Marawi was the will of Allah. **P25**

I cannot talk about it—I do not want to talk about it. What has happened has affected all of my family. I am angry with ISIS, cannot trust ISIS people, these people are from within our community. I am angry towards the bad people, I want to kill the bad people, I am full of rage. I worry for my children. **P2**

Multiple Levels of Loss

Subordinate themes:

- Home
- Money
- Status
- Community and spiritual resources
- Education
- Respect and dignity
- Self-esteem
- 'Way of life'

- Possessions
- Business

When the siege happened, I was still at work at the university. I was about to go home when the firefight started. I called all my children and told them to go home immediately. We live close by the university. The university President asked us to stay and not leave. We witnessed the airstrikes. We did not want to show our fear and anxiety to our children. We could see the bombs exploding in the city. We were on duty day and night—we were so worried about our children. We slept in shifts to guard our children. We knew of a wife of a neighbour taken hostage by ISIS. Fr. Chito negotiated her release. When we found out that Fr. Chito had also been taken hostage—this was one of the worst parts. We prayed. However, we also know of people who lost their lives. One neighbour was hit by a stray bullet and had to have his leg amputated. Every time I see him it is a painful reminder of what happened. Now very reluctant to have conversations with Muslims—tend to stick to my own community (RC). I am afraid that they may be ISIS sympathisers and therefore our lives may be in danger. **P34**

My home was not destroyed by the airstrikes—but it has been looted. I want to go back home, but I know there will be nothing there. I desperately want to go back to Marawi—but I'm being told that I cannot go there. **P45**

We had a big shop in Marawi. It was a family business, very successful. But we lost everything. We used to be respected in the community. Now we have nothing. **P28**

We had to leave everything behind—I miss my gadgets (electronic devices). We have nothing now really—we are surviving on my late mother's pension. **P31**

We have no work, no food, and no money to start our lives again. It is just not good enough. **P41**

I lived in Marawi for five years—I have very good memories of the city. My brother came and said, 'ISIS is coming'. At 3 pm, we heard gunshots. My father was not at home. We did not know what to do, or where to go. That evening we saw ISIS starting fires. My father had a second wife in another house and at the time, he was with them. We could see that ISIS were in control of the area. During the night, we escaped and headed for the mountains. We were all very afraid. Just before the siege, my mother died so we were all still grieving for her loss. It was a bad time. Leaving Marawi—leaving all my friends and our way of life. It was a place where we could practice our religion freely—I am very proud to be a Muslim. **P44**

Because of what happened in Marawi it has resulted in the discontinuation of my education—this saddens me. We have also lost all our money and have no financial help. My mother is very distressed—this is heart breaking. We saw pictures on the news, which showed our house, it was still intact, but we are not allowed to go back there. I feel helpless and hopeless. **P65**

Community Response

Subordinate themes:
Positive

- Altruism
- Heroism
- Protecting the more vulnerable

- Kindred spirit

Negative

- Community turning in on itself
- Phobic anxiety
- ISIS from within the community
- Scarcity of resources

> We have a disabled brother and I needed to get to him to rescue him, otherwise he would have been left behind. The most terrifying part was that people thought we were part of ISIS, and there was a point when people turned on us, but we were able to reassure them that we were not ISIS. We were very afraid. The bombings and airstrikes were very frightening. We also came across ISIS fighters and they started to follow us. We were terrified. As we were fleeing, we all started reciting words from the Quran—like in unison, and eventually ISIS left us alone. **P26**

> I have experienced evacuating more than once before—the Marawi siege, and previously during the first martial law. Twice before I have been an IDP. For this Marawi siege we were trapped for four days. I'd recently had a stroke, so our neighbours had to help us to escape. Many of our neighbours were not from Mindanao—but still they helped us. I feel strong feelings of guilt that I cannot be more supportive to my family. **P49**

> Now I am very reluctant to have conversations with Muslims. I tend to stick to my own Roman Catholic community. I am afraid that there may be ISIS sympathisers living amongst us, and therefore our lives are in danger. **P33**

> I blame ISIS, but not just them; I blame the whole Islam community. I feel angry at the Muslims who support ISIS and the Muslims that fight. **P36**

Impact on Children

Subordinate themes:

- Child mental health concerns
- The 'innocence of children'
- Aggressive play

> When I notice the children playing, their play is more violent and aggressive, they fight all the time—they pretend to be ISIS fighters, and this is very difficult. I try to play with the children to help them not play in such aggressive ways. **P17**

> My children are not the same as before. They often sit and stare. They are overthinking. Their minds are distracted. I feel guilty when I see them suffering. But, I'm helpless to know what to do for them. **P44**

> I am afraid for my children for the future that they may join ISIS. We know of children who attended the Madrasa and were never seen again. As a parent this is terrifying to lose one's children in this way. **P24**

My children have lost the desire to study. I'm afraid for their future. The children are finding it difficult to adjust to being here in the camp. **P61**

When the children hear helicopters flying over they get very scared and frightened. They talk about the bombings back in Marawi. **P51**

I am very concerned about my children—they are now very aggressive. **P24**

My children are irritated most of the time. When they play it is more violent and aggressive, they fight all the time—they pretend to be ISIS fighters, this is very difficult for me to handle. **P26**

My children are always fighting, and it is more aggressive and violent than it was before. This frightens me. **P35**

The children are playing ISIS with toy guns and pretending to shoot and kill other children. They sometimes even pretend to wear the ISIS masks. They witnessed the 'Black People' during the siege. **P51**

Religious Values and Beliefs

Subordinate themes:

- Siege taking place during Ramadan
- ISIS—good or bad Muslims
- Being recruited into ISIS through abduction
- Existential crisis and the role of Allah
- Strengthening in religious faith
- Complicated relationship with ISIS
- Not being able to keep the 'fast'

This is all God's will. What has happened has strengthened my faith, and the faith of my community. We have become more resolute. **P34.**

We directly witnessed the crossfire. That this was happening during Ramadan. When we evacuated I carried a 10 kg. bag of rice, which was bought to observe the fast and the prayer. **P45.**

I liked living in Marawi. It was a place where we could practice our religion freely—I am very proud to be a Muslim. Everybody is responsible for what has happened. Marawi was becoming not a very good place. Some people were not devout in their faith. What happened in Marawi was God's punishment. I blame ISIS and the military for what happened. I'm angry with the military as it was the military that destroyed our city. **P55.**

I know this experience has changed me. I try to connect more with my faith, but I am finding this difficult. I keep asking myself, why did this happen to us. **P20.**

Why is this happening to us—have I not been a good Muslim, is Allah disappointed in us, in me? **P24.**

I feel very, very angry. We always ensured that somebody stayed in the chapel to protect it from ISIS. When we got the text message to say that Fr. Chito had been taken hostage, we all felt a lot of pain and extremely powerless. **P34.**

Uncertainty About the Future

Subordinate themes:

- Wanting to go back home
- Lack of opportunity for reinvention
- Restrictions in wealth creation
- Poor communication about the future

My wife is very uneasy—traumatised—she is constantly angry with me. In Marawi I always knew what to do—but here in the camp nothing is certain. We have no money. **P59**

I get fever when some disturbance increases. If I have lots of worries, then I get lots of physical ailments—my BP increases. Feel very different. I'm lonelier. The food here is not good, and also not enough. We are uncertain about the future and worried all of the time. **P37**

A lot of worries when we think about the future, very anxious about our children, as our young children need to be fed and sent to school. I feel helpless as we have so few options. **P35**

We saw pictures on the news which showed our house, it was still intact, but we are not allowed to go back there. I feel helpless and hopeless. Nobody tells us anything. **P27**

I feel a lot of guilt since we have no source of income I feel ashamed as we have to either borrow or depend on others. This brings a lot of anger and shame to us, to me. **P36**

We are all scared and deprived of basic needs, which never happened before. We were always well provided for. Financial difficulties are the most problematic and have impacted on our lives the most. We do not know when life will become normal again. **P38**

Post-Traumatic Growth and Resilience

Since the siege I have become more reflective, more devout in my faith. I want to build a stronger community for the future. **P32**

Now I pray more every day. I am always reading the Quran. I have recently volunteered to work for an NGO as a facilitator. **P40**

I want to become a medical doctor in the future. Marawi was not a good place. There were females not wearing their veils—and doing bad things. The markets were not clean, and the water was dirty, waste management was not good. When it rained and the sun came out, the smell was terrible. It was so bad that it affected the health of the children. Having EMDR therapy with Fr. Cornelio was very helpful. It helped me understand my feelings, what I was encountering and experiencing. It helped me process the trauma through the drawing and BLS (Butterfly Hug). The memories are always there—but now they are more distant and feel in the past. We did a three-day training with Fr. Cornelio, which was good experience in sharing. I know for certain that I want to live my life by helping others. **P55**

There are times when I cry when I think of the happiness we had before. We have been taken into this Christian community—they have been very good and kind to us. I did not see good in Christian people before—I have always seen them as bad people. However, my view has changed—I see Christians differently now—I can accept help from my Christian neighbours. **P56**

> What has happened to us is hard, but it has brought my family closer together. We support one another. We will get through this—and be stronger again as a community. Marawi will be a stronger city in the future. **P1**

> My relationship with God is stronger now. Allah is the answer to all our problems. **P48**

Conclusion

These case studies highlight the substantial impact of the political, legal and sociocultural environment on both the prevalence of trauma as well as processes of psychosocial rehabilitation. Indeed, trauma among this population was also shown to be related to collective and historic trauma experienced on a community level. One of the key themes to emerge from the case of the Yezidi community was the significant emotional impact of having members still held hostage, lost or missing. On a collective level, this appears to have resulted in unresolved, ongoing trauma. For many, the uncertainty as to whether or not their loved ones were alive or dead appears to have complicated the mourning process. Some individuals in the project report feeling as though they are "frozen" in this liminal space, unable to start on the important and necessary work of grieving. Hope that loved ones may still be alive is a double-edged sword—keeping many stuck on a perpetual loop of acute and intense pain, unable to proceed along the emotional journey of mourning. Here, we think of the symbolic importance of mass memorials such as the case of countries such as Rwanda and Bosnia, where rituals of mourning have offered some possibility of healing from this complicated, collective grief. The trauma is irrevocably collective, symbolic and political—as are healing mechanisms. If trauma may be experienced collectively, it stands to reason that processes of healing should similarly be facilitated collectively.

This similarly speaks to a need to consider the political context in which the intervention takes place. For example, the Free Yezidi Foundation programme incorporates an advocacy strategy targeting those directly affected (notably enslaved women and girls), as well as the international community. A sense of justice being served through the social recognition of this suffering (Marková, 2016) is integral to the healing process. Collective and historic trauma does not occur in a sociopolitical vacuum, and neither should intervention strategies. As noted by Yassin et al. (2018), "although interventions at the micro and mezzo levels are extremely helpful, radical changes do not occur without implementing support and strategic interventions at the macro level" (p. 9).

Implications for interventions include utilising eco-social frameworks for research and practice, engaging in advocacy, and establishing agendas for mental health practice that emphasise individual and collective self-determination (Harvey, 2007; Sousa & Marshall, 2017). Understanding the collective impact of dislocation, trauma and loss, of political persecution and human malevolence, and social systems involving abuse, neglect, and ethnic and cultural rejection, is crucial in terms of guiding policy makers and clinicians to assist, and as advocates to address, the social, cultural and political perspectives of trauma. Furthermore, it is fundamental to the success of any mental health intervention targeting displaced populations. Attending to the mental health needs of trauma survivors, including interdisciplinary rehabilitation from trauma, is a key part of restoring dignity in the wake of human rights abuses and providing a form of justice for those who suffered harms.

References

Ainamani, H. E., Elbert, T., Olema, D. K., & Hecker, T. (2017). PTSD symptom severity relates to cognitive and psycho-social dysfunctioning–A study with Congolese refugees in Uganda. *European Journal of Psychotraumatology, 8*(1), 1283086.

Ba, O. B., & LeFrangois, B. A. (2011). Ethnic genocide, trauma, healing, and recovery: The case of identity ruptures and restoration among bosnian refugees. In T. Matyok, J. Senehi, & Byrne, S. (Eds), *Critical issues in peace and conflict studies: Theory practice and pedagogy* (pp. 81 - 96). Lanham: Lexington Books.

Becker, D. (1995). The deficiency of the concept of posttraumatic stress disorder when dealing with victims of human rights violations. In R. J. Kleber, C. R. Figley, & B. P. R. Gersons (Eds.), *Beyond trauma: Cultural and societal dynamics* (pp. 99–110). New York, NY: Plenum Press.

Becker, D. (2004). Dealing with the consequences of organised violence in trauma work. *Transforming ethnopolitical conflict* (pp. 403–420). New York: Springer.

Becker, D., Lira, E., Castillo, M. I., Gómez, E., & Kovalskys, J. (1990). Therapy with victims of political repression in Chile: The challenge of social reparation. *Journal of Social Issues, 46*(3), 133–149.

Bigfoot, D. S., & Schmidt, S. R. (2010). Honoring children, mending the circle: Cultural adaptation of trauma-focused cognitive-behavioral therapy for American Indian and Alaska Native children. *Journal of Clinical Psychology, 66*(8), 847–856.

Bracken, P., Giller, J. E., & Summerfield, D. (1997). Rethinking mental health work with survivors of wartime violence and refugees. *Journal of Refugee Studies, 10*(4), 431–442.

Ceri, V., Özlü-Erkilic, Z., Özer, Ü., Yalcin, M., Popow, C., & Akkaya-Kalayci, T. (2016). Psychiatric symptoms and disorders among Yazidi children and adolescents immediately after forced migration following ISIS attacks. *Neuropsychiatrie, 30*(3), 145–150.

Clark, J. N. (2008). The three Rs: Retributive justice, restorative justice, and reconciliation. *Contemporary Justice Review, 11*(4), 331–350.

Denborough, D. (2011). Resonance, rich description and social-historical healing: The use of collective narrative practice in Srebrenica. *International Journal of Narrative Therapy and Community Work, 3,* 27–42.

Drožđek, B., & Wilson, J. P. (2007). *Voices of trauma: Treating psychological trauma across cultures.* New York, N. Y.: Springer.

Du, B., & Witmer, J. (2020). Loss of Possessions, Identity, and Sense of Self. In J. Kottler, S. Banu, & S. Jani (Eds.), *Handbook of refugee experience: Trauma, resilience, and recovery* (pp. 35–42). San Diego, California: Cognella.

Eagle, G. (2014). From evolution to discourse: Key conceptual debates in the history and study of traumatic stress. *Psychology in Society, 47,* 1–20.

Eagle, G., & Kaminer, D. (2013). Continuous traumatic stress: Expanding the lexicon of traumatic stress. *Peace and Conflict: Journal of Peace Psychology, 19*(2), 85.

Eisenbruch, M. (1991). From post-traumatic stress disorder to cultural bereavement: Diagnosis of Southeast Asian refugees. *Social Science and Medicine, 33*(6), 673–680.

Erikson, K. T. (1976). Collective trauma: Loss of communality. In K. T. Erikson (Ed.), *Everything in its path* (pp. 186–245). New York: Simon and Schuster Inc.

Falicov, C. J. (2002). The family migration experience: Loss and resilience. In M. Suarez-Orozco & P. M. (Eds.), *Latinos: Remaking America* (pp. 274–288). Berkeley, CA: University of California Press.

Gerdau, I., Kizilhan, J. I., & Noll-Hussong, M. (2017). posttraumatic stress disorder and related disorders among female Yazidi refugees following Islamic state of Iraq and syria attacks—a case series and mini-review. *Frontiers in Psychiatry, 8,* 282.

Greene, M. C., Jordans, M. J., Kohrt, B. A., Ventevogel, P., Kirmayer, L. J., Hassan, G., et al. (2017). Addressing culture and context in humanitarian response: Preparing desk reviews to inform mental health and psychosocial support. *Conflict and Health, 11*(1), 21.

Groen, S. P., Richters, A., Laban, C. J., & Devillé, W. L. (2017). Cultural identity among Afghan and Iraqi traumatized refugees: Towards a conceptual framework for mental health care professionals. *Culture Medicine and Psychiatry, 42*(1), 69–91.

Harvey, M. R. (2007). Towards an ecological understanding of resilience in trauma survivors: Implications for theory, research, and practice. *Journal of Aggression, Maltreatment and Trauma, 14*(1–2), 9–32.

Hengst, S. M., Smid, G. E., & Laban, C. J. (2018). The effects of traumatic and multiple loss on psychopathology, disability, and quality of life in iraqi asylum seekers in the Netherlands. *The Journal of Nervous and Mental Disease, 206*(1), 52–60.

Jenkins, J. H. (1996). Culture, emotion, and PTSD In A. J. Marsella, M. J. Friedman, E. T. Gerrity, & R. M. Scurfield (Eds.), *Ethnocultural aspects of posttraumatic stress disorder: Issues, research, and clinical applications* (pp. 165–182). Washington, DC: American Psychological Association.

Kanyangara, P., Rimé, B., Philippot, P., & Yzerbyt, V. (2007). Collective rituals, emotional climate and intergroup perception: Participation in "Gacaca" tribunals and assimilation of the Rwandan genocide. *Journal of Social Issues, 63*(2), 387–403.

Karageorge, A., Rhodes, P., Gray, R., & Papadopoulos, R. (2016). Refugee and staff experiences of psychotherapeutic services: A qualitative systematic review. *Intervention, 15*(1), 51–69.

King, R. U. (2011). Healing psychosocial trauma in the midst of truth commissions: The case of gacaca in post-genocide Rwanda. *Genocide Studies and Prevention, 6*(2), 134–151.

Kira, I. A. (2010). Etiology and treatment of post-cumulative traumatic stress disorders in different cultures. *Traumatology, 16*(4), 128.

Kirmayer, L. J. (2019). Toward an ecosocial psychiatry. *World Social Psychiatry, 1*(1), 30.

Kirmayer, L. J., & Jarvis, G. J. H. (2019). Culturally responsive services as a path to equity in mental healthcare. *Healthcare Papers, 18*(2), 11–23.

Kirmayer, L. J., & Minas, H. (2000). The future of cultural psychiatry: An international perspective. *Canadian Journal of Psychiatry Revue Canadienne De Psychiatrie, 45,* 438–446.

Kirmayer, L. J., & Ramstead, M. J. (2016). Embodiment and enactment in cultural psychiatry. In C. Durt, T. Fuchs, & C. Tewes (Eds.), *Embodiment, enaction, and culture: Investigating the constitution of the shared World* (pp. 397–422). Cambridge, MA: MIT Press.

Kirmayer, L. J., Kienzler, H., Afana, A. H., & Pedersen, D. (2010). Trauma and disasters in social and cultural context. *Principles of Social Psychiatry, 2,* 155–177.

Kleinman, A. (1978). Concepts and a model for the comparison of medical systems as cultural systems. *Social Science and Medicine Part B: Medical Anthropology, 12,* 85–93.

Lindert, J., Carta, M. G., Schäfer, I., & Mollica, R. F. (2016). Refugees mental health—A public mental health challenge. *The European Journal of Public Health, 26*(3), 374–375.

Maercker, A., & Horn, A. B. (2013). A socio-interpersonal perspective on PTSD: The case for environments and interpersonal processes. *Clinical Psychology and Psychotherapy, 20*(6), 465–481.

Maier, T., & Straub, M. (2011). My head is like a bag full of rubbish: Concepts of illness and treatment expectations in traumatized migrants. *Qualitative Health Research, 21*(2), 233–248.

Makhashvili, N., & Tsiskarishvili, L. (2007). Lost in the Desert–from Despair to Meaningful Existence: A Chechen Refugee Family Crossing Borders. In B. Drožđek & J. P. Wilson (Eds.), *Voices of trauma: Treating psychological trauma across cultures* (pp. 233–256). New York, NY: Springer.

Marín Beristain, C., Paez, D., & González, J. L. (2000). Rituals, social sharing, silence, emotions and collective memory claims in the case of the Guatemalan genocide. *Psicothema, 12*(Su1), 117–130.

Marková, I. (2016). *The dialogical mind: Common sense and ethics*. Cambridge: Cambridge University Press.

Masade, I. (2007). Where is home? Transnational migration and identity amongst nigerians in cape town. In S. Field, Meyer, R. & F. Swanson (Eds.), *Imagining the city: Memories and cultures in Cape Town* (pp. 93–114). Cape Town: HSRC Press

Mattar, S. (2011). Educating and training the next generations of traumatologists: Development of cultural competencies. *Psychological Trauma: Theory Research Practice and Policy, 3*(3), 258–265.

Mohammadi, D. (2016). Help for yazidi survivors of sexual violence. *The Lancet Psychiatry, 3*(5), 409–410.

Nickerson, A., Bryant, R. A., Brooks, R., Steel, Z., Silove, D., & Chen, J. (2011). The familial influence of loss and trauma on refugee mental health: A multilevel path analysis. *Journal of Traumatic Stress, 24*(1), 25–33.

Nickerson, A., Cloitre, M., Bryant, R. A., Schnyder, U., Morina, N., & Schick, M. (2016). The factor structure of complex posttraumatic stress disorder in traumatized refugees. *European Journal of Psychotraumatology, 7,* 33253.

Papadopoulos, R. (2002a). Refugees, home and trauma. *Therapeutic care for refugees: no place like home, 9.*

Papadopoulos, R. (2002b). *Therapeutic care for refugees: No place like home*: Karnac Books.

Papadopoulos, R. (2007). Refugees, trauma and adversity-activated development. *European Journal of Psychotherapy and Counselling, 9*(3), 301–312.

Pearlman, A. L. (2013). Restoring self in community: Collective approaches to psychological trauma after genocide. *Journal of Social Issues, 69*(1), 111–124.

Rousseau, C., Guzder, J., Santhanam-Martin, R., & de la Aldea, E. (2014). Trauma, culture, and clinical work: The "House of Stories" as a pedagogical approach to transcultural training. *Traumatology: An International Journal, 20*(3), 191-198.

Ryder, A. G., Ban, L. M., & Chentsova-Dutton, Y. E. (2011). Towards a cultural–Clinical psychology. *Social and Personality Psychology Compass, 5*(12), 960–975.

Saul, J. (2013). *Collective trauma collective healing: Promoting community resilience in the aftermath of disaster*. London: Routledge.

Schweitzer, R., Melville, F., Steel, Z., & Lacherez, P. (2006). Trauma, post-migration living difficulties, and social support as predictors of psychological adjustment in resettled Sudanese refugees. *Australian and New Zealand Journal of Psychiatry, 2*(40), 179–187.

Somasundaram, D. (2014). Addressing collective trauma: Conceptualisations and interventions. *Intervention, 12*(1), 43–60.

Sousa, C., & Marshall, D. J. (2017). Political violence and mental health: Effects of neoliberalism and the role of international social work practice. *International Social Work, 60*(4), 787–799.

Staub, E., Pearlman, L. A., Gubin, A., & Hagengimana, A. (2005). Healing, reconciliation, forgiving and the prevention of violence after genocide or mass killing: An intervention and its experimental evaluation in Rwanda. *Journal of Social and Clinical Psychology, 24*(3), 297.

Volkan, V. D. (2004). From hope for a better life to broken spirits: An introduction. In J. P. Wilson & B. Drožđek (Eds.), *Broken spirits: The treatment of traumatized asylum seekers, refugees, war and torture victims* (pp. 7–12). New York: Brunner Mazel/Routledge

Watters, C. (2001). Emerging paradigms in the mental health care of refugees. *Social Science and Medicine, 52*(11), 1709–1718.

Wilson, J. P., & Drožđek, B. (2007). Are we lost in translations?: Unanswered questions on trauma, culture and posttraumatic syndromes and recommendations for future research. In B. Drožđek & J. P. Wilson (Eds.), *Voices of trauma: Treating psychological trauma across cultures* (pp. 367–386). New York: Springer.

Wind, T. R., & Komproe, I. H. (2018). Closing the gap between disaster mental health research and practice: Evidence for socio-ecological mental health interventions through multilevel research. *Intervention, 16*(1), 5.

Womersley, G., & Arikut-Treece, Y. (2019). Collective trauma among displaced populations in Northern Iraq: A case study evaluating the therapeutic interventions of the Free Yezidi Foundation. *Intervention, 17*(1), 3.

Yassin, N., Taha, A. A., Ghantous, Z., Atoui, M. M., & Forgione, F. (2018). Evaluating a mental health program for Palestinian refugees in Lebanon. *Journal of Immigrant and Minority Health, 20*(2), 388–398.

Chapter 7
Collective Resilience and Imagination

Collective Resilience Among Displaced Populations

While indeed the stories of forced displacement are often unfathomably difficult and layered with sometimes profound and traumatizing obstacles, they too are often stories of hope and human triumph (Neace, 2020). The past few decades have seen a substantial interest in the field of resilience among refugee communities in particular (Bäärnhielm, 2016; Bélanger-Dumontier & Vachon 2015; Laban, 2015; Lusk & Baray, 2017b; Goguikian Ratcliff, 2007; Roberto & Moleiro, 2016; Simich, 2014; Siriwardhana et al., 2015; Tummala-Narra, 2007)—as well as the related concepts of post-traumatic growth (Calhoun & Tedeschi, 2014; Drožđek & Wilson, 2007; Marsella, 2010; Tankink & Richters, 2007; Tedeschi & Calhoun, 2004; Uy & Okubo, 2018) and adversity-activated development (Papadopoulos, 2002a,2002b,2007) whereby people "not only survive the inhuman and cruel conditions they have endured with a significant degree of intactness but, moreover, they become strengthened by their particular exposure to adversity" (Papadopoulos, 2007, p. 306).

Resilience is a common trajectory following exposure to traumatic events. However, the mechanisms that facilitate resilience are not entirely clear. This is especially the case with cross-cultural populations. Scholars in this area have pointed to the individualistic nature of the concept and the absence of cultural factors in resilience research. They call for a social–ecological view of resilience that incorporates multiple factors, including indigenous ideologies and systems of meaning-making (Raghavan & Sandanapitchai, 2020). The burgeoning literature on resilience among displaced populations thus has begun to highlight the interaction of protective mechanisms with exterior risk factors. The more recent explicit focus is thus on the socio-ecological environment. Within this paradigm, resilience is not a fixed, individual trait. It is dynamic and variable. It reflects both the individual and the world around them. It's considered essentially as a social and environmental attribute (Lusk & Baray, 2017a), and the capacity of a person's "informal and formal social networks

G. Theisen-Womersley, *Trauma and Resilience Among Displaced Populations*,
https://doi.org/10.1007/978-3-030-67712-1_7

to facilitate positive development under stress" (Ungar, 2013, p.1). It is collective. As notably conceptualised by Ungar (2004, 2005, 2008, 2011),

> Resilience is both the capacity of individuals to navigate their way into psychological, social, cultural, and physical resources that sustain their well-being and their individual and collective capacity to negotiate for these resources to be provided and experienced in culturally meaningful ways (Ungar 2008, p. 225)

Such an understanding of resilience explicitly considers the ecological embeddedness of the individual within social, cultural and historical context in order to consider the complex interactions of protective mechanisms with exterior risk factors. Recent research on resilience in refugee contexts in particular focusses less on the construct as an intrinsic process (Song et al., 2015) but a dynamic one—inevitably context and time specific (Maercker & Hecker, 2016; Sleijpen et al., 2017). Furthermore, this understanding of resilience rejects an understanding of the concept as situated within an individual, but similarly considers the "collective resilience" of entire communities (Meili et al., 2019; Tummala-Narra, 2007).

In a recently published study on psychopathology among African unaccompanied refugee minors, Huemer et al. (2016) found a surprisingly low prevalence of PTSD They noted that "for the majority of subjects, resilience actually co-occurred with indicators of vulnerability." (p. 1, my emphasis). This echoes the findings of Sleijpen et al. (2016, 2017), whose results concluded that there was simply no statistically significant relationship found between post-traumatic growth (PTG) and PTSD Indeed, they appeared to be independent and co-occurring constructs. What the literature highlights, therefore, is the substantial resilience shown among refugee communities which co-exist with mental health challenges. As argued by Minihan et al. (2018), resilience is a common pathway among trauma survivors, and "even in the context of cumulative trauma and resettlement stress, psychosocial adaption is the normative response." (p. 257). Moreover, the degree of resilience displayed by a person in a certain context may be said to be related to the extent to which that context has elements that nurture this resilience (Gilligan, 2004). Goguikian Ratcliff et al. (2014) demonstrate that when faced with local professional social reality, migrant women in Quebec develop specific strategies of resistance and resilience that guide their choices relating to integration: accept unskilled jobs, back to school, favoring ties national or family community, give up work and stay at home, etc. Among Congolese refugees in Kenya, Tippens (2017) identified the following strategies of resilience: (a) relying on faith in God's plan and trust in religious community, (b) establishing borrowing networks, and (c) compartmentalizing the past and present.

In terms of a resilience in the face of ongoing stressors related to social marginalisation, there is increasing evidence in favour of what Kadianaki (2010) refers to as a "fluid and contextualized immigrant identity, negotiated and constructed in particular social contexts, forged through social representations, dominant social discourses and specific social structures, and affected by issues of power" (p. 438). She highlights several cases "cases of individuals who responded to the stigmatized representation of their ethnic identities by creating … 'symbolic spaces.' These spaces were 'furnished' with interconnected cultural elements and familiar national symbols, which sustained positive identities in the face of opposition, racism, and discrimination" (p. 443).

This further clouds an already murky picture of trauma among refugees: on the one hand, it is clear that refugees continue to suffer from a plethora of traumatic experiences—facing multiple inter-connected stressors pre-migration, during migration and post-migration. However, the evidence also points to the impossibility of remaining within a simplistic and reductionist discourse of "all refugees are traumatised." Do the multiple accounts of resilience among refugees serve to demonstrate that not people are affected by trauma, or does it simply highlight practical survival mechanisms put in place to defend against it? Furthermore, there is inconsistent evidence regarding the relationship between acculturation and mental health. As noted by Kartal and Kiropoulos (2016), some research suggests that higher levels of acculturation with the host culture are associated with better mental health, while others reported that higher levels of acculturation with the host culture is associated with worse mental health outcomes, a phenomenon named the "immigrant paradox" (Berry, 2003; Kartal & Kiropoulos, 2016; Sam & Berry, 2010). Likewise, post-migration resources were found to offer no contribution to mental health outcomes in multivariate analyses. While several large-scaled studies found associations between post-migration living difficulties and mental health status, findings on post-migration resources such as social support or language proficiency are inconsistent, one possible explanation being a declining influence of resources over the course of time after migration (Heeren et al., 2014). Many questions remain unanswered.

Imagination, Trauma and Migration

The act of migration itself is inherently imaginative (Salazar, 2010; Salazar & Smart, 2011). It is motivated by an (often collective, culturally-informed) imagination of a future beyond the here-and-now. As argued by Zittoun and Gillespie (2015), "indeed, all human travel, and exploration in particular, is motivated by an imagination of a future that lies beyond the horizon of the present and which is as-yet not actualized" (p. 113). It may be perceived as an act of agency on the part of the individual, who turns imagined possibilities into actuality. Due to the constantly evolving nature of imagination, continually developing in relation to the sociocultural environment, the period of transition following migration in and of itself may trigger the imagination of new possibilities. Upon arrival in Greece and first encounters on European soil, asylum seekers may find themselves imagining the possibility of life in a particular town in Sweden, for example.

Yet at the same time, and particularly in the case of forced migration, migration may similarly be perceived as a traumatic rupture: an "a-temporal space"—a transitional and disconnected period wherein experiences, skills, connections acquired and built in the past are rendered inaccessible (Métraux, 1999b). In the specific context of forced migration in particular, itself characterized by a rupture in connection to "home" (and all the social, cultural, professional and linguistic connections that this implies)—the physical, social and political isolation so typically experienced by asylum seekers upon arrival to host countries and often imposed by the state through legal requirements, serves only to feed monstrous feelings of disconnection (Bhimji, 2015). Disaffiliation, de-culturation and de-linking both in terms of family and social ties similarly affects the internal capacity to make links between different events and moments in life. Without the container of home-as-it-was, there is little membrane to hold the symbolic (Goguikian Ratcliff, 2012). In other words, there may be no or little capacity to imagine. As such, trauma begets trauma. Exposure to trauma, itself connected to a breakdown in social connection and exacerbated by the process of migration, risks the individual being caught up in a vicious cycle where no addressee may be found, no language exists to form a coherent narrative whereby trauma may itself be collectively represented and made sense of.

Here, the notion of trauma is understood to straddle both intrapsychic and interpersonal spaces, and is theorized as creating ruptures in time, memory, language and social connection. It is a freezing in non-dialogical space, a shattering of the capacity to generate meaning, and a severe disruption of those relational processes in which meaning is formed (Sucharov et al., 2007). The result is a significant disconnect between the traumatic events and the current sphere of experiences. The consequent lack of connection between past and present can also be understood as preventing the emergence of possible futures. Put simply, trauma may impede processes of imagination. It has even been defined as a state of "limited or constrained modalities of imagining" (Zittoun & Sato, 2018). As conceptualized in Zittoun's "loop" model of imagination which I explore here in this chapter, trauma may similarly impede the movement of *coming back* to the actual, ongoing present. In this case, imagination would be locked in the past, or in an alternative reality.

The position of applicant for refugee status is paradoxical because of its transitional nature—one can either be accepted as a refugee or denied the status and returned home—and, at the same time, its long, indeterminate duration. It is quintessentially the position of someone on the move, yet someone who cannot effectively move anywhere or anything in his or her life. In this context, hope reveals a wide range of opportunities while despair makes them all look impossible or distant. However, things are not again as simple. It is through anxiety and despair that refugees discover the fundamental openness of their existence (Collins & Shubin, 2015). Hope, on the other hand, might not be experienced as empowering by every migrant but potentially frustrating (Collins, 2018a, b). Contrasting emotions are not necessarily confusing; they help refugees understand their position in the world while, at the same time, enable the imagination of new positions and ignite the movement towards them.

Hope, and the ability to imagine a better future for oneself, is intrinsically related to the ways in which we either position ourselves in the world or are being positioned by others. It colours all of the perspectives or action orientations we develop, and prompts and accompanies changes of physical, social, and symbolic position. Some of these states are possibility-enabling, others possibility-reducing in how they either facilitate or inhibit mobility both geographically as well as between perspectives and positions. The emotional life of refugees facing potentially traumatic events is marked primarily by ambivalence and conflict. The position of refugee is associated, at once, with hope and despair, possibility and impossibility, mobility and immobility.

It is important to highlight the concepts of possibility and impossibility into this discussion. They are intimately connected to imagining and hoping for a better future. They ultimately frame the way we feel about and move between positions and perspectives. Acts of repositioning—physical, social and/or symbolic—transform our relation to the world and how we perceive and understand it. New affordances for action can be discovered, new constraints encountered. In the end, movement develops, at all times, slightly different *horizons of possibility (and impossibility)* that are experienced emotionally as rewarding, exciting, painful or frightening. In their study of pre-reflective and affective mobilities, Collins and Shubin (2015) discuss the unexpectedness of migration and the uncertainty about the present felt by English teachers in South Korea. Following Heidegger's ideas, they stress the fact that anxiety is not only a challenging emotional state—it is one that opens the person up to other possibilities for being in the world. The radical change of position involved by migration and inhabiting a new environment can and does transform how these teachers view themselves and gives them, to some extent, an opportunity to re-invent themselves. These possibilities of "being otherwise" irrupt into normal existence and are intensely experienced. Encountering the unknown can threaten one's current self-understanding but it also shows that something else might become possible, even as that final destination remains unknown. In the words of the two authors:

> This highlights the value of celebrating ambiguity and excess in mobile lives and challenges the reduction of life events to specific paradigms, which claim to explain and shape how life transitions come about. (…) Indeed, there is a wider need in migration studies to explore the possibility that the time–spaces of migration emerge in ways that do not come from the acts of migrants themselves or the broader systems they are situated within. The Heideggerian approach deployed in this paper offers considerable potential for this task, highlighting the situatedness of migrants and the complex more-than-subjective dimensions of migration while recognising the enduring openness of the world and its possibilities for generating different ways of being and being mobile (Collins & Shubin, 2015, p. 104).

In focussing on hope, and imagination of a better future, the chapter thus examines the development of individual refugee lives and the ways in which they emotionally dis-connect and re-connect to other people, places, and homes. As noted by Boccagni and Baldassar (2015):

> At all of its 'stages', the migration process is characterized by important transformations along the migrants' life course involving the transmission, reproduction and evolution of emotions in relation to belonging, identity and 'home'. Indeed, the notion of 'the migrant condition' is a reference to the characteristic ambiguities and tensions around emotional connections to 'here' and 'there' (p. 2).

Through this emphasis, the chapter explores how all acts of migration, independent of what motivates them, present us with ambivalence, uncertainty, and a new sense of what is possible and impossible. Mobility itself open and close spaces of possibility and ways of being in the world. These subjective configurations, associated with a given perspective or relation to the world, contribute to widening or narrowing one's perception of what is (im)possible. Hope and despair stand out as contrasting examples of this dynamic, with the former raising the possibility of a different future, the latter trapping the person within an unchangeable past and present. Furthermore, it should be noted that all of these emotional states are experienced subjectively by the individual, yet inextricably connected to the sociocultural environment—including social networks and cultural systems wherein the individual is embedded. Indeed, entire communities may collectively experience emotional states connected to mobility. The hopes of an entire village for economic prosperity may rest on the shoulders of one individual migrant. The fear of persecution may restrict movements of entire groups of ethnic minorities. Mixed and contrasting emotions colour refugee trajectories, alternating or combining hope and nostalgia, guilt and ambition, affection and disaffection, and the possibility to imagine better futures.

The theoretical background of sociocultural psychology allows for an exploration of this ever-changing and dynamic development of imagination over time, and within sociocultural context. It evokes a methodology incorporating an exploration "not only of the subjective perspective, but also the dynamics by which the social and cultural environment guide and enable the person's development" (Zittoun, 2017). Of particular interest in this study is the way in which the imagination of refugee populations is influenced by the encompassing fabric of the cultural collective—and the complex interplay inherent to the trauma-(im)mobility-(un)imagination nexus. This includes a focus on the processes inherent to changes in imagination as (im)mobile individuals configure, reconfigure, and made meaning of ever-changing new realities. The approach similarly highlights the societal, institutional, and individual conditions that form and shape imagination in constantly changing contexts (Adams & Fleer, 2017).

Imagination from a Sociocultural Perspective

To explore the (un)imagination-(im)mobility nexus, I draw on an expansive and developmental view on imagination from a sociocultural perspective as developed by Zittoun (2012a; Zittoun & Cerchia, 2013; Zittoun & Gillespie, 2015; Zittoun & Sato, 2018), Valsiner (Valsiner, 2000; Valsiner & Rosa, 2007), and others. They define imagination as the process of temporarily disengaging from the here-and-now, a process which demands the use of various resources, so as to take some distance from the current present and situated experience. Such an approach emphasizes the importance of non-linear temporality in the context of migrants' changing subjective current realities—as individuals weave together images of the past, present and future to cope with situations of trauma, confer meaning to their current situation and redefine-reposition themselves toward the future. This includes tracking the processes of change in imagining alternative possible lives. From a sociocultural perspective, imagination is understood necessarily to be culturally-informed and shared. In other words, it may be distributed among communities. Imagination is thus theorized as being significantly shaped or contested by the collective imagination of entire communities: for example, from the shared imaginary expectations of life in Europe among communities in countries of origin, to the constantly developing situated imaginaries of refugee communities upon arrival in Europe. As such, imagination is inherently cultural (Zittoun & Glăveanu, 2017). Indeed, "communities of imagination can become galvanized by a vision of the future and seek to institute it, leading to sociogenesis, that is, the development of society itself" (Zittoun & Gillespie, 2015). It has similarly been argued that it is culture which constitutes the basis for the "collective aspirations" of migrants (Appadurai, 2004).

Individuals who imagine life elsewhere, for example, are seen within this framework as drawing on communal cultural resources which form part of a collective semiotic guidance system (Valsiner, 2007)—the process is considered to be co-constructed and dialogical. This includes drawing on cultural symbols, patterned practices such as storytelling, mental time travel and other forms of mental projection in order to imagine (Kirmayer & Ramstead, 2016). Imagination among individuals therefore is constantly evolving across the life course in relation to the sociocultural environment. It is "culturally guided and personally-semiotically reconstructed" (Valsiner, 2000).

This perspective is captured in Zittoun's model of imagination as a process which creates "loops" out of the present, here-and-now of experiences connected to the material reality of the current environment. As illustrated in her model, she conceptualises the process as being triggered by some disrupting event, which generates a disjunction from the person's unfolding experience of the "real" world, and as unfolding as a loop, which eventually comes back to the current, actual experience (Zittoun & Cerchia, 2013) Fig. 7.1.

Thus, what is conceptualised as triggering imagination is a "rupture," "disruption" or "misfit" between the given experience of the world and one's ongoing flow of thinking—a situation requiring new solutions and experiences (Glăveanu et al., 2018). This developmental perspective views imagination as a process that allows the individual to take distance from the here-and-now of current experience to consider alternative possibilities: for example, rereading the past or opening possible futures. A rupture in one's life in Africa, for example, may trigger an individual to imagine a life for themselves in Europe, as a solution. Imagination is therefore a resource for individuals to draw upon to make meaning of—and act upon—the world: an important component of development and a way to expand one's experience (Vygotsky,

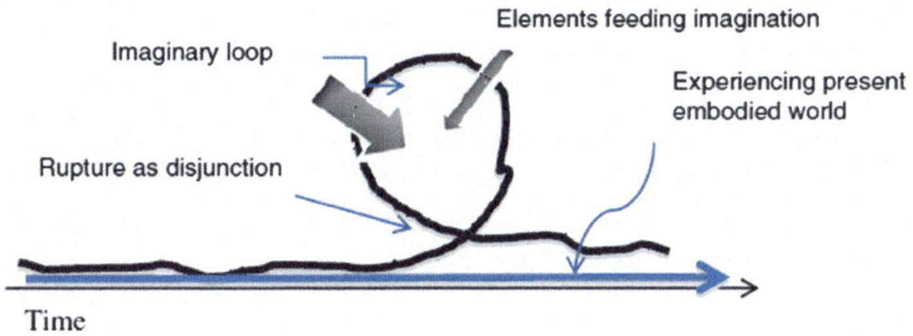

Fig. 7.1 Imaginary loop: expansion version

1980, 1997). It allows for the implementation of social and cultural affordances, that is, expectancies, prescriptions, and possibilities for action in context (Kirmayer & Ramstead, 2016). It is a "freedom" which expands experience beyond the here-and-now, allowing humans to reimagine themselves and their future choices, coming to radically new perspectives, ideas and modes of acting (Zittoun & Cerchia, 2013; Zittoun & Gillespie, 2015; Zittoun & Sato, 2018).

Case Study: Resilience and Imagination Among Victims of Torture in Athens, Greece

To explore the way in which the complex imagination-mobility-trauma nexus unfolds in the context of the so-called "refugee crisis" in Greece, I present the results of 12 months of research among asylum seekers and refugees in a center for victims of torture in Athens. This involved 3 months of participant observation in the centre (including attending daily team meetings and co-facilitating sessions with the beneficiaries). Furthermore, 125 in-depth, qualitative interviews with refugees, health professionals, interpreters, and refugee community leaders across Athens. In particular, multiple qualitative interviews were carried out with 10 individual refugee victims of torture, identified as suitable participants by the health professionals of the centre. These individuals were followed over the course of a year, with an average of five in-depth qualitative interviews being conducted with each participant, in order to explore their subjective experiences of migration and their aspirations for the future. 64 health professionals and community leaders were also interviewed, including religious leaders, leaders of refugee associations as well as doctors, psychologists, social workers and cultural mediators working with this population.

A key proposition of analysis from the perspective of sociocultural psychology is to use case studies to explore individual migration trajectories within unique, specific, and ever-developing contexts. The analytic focus therefore is on individual trajectories unfolding in relation to the sociocultural environment (including material realities as well as connection to social others), specifically with a view of tracking dynamic processes of "trauma" and "imagination" within these trajectories. In other words, the vignette presented here as a case study serve to illustrate the complex realities and interrelatedness of migration trajectories, trauma and imagination. In particular, a case of a refugee victim of torture who participated in the research over the course of a year is presented. The intention is to detail how imagination "may be thwarted, and how, through considerable resistance and struggle, it may nevertheless help to overcome the consequences of radical sociocultural disruption" (Keightley & Pickering, 2018). The case described here also appears in a scientific article published in *Culture and Psychology* (Womersley, 2020).

The Case of Jules

Jules is a 45-year Congolese man who was arrested and tortured after engaging in anti-government protests. After being released, he fled the country imagining France to be his ultimate destination. He arrived in Athens in December 2015. Our first interview took place in August 2016, nine months after his arrival. During this first interview, he refers to his motivation to continue his journey to Western Europe, stating:

> In any case, all the Congolese know that in France, Belgium, Germany or Austria—that if you ask for asylum they will give you money… someone could sacrifice themselves or a family could sell one person of the family to come to Europe. Europe is the dream of Africans

His words highlight aspects of the collective nature of the imagination of refugees dreaming of Europe. It's not only him, but all Congolese who know (imagine?) that they will receive money upon entering Western Europe. Furthermore, the motivation to migrate is not necessarily driven by the individual alone, but linked to the aspirations of an entire family who collectively take the decision for one person to migrate on behalf of the others. Europe is a "dream" shared by "Africans."

According to the imagination "loop" model, it could be argued that this collective "dream" of Africans serves as the sociocultural elements fuelling Jules' imagination of life in Europe, a dream which he goes on to actualise through the embodied experience of migrating (Fig. 7.2):

As illustrated in the figure above, Jules' imagination is nourished by the collective dreams of others within his sociocultural environment, allowing him momentarily to depart from the "here and now" of his life in the Democratic Republic of Congo, in order to imagine a better life elsewhere. It is this figurative departure which allows for a subsequent literal departure to Europe.

In a subsequent interview conducted six weeks later, in September 2016, this initial "dream" to which Jules had so enthusiastically referred, seems somewhat to have been shattered:

> We are human beings, but I am an adult without a wife, without a child. My life is bloody ruined, everyone is in the same hole, who can change it? Nobody. Nobody cares about us… [these problems] devour us. If I was well, you could see that I was well, but I'm sick, I'm not in good health. I'm physically fine, but in my interior—I'm not at all okay […] I'm with the others but not in spirit

He is confronted with a reality different to that which he had initially imagined—rupturing the sense of social connectedness and identity as a member of a community. He is not a husband, nor a father. Rather, the social fabric within which he was located has fragmented. From a sociocultural perspective, ruptures created by trauma are embedded within an intersubjective context wherein severe emotional pain cannot find a relational home in which to be held and integrated (Atwood et al., 2002; Stolorow, 2011). These traumatic ruptures lie at the intersection of the individual and their social context and are related to safety, trust, independence, power, esteem, intimacy as well as spiritual and existential beliefs. Jules finds himself feeling alone,

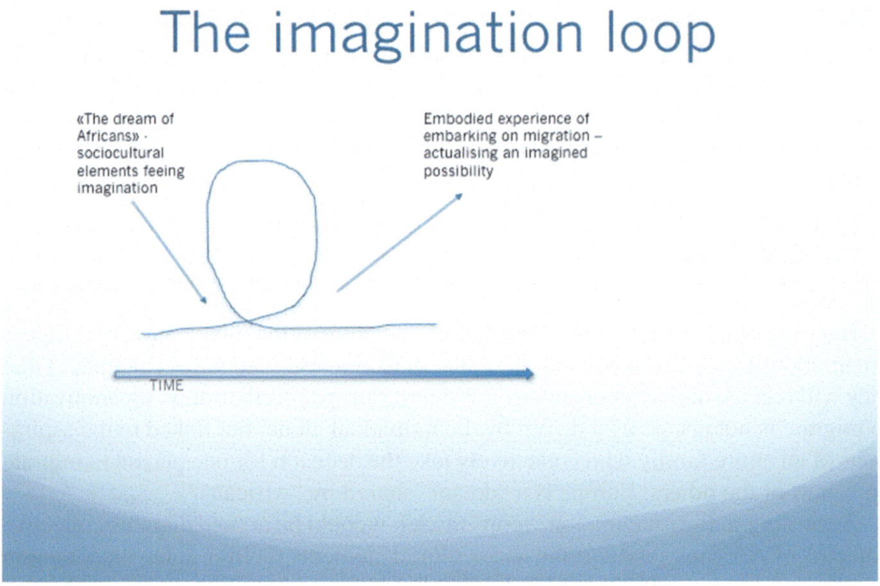

Fig. 7.2 The Imagination loop

"not with the others," and with the perception that nobody cares. Furthermore, this rupture has an impact on his ability to imagine a life for himself in Europe, as depicted in Fig. 7.3.

As illustrated in the figure above, the experience of migration itself is a traumatic rupture isolating Jules' from his sociocultural environment. However, a few months later, in an interview conducted in January 2017, he refers to new social connections having been formed. There are some repairs to the rupture experienced in the social fabric of his life. He has started to relate more to his neighbours, members of his church congregation, and his psychologist. Notably, he also reports falling in love with his Greek social worker and wanting to marry her:

> And my psychologist asked me 'and if you aren't granted asylum, what are you going to do?' I replied, 'I will ask my social worker to marry me.' She asked me why, and I replied 'why not?' … I don't say anything but she knows that I love her. I've told my whole entourage

Compared to prior periods, he increasingly refers to others in his social world—for example, reporting discussions that he has had with his psychologist as well as members of the Congolese community in Athens. He has a "whole entourage" to tell about his newfound wish to marry his social worker. Similarly, it is during this time that new life projects start to be imagined. He is able to envisage a future as a husband, married to a Greek women and constructing a life together in Greece. Imagination flourishes, as depicted in Fig. 7.4,

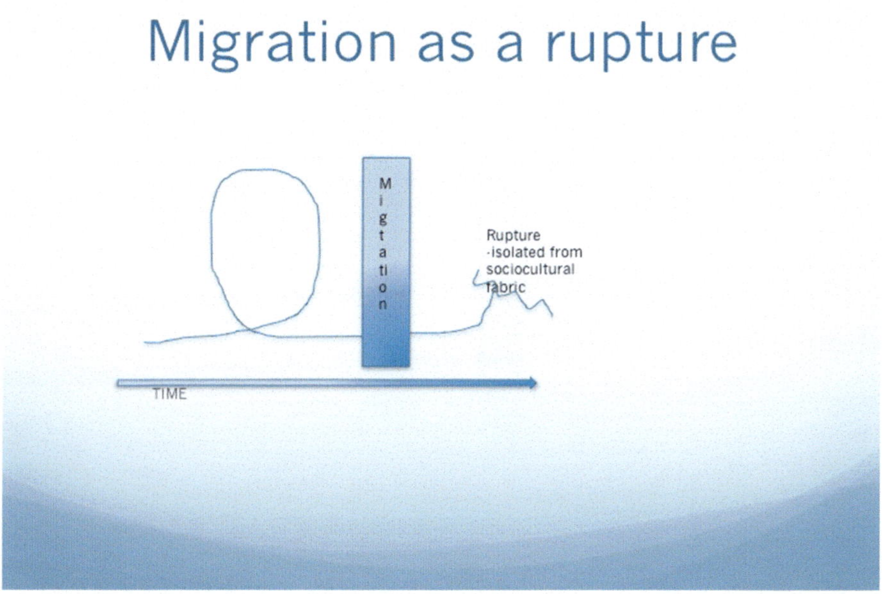

Fig. 7.3 Migration as a rupture

His first asylum interview takes place in September 2017 during which he has to speak about the torture he endured. He describes this event as having "retraumatized" him:

> It's a story that hurts you and causes a lot of emotions […] the pain that I felt that day, that could be at 10%, if the pain has passed, but if you have to repeat the story, you feel it at 100% […] it hurts you to have to tell your story, yes it hurts. Even during the interview, it hurts you.

His claim to asylum is ultimately rejected a few weeks later. The news devastates Jules. When asked about his future plans following this court decision, he states that:

> My vision is to go somewhere or stay here, I really don't know…but if I had the idea of going somewhere else, I couldn't ask for asylum here. Some have their families over there [in Western Europe] already, but I am the only one in my family. So if I had to go to France, well, where would I sleep? I don't have a place there. It's hard, but what can I do? I don't see any solutions

It can be argued that the negative decision on his asylum claim is a traumatic rupture in his life, impeding his ability to imagine. He "really doesn't know" what his "vision" is. There are simply no solutions, no clear idea of a future. Notably, he associates the lack of being able to imagine a future for himself with a lack of social connections: others have families "over there" (in Western Europe), whereas he does not. He cannot imagine having "a place" in Western Europe as he does not have any

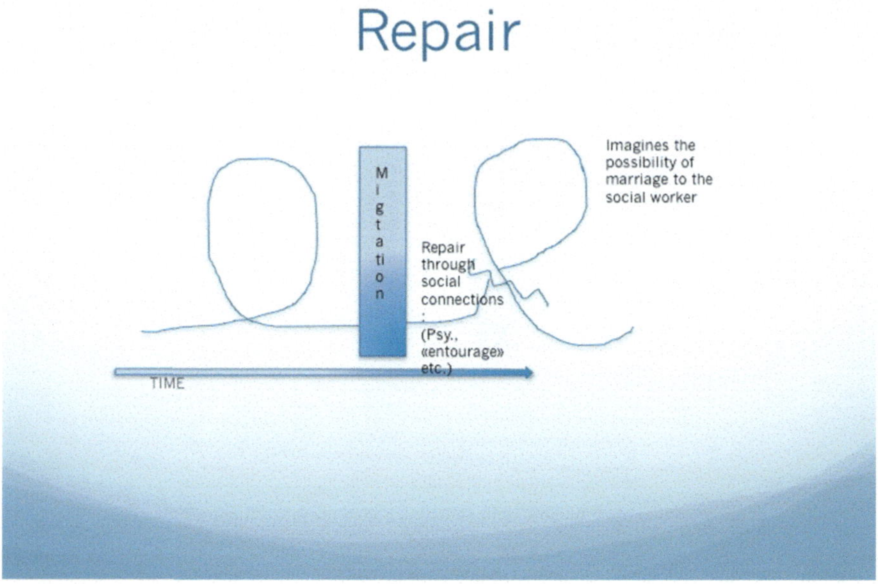

Fig. 7.4 Repair

family or friends to accommodate him. In other words, as depicted in Fig. 7.5, the traumatic rupture of being denied asylum echoes a social disconnection, impeding his capacity to imagine a future for himself:

Elsewhere (Womersley & Laure Kloetzer, 2018a), we have conceptualised the trauma of migration as a "double" rupture—one rupture related to traumatic events experienced in the country of origin and subsequent forced migration, the second related to issues of displacement and social isolation experienced by displaced population. Particularly for those whose claims to asylum are rejected, this "double rupture" invokes a vicious cycle of trauma and isolation, a series of disruptions to the relational processes nourishing imagination.

In July 2017, a few months subsequent to his asylum claim being denied, Jules reports that:

> There have been some big changes because when you cry a lot, there's a moment where you stop crying. You see the reality in front of you. I have already suffered a lot from thinking, thinking. I must think until where and until when? Must I spend my whole life crying? [...] since being here, the pain has changed form [...] The essential is that I'm in good health. I'm alive. It's not the end of the world. Life continues.

There is evidence of repair to the rupture of being denied asylum. His words highlight him having a new sense of perspective—of past, present and future. He projects himself into the future and decides that he does not want to "spend [his] whole life crying." Rather, he refers to being able to "see the reality in front of

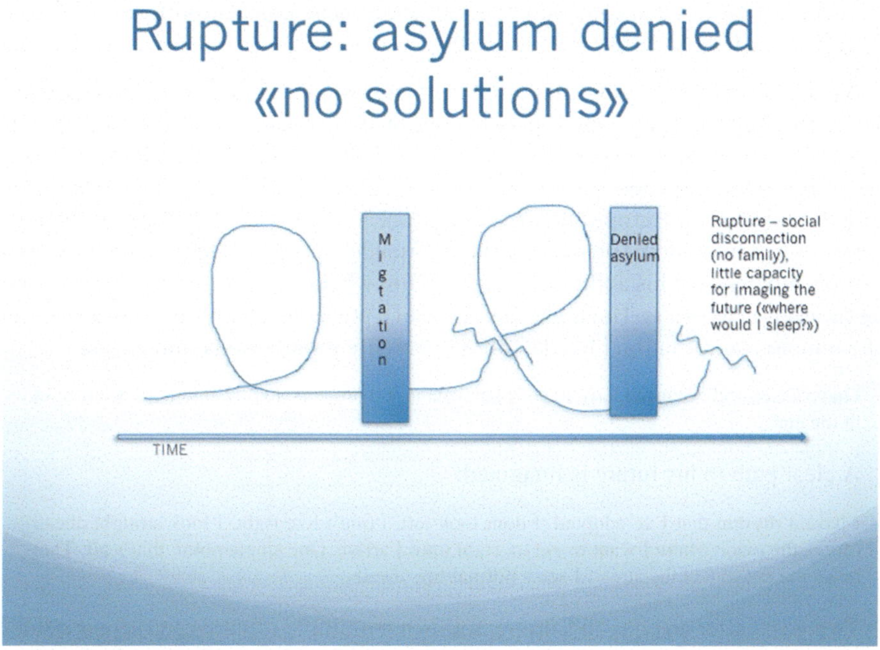

Fig. 7.5 Rupture: asylum denied «no solutions»

[him]." A new, clear vision for the future appears to have emerged. He imagines a new life for himself—not in Athens but in "other European countries":

> In other European countries, they easily give you papers [refugee status]. Like in France, papers or not, I'd have work there. In France, anything is authorized. I want to spend the rest of my youth and my old age next to the white people, the Europeans. I need to learn their habits—how do they speak? How do they walk?...

He imagines a life in France, a life where "anything is authorized," where he will easily be granted asylum. He imagines being able to work easily, regardless of refugee status. This would be for him the metaphorical land of milk and honey, echoing the dream which initially fueled his desire to come to Europe. This dream similarly includes a newly imagined form of social connectedness —that of being connected to "white people, the Europeans." He imagines being able to build these social connections through studying their habits, down to the way in which they speak and they walk. This, he imagines, would enable a seamless integration into Western Europe, and would be the key to a rich and successful future.

> I know that the beginning is difficult, but it will be better with time… with friends, with people, with a little help. You can have no money but if you have travel documents and your ideas, you can go anywhere… I'm poor in money but rich in spirit. I know that with my ideas, I can go anywhere…there are people who are here, but who are like a television with the remote control somewhere else. Anything and anybody can change the channel. But

> me, I'm not like that. I'm here—the television and the remote control in my hands… I'm a visionary, by the grace of god I'm a visionary

As stated by Pelaprat and Cole (2011), "imagination is the process of resolving and connecting the fragmented, poorly coordinated experience of the world so as to bring about a stable image of the world" (p.399, as cited in Zittoun & Cerchia, 2013). Jules describes being a "visionary"—having a clear idea of what he imagines for his future life in Europe. What is important to note is that he does not believe this imagined future to be possible without "friends…people." Once again, there is a relationship between his ability to imagine a life where he "can go anywhere"—and the connection to others. Having a new sense of a power to act over his future, having "the remote control in [his] hands," allows new life projects to be imagined:

> I have ideas, and because I have ideas, I have plans and projects. I know it will all be all right in the end…

A clear path to his future is imagined:

> I have a rhythm that I've adopted. I dont look left, I don't like right. I look straight ahead of me, the place where I want to get to, right until I arrive. One single point, that's all. That helps me not to feel the stress. I see a normal life ahead

Two years after arriving in Europe, following multiple ruptures and repairs, Jules has a rich capacity to imagine a future for himself in Europe, as depicted in Fig. 7.6.

As illustrated in the figure above, the repair to the traumatic rupture of being denied asylum lies in the "imagination loop" being completed. The future is once again rich in new imagined possibilities. In our last interview, he boldly concludes that:

> "It's Europe, Europe is miracles"

Discussion

What is revealed through an analysis of Jules' migration trajectory is the importance of socio-cultural resources which shape and define his imagination. The imagination of a "brighter" future in Europe may never wholly be considered "his" alone but collectively shared and distributed. He is not alone in having arrived in Europe after an arduous migration journey fueled by "geographical imaginaries" (Salazar, 2010; Salazar & Smart, 2011) of a better life in Europe. In sharp contrast to the initially imagined "dream" of a "miracle" life in Europe, he felt disillusioned by the every-day reality of Athens—a disillusion seemingly shared by the vast majority of refugees encountered over the course of the research. Many participants reported experiencing a similarly sense of disillusion:

> We had another vision of Europe… Europe is different from Africa. For me, at least, Europe is even more complicated than Africa…
>
> We came because we had different dreams, we came to see the reality

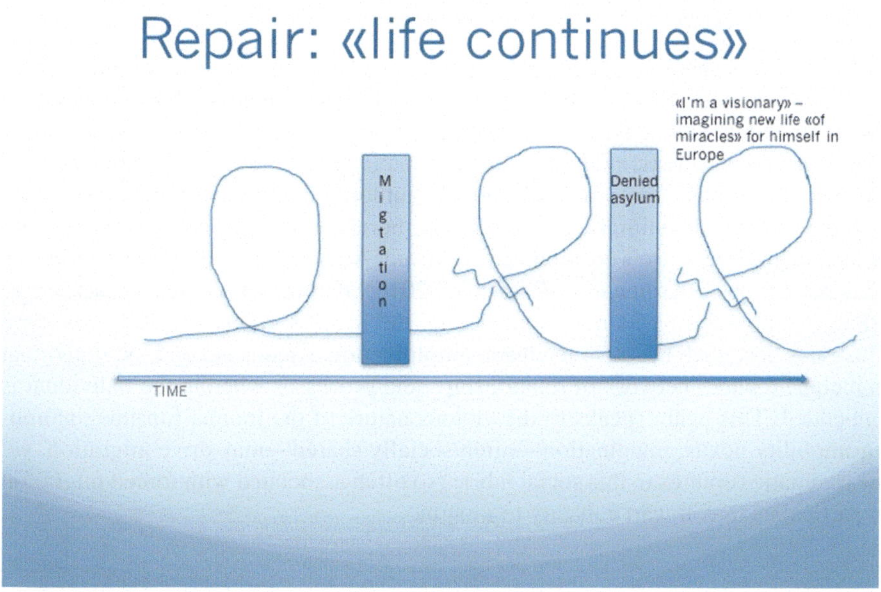

Fig. 7.6 Repair: «life continues»

> When we dreamed, we then later understood that life is something else
>
> Often we had Europe in our minds like the films that we saw. When you watch a film, it's just a scene that they created. You forget that there's a reality behind it. There's an actor, a director, interpretors to make it all look real. Now it's only when you come to Europe that you see that reality

Note the frequent use of the collective pronoun "we," instead of the singular "I," in the above quotes—alluding to the collective nature of the aspirations of many refugees and a culturally shared imagination of life in Europe.

Jules' case is illustrative of the dynamic interplay between trauma, migration and imagination. However, it is not representative of all research participants. His imagination continues to thrive despite the multiple traumatic ruptures he faces. Among other participants, however, this rich capacity to imagine the future appears to have been thwarted by ongoing traumatic ruptures to their lives. Social isolation, harsh living conditions, insecure residency status and continual exposure to violence and trauma characterises the daily lives of so many of the participants encountered. Without a connection to a meaningful past or a beckoning future, and without a sense of connection to others, they report feeling "trapped" in a traumatic present—as evidenced in the following statements:

> I can't think properly what to do in my future. I'm not able to think about my future, what is going to happen next in my future. I don't know what is going to happen.

> I'm trapped here.
>
> I don't know when will my life going to take me. I don't know what is going to happen next with me now…I don't want to stay here because there is no life.

We have presented a detailed analysis of a case elsewhere (Womersley & Kloetzer, 2018c), wherein an Indian asylum seeker and victim of torture finds himself in shared accommodation with Pakistani nationals. He accuses his Pakistani roommate of spying on him. Psychotic symptoms start to emerge, including auditory hallucinations and paranoia. Many of the voices are those of authority figures, including the torturers in India and, rather tellingly, police officers, bureaucrats and judges in the asylum procedure in Greece. He's hospitalized as a result. All of these ruptures create negative "feedback loops" (Kirmayer & Ramstead, 2016), defined as a process whereby an effect is reinforced by its own influence on the process giving rise to it. The case illustrates how such negative feedback amplification extends beyond the individual to include a wider network of relationships and processes wherein the individual is embedded. This again speaks to the vicious nature of the trauma-(un)imagination-(im)mobility nexus: imagination—often socially shared—may drive migration, yet the traumatic ruptures to this social fabric (so often associated with forced migration in particular) may thwart capacity to imagine.

Conclusion

An in-depth analysis of the case of Jules from within a sociocultural framework highlights the complex interplay between imagination, trauma and migration. Imagination is a powerful motivating force driving migration. However, this is not a static, once-off process. There is no singular moment of deciding to migrate. Not only is the imagination of individuals constantly transforming in relation to the ever-changing sociocultural environment: it is significantly shaped and contested by shared or collective imaginings of entire communities. This starts, for example, with collective imagination of life in Europe among communities in the country of origin, and extends to the constantly developing shared imagination of refugee communities as they arrive in Europe. Yet migration, and particularly forced migration, inevitably brings changes which are likely to be experienced as ruptures which radically affect one's subjective sense of self and sense of connection to others. The capacity to imagine, and consequently heal from traumatic ruptures, may only be restored within the context of the sociocultural environment surrounding the individual, and their relation to their social world. As Zittoun and Sato (2018) convincingly conclude, "imagination is facilitated by both [social] recognition and material resources that have cultural meaning and is, in this sense, the process by which post-traumatic growth occurs" (p. 203). If trauma is healed, imagination may be restored. If imagination is restored, trauma may be healed.

The research highlights the important value sociocultural psychology may bring to the field of (im)mobility and migration studies by enriching understandings of trauma and imagination among refugee populations, with an emphasis on the socio-cultural location of human subjects. From within this perspective, what is highlighted are the ever-changing cultural and social systems which are in continual interaction with the various forms of an individual subjective experiences of (im)mobility. Furthermore, it highlights how "immobility may transform transnational and transcultural categories, praxis, imaginaries, and subjects" (Khan, 2016). Sociocultural psychology allows for this urgent and critical reconsideration of trauma and imagination as dynamic processes influenced by the interplay of changing social, historical, material, economical, political and subjective dimensions, in populations fighting to construct their new lives in Europe.

References

Adams, M., & Fleer, M. (2017). International transitions: Generating subjective sense and subjective configuration in relation to the development of identity. *Mind Culture and Activity, 24*(4), 1–15.

Appadurai, A. (2004). The capacity to aspire. *Culture and Public Action, 1,* 59–84.

Atwood, G. E., Orange, D. M., & Stolorow, R. D. (2002). Shattered worlds/psychotic states: A post-Cartesian view of the experience of personal annihilation. *Psychoanalytic Psychology, 19*(2), 281.

Bäärnhielm, S. (2016). Refugees' mental health-a call for a public health approach with focus on resilience and cultural sensitivity. *European Journal of Public Health, 26*(3), 375–376.

Bélanger-Dumontier, G., & Vachon, M. (2015). Review of refuge and resilience: promoting resilience and mental health among resettled refugees and forced migrants. *Transcultural Psychiatry, 52*, 274-275.

Berry, J. W. (2003). Conceptual approaches to acculturation. In K. M. Chun, P. B. Organista, & G. Marín (Eds.), *Acculturation: Advances in theory measurement and applied research* (pp. 17–37). Washington D.C.: American Psychological Association.

Bhimji, F. (2015). Collaborations and performative agency in refugee theater in Germany. *Journal of Immigrant and Refugee Studies, 1,* 1–23.

Boccagni, P., & Baldassar, L. (2015). Emotions on the move: Mapping the emergent field of emotion and migration. *Emotion Space Society, 16,* 73–80.

Calhoun, L. G., & Tedeschi, R. G. (2014). *Handbook of posttraumatic growth: Research and practice.* London: Routledge.

Collins, F. L. (2018). Desire as a theory for migration studies: Temporality assemblage and becoming in the narratives of migrants. *Journal of Ethnic and Migration Studies, 44*(6), 964–980.

Collins, F. L. (2018). Keeping bodies moving: Hope disruption and the possibilities of youth migration. *Journal of Intercultural Studies, 39*(6), 626–641.

Collins, F. L., & Shubin, S. (2015). Migrant times beyond the life course: The temporalities of foreign English teachers in South Korea. *Geoforum, 62,* 96–104.

Drožđek, B., & Wilson, J. P. (2007). *Voices of Trauma: Treating psychological trauma across cultures.* New York, N.Y.: Springer.

Gilligan, R. (2004). Promoting resilience in child and family social work: Issues for social work practice education and policy. *Social Work Education, 23*(1), 93–104.

Glăveanu, V. P., Karwowski, M., Jankowska, D. M., & de Saint Laurent, C. (2018). Creative imagination. In T. Zittoun, & V. P. Glăveanu (Eds.), Handbook of Imagination and Culture (pp 1–39). New York, NY: Oxford University Press.

Goguikian Ratcliff, B. (2007). Traumatismes et résilience chez l'enfant migrant: Le rôle de l'ancrage culturel et familial. *L'Autre, 8*(2), 249–256.

Goguikian Ratcliff, B. (2012). Repenser les liens entre migration, exil et traumatisme. *(Re)penser l'Exil, 1,* 1–8.
Goguikian Ratcliff, B., Bolzman, C., & Gakuba, T. (2014). Déqualification des femmes migrantes en Suisse: Mécanismes sous-jacents et effets psychologiques. *Alterstice, 4*(2), 63–76.
Heeren, M., Wittmann, L., Ehlert, U., Schnyder, U., Maier, T., & Müller, J. (2014). Psychopathology and resident status–comparing asylum seekers refugees illegal migrants labor migrants and residents. *Comprehensive Psychiatry, 55*(4), 818–825.
Huemer, J., Nelson, K., Karnik, N., Völkl-Kernstock, S., Seidel, S., Ebner, N., et al. (2016). Emotional expressiveness and avoidance in narratives of unaccompanied refugee minors. *European Journal of Psychotraumatology, 7*(1), 29163.
Kadianaki, I. (2010). Making sense of immigrant identity dialogues. *Culture and Psychology, 16*(3), 437–448.
Kartal, D., & Kiropoulos, L. (2016). Effects of acculturative stress on PTSD, depressive, and anxiety symptoms among refugees resettled in Australia and Austria. *European Journal of Psychotraumatology, 7*(1), 28711.
Keightley, E., & Pickering, M. J. (2018). The Mnemonic imagination and second-generation migrant experience. In T. Zittoun & V. P. Glaveanu (Eds.), *Handbook of imagination and culture* (pp. 167–185). Oxford: Oxford University Press.
Khan, N. (2016). *Immobility In Keywords of mobility: Critical Engagements* (pp. 93–112). New York, Oxford: Berghahn.
Kirmayer, L. J., & Ramstead, M. J. (2016). Embodiment and enactment in cultural psychiatry. In C. Durt, T. Fuchs, & C. Tewes (Eds.), *Embodiment enaction and culture: Investigating the constitution of the shared World* (pp. 397–422). Cambridge, MA: MIT Press.
Laban, C. J. (2015). Resilience-oriented treatment of traumatised asylum seekers and refugees. In M. Schouler-Ocak (Ed.), Trauma and migration (pp. 191-208). Cham: Springer.
Lusk, M., & Baray, S. C. (2017). Mental health and the role of culture and resilience in refugees fleeing violence. *Environment and Social Psychology, 2*(1), 1–13.
Lusk, M., & Baray, S. C. (2017b). Mental health and the role of culture and resilience in refugees fleeing violence. *Environment and Social Psychology, 2*(1).
Maercker, A., & Hecker, T. (2016). Broadening perspectives on trauma and recovery: A socio-interpersonal view of PTSD. *European Journal of Psychotraumatology, 7*, 29303.
Marsella, A. J. (2010). Ethnocultural aspects of PTSD: An overview of concepts issues and treatments. *Traumatology, 16*(4), 17.
Meili, I., Heim, E., Pelosi, A. C., & Maercker, A. (2019). Metaphors and cultural narratives on adaptive responses to severe adversity: A field study among the Indigenous Pitaguary community in Brazil. *Journal of transcultural psychiatry*, 1363461519890435.
Métraux, J.-C. (1999). Dons de mémoire: Lecture anthropologique et sociale d'une psychothérapie interculturelle. *Psychothérapies, 19*(4), 225–234.
Minihan, S., Liddell, B. J., Byrow, Y., Bryant, R. A., & Nickerson, A. (2018). Patterns and predictors of posttraumatic stress disorder in refugees: A latent class analysis. *Journal of Affective Disorders, 232*, 252–259.
Neace, R. T., Thaier, C., & Nasir, S. (2020). Understanding refugees: A complex discussion. In J. Kottler, S. Banu, & S. Jani (Eds.), *Handbook of refugee experience: Trauma, resilience, and recovery* (pp. 9-20). San Diego: California Cognella Academic Publishing
Papadopoulos, R. (2002b). *Therapeutic care for refugees: No place like home*: Karnac Books.
Papadopoulos, R. (2002a). Refugees home and trauma. *Therapeutic care for refugees: No place like home, 9.*
Papadopoulos, R. (2007). Refugees, trauma and adversity-activated development. *European Journal of Psychotherapy and Counselling, 9*(3), 301–312.
Pelaprat, E., & Cole, M. (2011). "Minding the gap": Imagination, creativity and human cognition. *Integrative Psychological and Behavioral Sciences, 45*, 397–418.

Raghavan, S., & Sandanapitchai, P. (2020). *The relationship between cultural variables and resilience to psychological trauma: A systematic review of the literature.* Traumatology: Advanced Online Publication.

Roberto, S., & Moleiro, C. (2016). Looking (also) at the Other Side of the Story. Resilience Processes in Migrants. *Journal of International Migration and Integration, 17*(3), 929–946.

Salazar, N. B. (2010). Towards an anthropology of cultural mobilities. *Crossings: Journal of Migration and Culture, 1*(1), 53–68.

Salazar, N. B., & Smart, A. (2011). Anthropological takes on (im) mobility. *Identities, 18*(6), 1–9.

Sam, D. L., & Berry, J. W. (2010). Acculturation when individuals and groups of different cultural backgrounds meet. *Perspectives on Psychological Science, 5*(4), 472–481.

Simich, L. & Andermann, E. (2014). In *Refuge and resilience: Promoting resilience and mental health among resettled refugees and forced migrants.* Dordrecht: Springer.

Siriwardhana, C., Abas, M., Siribaddana, S., Sumathipala, A., & Stewart, R. (2015). Dynamics of resilience in forced migration: A 1-year follow-up study of longitudinal associations with mental health in a conflict-affected, ethnic Muslim population. *British Medical Journal Open, 5,* e006000.

Sleijpen, M., Haagen, J., Mooren, T., & Kleber, R. J. (2016). Growing from experience: An exploratory study of posttraumatic growth in adolescent refugees. *European Journal of Psychotraumatology, 7*(1), 28698.

Sleijpen, M., Mooren, T., Kleber, R. J., & Boeije, H. R. (2017). Lives on hold: A qualitative study of young refugees' resilience strategies. *Childhood, 24*(3), 348–365.

Song, S. J., Kaplan, C., Tol, W. A., Subica, A., & de Jong, J. (2015). Psychological distress in torture survivors: Pre-and post-migration risk factors in a US sample. *Social Psychiatry and Psychiatric Epidemiology, 50*(4), 549–560.

Stolorow, R. D. (2011). *World affectivity Trauma.* New York: Routledge.

Sucharov, M. S., Buirski, P., & Kottler, A. (2007). Kafka's window and Kohut's mirror: A dialogic journey to the center of traumatic worlds. In P. Buirski & A. Kottler (Eds.), *New developments in self psychology practice* (pp. 193–206). Lanham: Jason Aranson.

Tankink, M., & Richters, A. (2007). Silence as a coping strategy: The case of refugee women in the Netherlands from South-Sudan who experienced sexual violence in the context of war. In B. Drožđek & J. Wilson (Eds.), *Voices of trauma: Treating psychological trauma across cultures* (pp. 191–210). New York: Springer.

Tedeschi, R. G., & Calhoun, L. G. (2004). Posttraumatic growth: Conceptual foundations and empirical evidence. *Psychological Inquiry, 15*(1), 1–18.

Tippens, J. A. (2017). Urban congolese refugees in Kenya: The contingencies of coping and resilience in a context marked by structural vulnerability. *Qualitative Health Research, 27*(7), 1090–1103.

Tummala-Narra, P. (2007). Conceptualizing trauma and resilience across diverse contexts. *Journal of Aggression Maltreatment and Trauma, 14*(1–2), 33–53.

Ungar, M. (2004). A constructionist discourse on resilience: Multiple contexts, multiple realities among at-risk children and youth. *Youth and Society, 35*(3), 341–365.

Ungar, M. (2005). *Handbook for working with children and youth: Pathways to resilience across cultures and contexts.* London: Sage Publications.

Ungar, M. (2008). Resilience across cultures. *The British Journal of Social Work, 38*(2), 218–235.

Ungar, M. (2011). The social ecology of resilience: Addressing contextual and cultural ambiguity of a nascent construct. *American Journal of Orthopsychiatry, 81*(1), 1–17.

Uy, K. K., & Okubo, Y. (2018). Re-storying the trauma narrative: Fostering posttraumatic growth in cambodian refugee women. *Women and Therapy, 41*(3–4), 1–18.

Valsiner, J. (2000). *Culture and human development.* London: Sage.

Valsiner, J. (2007). *Culture in minds and societies: Foundations of cultural psychology.* India: Sage.

Valsiner, J., & Rosa, A. (2007). *The Cambridge handbook of sociocultural psychology.* Cambridge: Cambridge University Press.

Vygotsky, L. S. (1980). *Mind in society: The development of higher psychological processes*. Cambridge, MA: Harvard University Press.

Vygotsky, L. S. (1997). *The collected works of LS Vygotsky: Problems of the theory and history of psychology* (Vol. 3). London: Springer Science and Business Media.

Womersley, G. (2020). (Un)imagination and (im)mobility: exploring the past and constructing possible futures among refugee victims of torture in Greece. Culture & Psychology, 1354067X19899066.

Womersley, G., & Kloetzer, L. (2018). Being Through doing: The self-immolation of an asylum seeker in Switzerland. *Frontiers in Psychiatry, 9,* 110.

Womersley, G., & Kloetzer, L. (2018c). « En Afrique, "aller voir le psychologue," je n'ai jamais entendu ça »: Médiation culturelle chez les réfugiés victimes de torture en Grèce. *Revue Européenne des Migrations Internationales, 34(2),* 29–54.

Zittoun, T. (2012a). Life-course: A socio-cultural perspective. In Vaalsiner. J (Ed.), *Oxford library of psychology: The Oxford handbook of culture and psychology* (Vol. 60, pp. 513–535). Oxford: Oxford University Press.

Zittoun, T. (2017). Modalities of generalization through single case studies. *Integrative Psychological and Behavioral Science, 51*(2), 171–194.

Zittoun, T., & Glăveanu, V. P. (2017). *Handbook of imagination and culture*: Oxford University Press

Zittoun, T., & Cerchia, F. (2013). Imagination as expansion of experience. *Integrative Psychological and Behavioral Science, 47*(3), 305–324.

Zittoun, T., & Gillespie, A. (2015). *Imagination in human and cultural development*. London: Routledge.

Zittoun, T., & Sato, T. (2018). Imagination in adults and the aged person. In T. Zittoun & V. P. Glăveanu (Eds.), *Handbook of imagination and culture* (pp. 187–208). New York, NY: Oxford University Press.

Chapter 8
Collective Aspirations

Europe has faced an unprecedented influx of asylum seekers– with over one and a half million sea arrivals reported since 2015 by the United Nations High Commissioner for Refugees (UNHCR).[1] As the "reception crisis" continues unabated, Greece remains one of the first ports of sanctuary. According to recent statistics provided for March 2018 by the UNHCR,[2] over 50,000 asylum seekers and refugees currently remain in Greece following this mass flow. The majority of the one million asylum seekers arriving in the country appear to have seen Greece as a transit country, yet neither of the refugees' legal routes out of Greece are functioning as anticipated: the scheme to relocate people to other member states failed to meet one-tenth of its target and has been scaled back; reunification with family elsewhere in Europe proceeds slowly; returns to Turkey have no more than trickled after legal challenges; while voluntary returns to countries of origin remain modest so far (Howden, 2017).

Greece therefore represents a unique context in which to explore the aspirations of asylum seekers entering Europe: perceived both as a country of transit as well as a final destination. Currently, many asylum seekers find themselves "stuck" in limbo in this context, unable to proceed with their asylum claim or continue their journey to the destination countries of Western Europe to which they continue to aspire. Such a situation of "protracted displacement" or "protracted refugee situations" has been characterised by Brun (Brun, 2015; Brun & Fábos, 2015) as related to "the permanence of temporariness" (Brun, 2015)—an enduring liminal state wherein people may feel trapped in the present yet actively relate to alternative notions of the future. Within this space, aspirations of returning home contend with hopes to achieve a more stable exile through staying or moving elsewhere. Despite these hopes, aspirations may thwarted bureaucratically, thwarted physically, thwarted psychically. Should this be the case, energy may be focused on short-term survival, and there is often limited projection into the future (Métraux, 2017).

[1] https://data2.unhcr.org/en/situations/mediterranean#_ga=2.128715788.1601678871.1525327989-1029508152.1512727845, accessed the 03rd of May 2018.

[2] https://reliefweb.int/sites/reliefweb.int/files/resources/62950.pdf

G. Theisen-Womersley, *Trauma and Resilience Among Displaced Populations*,
https://doi.org/10.1007/978-3-030-67712-1_8

In the context of a growing interest in emotions and temporalities linked to migration aspirations (Carling & Collins, 2017), this chapter focusses on the Greek context to explore the "changing notions of hope…in order to understand the role that an uncertain future plays and the potential for agency that people develop during displacement" (Brun, 2015). To do so, I draw on the theoretical framework of sociocultural psychology (Bruner, 1990; Cole, 1998; Valsiner, 2007; Valsiner & Rosa, 2007; Vygotsky, 1987, 1980; Wagoner, Chaudhary, & Hviid, 2014; Wagoner et al., 2011; Zittoun, 2012a, 2012b; Zittoun & Gillespie, 2015). Such an approach examines how individuals develop within sociocultural context, specifically in situated interactions with others as well as with material and symbolic objects within their environments. From within this theoretical framework, aspirations are understood to be necessarily distributed among communities. In other words, they are culturally informed and shared. In order to hope, to dream, to imagine, to plan, individuals draw on communal cultural resources as part of a semiotic guidance system, including "cultural symbols, patterned practices such as storytelling, mental time travel, and other forms of mental projection" (Kirmayer & Ramstead, 2016). Within this framework, the individual constructs the social and at the same time is constructed by the social (Zepke & Leach, 2002). Three concepts based on this theoretical framework in relation to migration aspirations will be highlighted: (i) the role of imagination as a resource for aspiring, (ii) non-linear temporalities of aspirations and ever-changing subjective realities, and (iii) the collective nature of aspirations.

As explored in chap. 7, imagination is seen as a resource for aspiration, an important component of development and a way to expand one's experience (Vygotsky, 1987, 1980). Imagination facilitates aspirations and the implementation of social and cultural affordances—including expectancies, prescriptions and possibilities for action (Kirmayer & Ramstead, 2016). It is a "freedom" which expands experience beyond the here-and-now, allowing humans to reimagine themselves and their future choices, coming to radically new perspectives, ideas and modes of acting (Zittoun & Cerchia, 2013; Zittoun & Gillespie, 2015; Zittoun & Sato, 2018). As such, migration itself is inherently imaginative (Salazar, 2010; Salazar & Smart, 2011), an act of agency which turning imagined possibility into actuality, and in turn triggering the imagination of new possibilities (Zittoun & Gillespie, 2015).

Another key theoretical tenant of sociocultural psychology is that of the dynamic, temporal, and non-linear nature of experience. Past, present and future interweave to produce experiences that do not necessarily follow chronological time. This speaks to the "the potentially transient nature of aspirations" (Carling & Schewel, 2017), "the multiple temporalities of migrant lives and future potential; the assemblage of spatialities and relations articulated in migration; and the politics of migration that is generated through the enlisting of migrants by states and migrants' own desire for becoming through migration." (Collins, 2018). This "becoming" (Collins, 2018) refers to a continual process of resubjectification. Subjective configurations are flexible, changing forms that are shaped by the context of the situation, the state of mind of the individual during the lived experience, and their participation in various social networks where actions are expressed and undertaken. Such an approach contests the idea that migrant "decision-making" occurs at a singular moment in time (Carling

& Collins, 2017). Instead, aspirations represent "dynamic and reciprocal systems influenced not only by the past subjective sense and the social context, but also the current subjective sense and environment" (Adams & Fleer, 2017, p. 4). As people develop, so do their aspirations.

Aspirations are therefore part of an ongoing process of transformation—related to individuals, as well as their sociocultural histories and resources (Goulart, 2017; Goulart & González Rey, 2016). To understand this process of dynamic, subjective transformations, I draw on González Rey's (2008) definition of subjectivity as a "nonlinear, non- universal, non-deterministic and a context-sensitive process, whose main subjective configurations are part of an ongoing process... related, first and foremost, to the way in which the history and current contexts of individuals and social instances turn into symbolical emotional processes" (p. 5). His notion of a "future subjective sense" captures the interrelated and nonlinear movements of past, present, and the future imagined events and spaces. As the individual moves into new spaces, new realities are produced through a dynamic integration of these internal and external experiences (González Rey, 2008, 2016).

An aspiration to migrate reflects the transformative potential of ever-changing subjective realities, implying that this imagined transformation is not only viewed positively by the prospective migrant, but is also institutionally and culturally embedded. Indeed, entirely collective "communities of imagination can become galvanized by a vision of the future and seek to institute it, leading to sociogenesis, that is, the development of society itself" (Zittoun & Gillespie, 2015). Culture constitutes the basis for "collective aspirations" (Appadurai, 2004). As argued by Carling and Schewel (2017)

> The context of migration aspirations includes social norms and expectations about migrating or staying, opportunities for migration and the more general structural forces facilitating or constraining particular migration trajectories. The environment not only affects the level of migration aspirations, but also their inherent meaning." (p. 8).

They define migration aspirations as "a comparison of culturally defined projects...a socially constructed entity that embodies particular expectations" (p. 9). Aspirations are therefore necessarily infused with "culturally rooted imagineries of mobility" (Salazar & Smart, 2011), including informed social norms and expectations as to what may or may not be possible. Thus, normative expectations of migration often originate from entities other than the subject himself or herself (Meyer, 2017). Furthermore, those who migrate may equally be the objects of desire or aspiration by a social collective. The sociocultural context in which migration occurs therefore cannot be ignored.

Highlighting the collective nature of aspirations contests notions which "reifies the individual migrant as a decision maker who chooses to migrate in a relatively autonomous or individualistic way" (Collins, 2018). To examine this individualistic-collective dichotomy of migration decision making, I turn to Carling's (Carling & Collins, 2017; Carling & Schewel, 2017; Carling, 2002) aspiration/ability model. The model distinguishes involuntary non-migrants (those who aspire to migrate but lack the ability to do so) from voluntary non-migrants (those without migration aspirations who would prefer to stay). Those who migrate, the model suggests, are those with both the aspiration and the ability to do so—in other words voluntary migrants. What the model doesn't seem to allow for, however, is the fourth quadrant of the aspiration/ability spectrum: involuntary migrants (those who do not aspire to migrate yet have the ability to do so, and do). In the context of the current influx of asylum seekers into Europe, what needs to be highlighted is the involuntary nature of much of this migration. Not only are many forced to leave due to circumstances beyond their control (for example, war, torture and other violent atrocities), we similarly need to bear in mind the collective nature of aspirations: often entire communities take the decision to pool resources in order for one individual to migrate in order to eventually be able to financially support those back home. The extent to which this would be a voluntary or involuntary decision to migrate on the part of the individual would appear to fall along a much more nuanced continuum than that for which dichotomous categories would allow.

The theoretical background of sociocultural psychology allows for an exploration of these nuances—of the ever-changing and dynamic development of aspirations over time, and within sociocultural context. It evokes a methodology incorporating an exploration not only of the subjective perspective, but also the dynamics by which the social and cultural environment guide and enable the person's development (Zittoun, 2017). Of particular interest in this study is the way in which aspirations are influenced by the encompassing fabric of the cultural collective, related both to the country of origin as well as the Greek context of protracted displacement and a liminal permanent temporariness.

Case Study: Collective Aspirations of Refugees in Europe

In order to explore the aspirations of refugee communities within the Greek context, a case study is presented which is taken from a larger yearlong research project I conducted among asylum seekers and refugees in a center for victims of torture in Athens. This research involved 3 months of participant observation in the centre (including attending daily team meetings and co-facilitating sessions with the beneficiaries). Furthermore, 125 in-depth, qualitative interviews with refugees, health professionals, interpreters, and refugee community leaders across Athens. In particular, multiple qualitative interviews were conducted with 10 individual refugee victims of torture, identified as suitable participants by the health professionals of the centre. These individuals were followed over the course of a year, with an average of five in-depth qualitative interviews being conducted with each participant, in order to explore their subjective experiences of integration and their aspirations for the future. All interviews were conducted in French or English without the assistance of a translator. 64 health professionals and community leaders were also interviewed, including religious leaders, leaders of refugee associations as well as doctors, psychologists, social workers and cultural mediators working with this population.

Analysis

To analyse the data, emphasis was placed on the importance of non-linear temporality in the context of individual's changing subjective current realities—as they weave together images of the past, present and future. Thus, the focus was on the ever-changing subjective constellations surrounding aspirations—namely those of the refugee victims of torture who participated in the research. This includes tracking the processes of change in aspirations as individuals configured, reconfigured, and made meaning of their new realities encountered in Greece. Such an approach highlights the societal, institutional, and individual conditions that form and shape individual aspirations, which is understood as constantly changing as the individuals moves across countries, societies, and institutions (Adams & Fleer, 2017).

The analysis draws on a dialogical approach, based on Bhaktinian (Bakhtin, 1978, 1981, 1986) notions of polyphonization (opposition and subvoices within the dialogical self) to draw out the conflict and tensions of ever-changing aspirations which are socially and culturally contextualised. This is because a sociocultural perspective on migration sees it as not an individual's isolated action but as happening in "discursive fields that push migrants to develop specific views of themselves" (Silvey, 2004), discursive fields which in turn act as resources to nourish aspirations. Within this dialogical matrix, symbolic elements in socio-cultural practices emerge as resources, providing a time orientation, and, consequently, a self-continuity between past and future (Kadianaki & Zittoun, 2014).

The proposition of a dialogical analysis within a socio-cultural framework is thus to use case studies to explore individual migration trajectories within specific situations, including analysing the relevant social and cultural elements, dialogical others, specific bodies of shared knowledge, social representations, cultural elements and tools, and so on: "in each situation, the relative strength of these elements, or the tension they generate, are negotiated by the person; the unique ways of dealing with that situation and inviting solutions can be seen as the emergent subjectivity" (Zittoun, 2012a). The vignette presented here as a case study therefore serves to illustrate the complex realities and interrelatedness of migration, the sociocultural environment and "potentially transient aspirations" (Carling & Schewel, 2017).

The Case of Mr B

Mr B is a 34 year old refugee, who had been imprisoned and tortured for one year and seven months in his native Sudan as a result of his political activism. He was referred to the centre for victims of torture for medical and psychological care upon his arrival in Athens in June 2016. His leg in particularly had been badly broken as a result of the torture, requiring multiple operations and ongoing physiotherapy. During our first meeting in August 2016, he describes the period wherein he managed to escape and make his way to Europe:

> I decided for myself, or I say to myself what can I do for my future. A, I have no future. B, I have no freedom. C, I have no education. I have nothing. What can I do? I have many relations. I have many friends. I talk with them [...] I just see some opportunities, I see some chances, I fill in...

By firstly drawing on his own internal resources (a dialogue with "myself"), plans for his future are elaborated upon by talking with his "many friends"—the dialogues within this social interaction serving as a resource which allows him to imagine opportunities for the future. It was through these social connections that he was able to escape and make his way to Europe. This continues to be evident in his recounting of his escape from Sudan into Libya, where interactions with others allowed him to construct plans for the future:

> The situation in Libya was really difficult for me. I didn't know other people [yet I thought to myself that] I can do some things for myself. After all, what can I do? I just listened. Some people were saying that they're going to other places. They're going to Egypt, after Egypt they're going to take the ship to come to Turkey, then to Greece, Greece to Italy, Italy to somewhere else. The people just talked about all of this information. I had no idea about these things. I just listened.

Throughout our interview, his narrative continues to highlight the importance of his ongoing internal dialogue as a resource for constructing plans for the future. A tension exists between the realisation of his own social disconnection ("I don't know other people") and his need for social connection in order to rely on others for information. The strategy he appears to develop around this tenson is to "just listen"—without a clear vision of what steps to take next, plans are developed along the way. He reports having no end destination in mind before leaving Sudan, "no idea about these things." As the migration journey continued, he describes having very little choice but "to try," his migration aspirations in a continual state of transformation:

> I'm thinking that I just need to have a chance, I want to leave. I want to go to other places. What can I do really? I tried the first time, I succeeded. I went to Turkey, Istanbul. I stayed in Istanbul for three months. I went to Izmir... [There's] no other way. Yes you have two choices. You go to prison or get deported. What can I do? I try [...] I have no choice. I came back to Italy...What can I do? [...] What can I do? I come here to Greece

The repetition of the words "what can I do?" highlights how little choice he felt he had in constructing plans for the future. His ever-changing aspirations adapt according to the conditions in which he finds himself. However, once settled in Greece and embarking on a process of physical and psychological rehabilitation, new aspirations begin to emerge. He forms new social connections with refugee communities of Athens, where seemingly overly romanticized discourses of "success" are linked to those who manage to make their way to Western Europe, the apparent metaphorical land of milk-and-honey:

> There are people that go over to that place [Western Europe], get the resident permit, go to school, go to England, go to University to learn the English language, go to France, learn the French language. Go to Sweden, learn the Swedish language. These are people who <u>succeed</u> [our emphasis]. In England, all the people have jobs, they're working.

Like many in his community, he feels increasing trapped in Greece. Aspirations for migration to Western Europe abound, nourished by stories of those who have already "succeeded" there:

> I want to do something for my future. This is not something easy but I need, you know, more time…The Greek situation really, is not easy […] I think I want to go somewhere else, but where? I don't know exactly …
>
> Some people have a lot of things happening, they have many dreams, they want to study. Other people want to go to another place. For my future, I want to go somewhere. Really. Somewhere, I don't know exactly where. There are two countries—maybe it's Germany, maybe it's France. I must choose between these two countries, which one is better? Can I easily get the paper [permit] to visit? Afterwards I'll learn German or French… To the future's future, I don't know what is happening [laughs] I have many dreams

The frustration increases as his feeling of being trapped in Greece is strongly related to his poor medical condition limiting his mobility:

> Every week I wait, you know. For example, on Monday I have an appointment, on Tuesday or Wednesday I have an appointment. Today I come, I also came on Friday, I come around two or three days a week. I talk more and more with other doctors, about surgery, about many things […] How many times, or how many days or how many months or how many hours I can wait? This is a question mark.

Thwarted both legally and medically from being able to migrate to Western Europe, he compares himself to others whom he imagines have succeeded in terms of migrating to Western Europe. There is a sense of him being stuck in Greece and loosing what Hviid (2008) has refered to as "social time"—lagging behind a culturally informed timeline dictating various milestones of social identity development such as getting married or having children:

> I want to work, I can get work far away [in Western Europe], for my future. I have a lot of friends, the same generation as me. We grew up together, but those people now have families, have children, have many things. But until now I have nothing. I am thinking that I want to do something. I can get married [but here in Greece] I lose my time

During a second interview, a month later in July 2017, he describes an increasing determination to migrate to Western Europe. He doesn't have a particular country in mind to which he aspires, but reports feeling optimistic for the future, wanting to "try" in one country and move on to "somewhere else" if it's "not better":

> I decided for myself that I want to leave to Greece, I will go try somewhere better. It's not something easy, for a human being, it's not easy to decide to stay or to wait. I'll go to that place and it's better, okay. If it's not better, I'll go to another place [...] I'll just go to try, I want to try. I want to fight for myself. I can do something better. Until now, the door is not closed. Until now, the time is early, not evening.

This optimism for a "better" future is placed in sharp contrast to the deception he felt upon arriving in Athens and discovering that his expectations of life in Greece did not meet the reality which met him upon arrival:

> I couldn't wait to get to Athens. Then I couldn't believe it when I arrived. I thought to myself "this is not Athens." I thought Athens was a shiny country [my emphasis]. The road doesn't look like this. Before coming, we had many dreams, you know. We were saying "This is Turkey, okay, how about Athens? Berlin? Sweden? UK? Germany?" We're thinking [it'll be] something like Las Vegas [laughs] Really, now our dreams are destroyed.

What he refers to is not only his individual aspirations, but the collective aspirations of entire migrant communities. It is not only "I" but "we" refugees who had many dreams that are now "destroyed." He wasn't the only participant of the research who referred to Europe as "Las Vegas"—three other participants did so as well. Many indicated having images of Europe in their mind based on what they had seen on television and in films—evoking a notion of success based on wealthy, excessive and luxurious lifestyles.

As was the case for the majority of refugees encountered in the course of the research, his deception surrounding the reality of life in Athens is offset by continuing aspirations for still being able to find "Las Vegas" in Western Europe. The goalposts of reaching the "shiny country," a metaphorical Eldorado, have been moved. Instead of aspiring to a better life in Europe, it is now a question of aspiring to a better life in Western Europe. Aspirations are geographically determined. For Mr B, these aspirations are both a source of hope and optimism, as well as of deep frustration. Rather than focusing his efforts on creating a more or less satisfactory life for himself in Greece, he feels trapped in a state of permanent temporariness, constantly trying to reach Western Europe but not succeeding:

> I go to battle. I try, I want to go somewhere—but I've not succeeded. I have no chance. I try to go to somewhere else. I try. Really, now I'm tired. Not tired in my body, tired in my mind.

In response to this state of mental exhaustion, his psychologist attempts to dissuade him from leaving Greece. Again and again, she states the legal reality of his situation: he has been recognised as a refugee in Greece, and therefore cannot apply for asylum elsewhere in Europe. In an interview with this psychologist in January 2017, she reports:

> He doesn't realize that he cannot very easily live in another European country since he's denying this reality. [I'm worried] that he will be very disillusioned. He's very smart but he seems to disregard this part of reality because it's unthinkable to him

In response to her attempts at dissuading his aspirations for migration to Western Europe, Mr B remains undeterred:

> You know, the human being dreams [...] I want to go somewhere, you know that in Greece here, there's no future here, really ... I want to open a new chapter. I want to do something ...after I get better I want to move, I want to change this weather, I want to see something new.

Aspirations for migration appear to be deeply connected to a sense of who he is as an individual human being. As observed by his psychologist:

> When he believes that the dream is still on then he can go, he's okay. Whenever something goes wrong, he feels that this pain goes on and on. And he cannot go on to realize his plans

Her words attest to the psychological and physical pain from which he suffers in Greece, a pain seemingly amplified by his ambitions being legally and medically thwarted. As Mr B himself reports:

> You know, my future has contact with my leg

In other words, plans for the future are inevitably intertwined with his medical rehabilitation. Interestingly, his physiotherapist takes a difference stance to that of his psychologist. Rather than dissuading his migration aspirations, he reports in an interview in July 2017:

> There are two possibilities for him: one, it is to go to England. One, it is to stay in Greece. He would think deeply. He has many very good advantages in going to England. He has a big Sudanese community there. He has people that he knows who speak the language.

Rather than focusing on legal restraints, the physiotherapist highlights the many cultural resources upon which Mr B could draw in England. However, he notes a change in Mr B's aspirations, which he links to the recent news of Britain voting to leave the E.U.:

> But I notice that between the first and last operation … he's increasing very, very much his efforts to learn Greek… Before, every two three times that we will meet, he will mention something about England and Britain. Now, I haven't heard him say something about Britain for months…

Indeed, following the news of the Brexit referendum, Mr B begins to set his sights on France, rather then England:

> France is better. After you take residence there, you're free. You take your refugee card, it's easy […] You go to learn French, after you learn French it's easy to get a job.

In August 2017, he reports experiencing increasing instances of racism and hostility towards refugees in Greece. He no longer feels comfortable walking on the streets of Athens as an African man, encountering instances of hostility by the Greek community in general, and arrests by the police in particular. Aspirations are therefore similarly determined by a need to remove himself from this social context:

> How can a migrant stay in this country when nobody respects me?

A year on from the first interview conducted, Mr B continues to aspire to a life in Western Europe, remaining steadfast in his hopes for a "shiny" future there:

> I have a lot of things I want to do. My dreams—I don't know for sure if it'll come true or not. But as I finish here, I want to go somewhere [where there are] possibilities, possibilities. After I leave to Greece, I want to go to France and Italy and Germany where everybody respects you. People there respect your skin colour, they respect your mind […] I can move all the countries [of Western Europe], no one will say "stop and do not go there." I can easily get a job, and I can marry

Despite being dissuaded to migrate by his psychologist, despite the knowledge of the legal impossibility of being received as a refugee outside of Greece, despite being in contact with friends in the Sudanese community who attest to the hardships encountered in other European countries, he aspires to migrate. As he himself concludes in our final interview:

> My dream still exists

Discussion

Mr B's story is representative of so many of the refugees who participated in the study. What is revealed through a dialogical analysis of his trajectory is the importance of socio-cultural resources, which he draws upon to shape and define his aspirations—aspirations which may never wholly be considered "his" alone, in their entirety, but which are collectively shared and distributed. He is not alone in having arrived in Europe after an arduous migration journey fueled by "geographical imaginaries" (Salazar, 2010; Salazar & Smart, 2011) of a better life in Europe. As stated by other participants:

> It's Europe, Europe is miracles
>
> [Europe] is the dream of any African
>
> In any case, all the Congolese know that in France, Belgium, Germany or Austria—that if you ask for asylum they will give you money... someone could sacrifice themselves or a family could sell one person of the family to come to Europe. Europe is the dream of Africans

What is similarly highlighted of the collective nature of these aspirations is the fact that many were sent to Europe by the family or even in certain cases by the extended community, with the responsibility of being able to offer financial support to those left in their countries of origin. Mr B made the decision to migrate to Europe himself. Often, however, the choice is not an individual one yet the result of the collective decision-making of entire communities. It is also worth noting that aspirations appeared to be largely based on taking advantage of the material circumstances—moment-by-moment decisions made on the spot, and changing on the spot. Like many others, Mr B had no clear pathway or destination in mind before setting out on his migration journey. Rather, he "just listened." Aspirations were transient and context-dependant, largely influenced by the ever-changing sociocultural and political context. This contests the notion that the decision to migrate is a once-off decision taken at a single moment in time by a single individual.

In sharp contrast to the "dream" of a "miracle" life in Europe, Mr B felt disillusioned by the every-day reality of Athens, a disillusion seemingly shared by the vast majority of refugees encountered over the course of the research:

> We had another vision of Europe... Europe is different from Africa. For me, at least, Europe is even more complicated than Africa...
>
> We came because we had different dreams, we came to see the reality
>
> When we dreamed, we then later understood that life is something else

For one of the other participants in the research in particular, the disillusion was amplified by the stark contrast of the poor economic reality of his life as a refugee in Greece, and collective expectations on the part of the family:

> Because in Africa, they think that when you're in Europe, you'll have enough money to send back home to Africa at any moment

He reported eventually losing contact with his family, seemingly overwhelmed by the shame of not having "succeeded" economically, the expectation all the greater given the substantial economic investment made in him by the extended family. He described his disillusion thus:

> Often we had Europe in our minds like the films that we saw. When you watch a film, it's just a scene that they created. You forget that there's a reality behind it. There's an actor, a director, interpretors to make it all look real. Now it's only when you come to Europe that you see that reality

He starts describing the Europe that "we" (collectively) imagined in "our" minds, yet switches to the single "you" who alone and individually "sees that reality." As was the case for Mr B, many felt trapped in this reality, with aspirations thwarted by the politico-legal reality of not being able to leave Greece:

> I know only one thing, that my world is just only this room... I'm just killing my time here until I'm getting my papers
>
> I can't think properly what to do in my future. I'm not able to think about my future, what is going to happen next in my future. I don't know what is going to happen.
>
> I'm trapped here.
>
> I don't know when will my life going to take me. I don't know what is going to happen next with me now...I don't want to stay here because there is no life.

Despite these thwarted ambitions, romanticized notions of Western Europe abounded among participants. The majority of French-speaking African participants, for example, referred to migrants in Western Europe as those "dévant la-bas": loosely translated into English, those "ahead over there." This "aheadness" was not only conceptualised in terms of having continued along their aspired migration journey, but speaks more deeply to a felt sense of geography, "social time" (Hviid, 2008), and socioeconomic success being inextricably combined. Those who were ahead geographically were also considered ahead in life. Aspirations were not pinned on particular indices of socioeconomic success, but rather on geographic location. A common Utopic belief of life "ahead there" was expressed in the words of one participant:

> In other European countries, they easily give you papers [refugee status]. Like in France, papers or not, I'd have work there. In France, anything is authorized

Paradoxically, it is perhaps these aspirations to a better life in Western Europe which allowed many, including Mr B, to hope and dream of the future, and therefore to survive. In Mr B's own words, his "dream still exists." These aspirations appeared to inject a sense of vitality and agency into a situation of permanent liminality. As one participant stated:

> I have ideas, and because I have ideas, I have plans and projects. I know it will all be all right in the end [...] I have a rhythm that I've adopted. I dont look left, I don't like right. I look straight ahead of me, the place where I want to get to, right until I arrive. One single point, that's all. That helps me not to feel the stress. I see a normal life ahead

Conclusion

A dialogical analysis of the case of Mr B, within the theoretical framework of sociocultural psychology, highlight aspirations as a powerful motivating force driving migration. These aspirations transform continually, part of a perpetually generative system wherein ever-changing subjective realities collide with the ever-changing sociocultural environmental. Not only are the aspirations of individuals constantly transforming as a result of sociopolitical developments; they are significantly shaped and contested by shared or collective aspirations of entire communities. This starts with collective aspirations of communities in the country of origin, and extends to the constantly developing shared aspirations of refugee communities in Europe.

In protracted refugee situations in particular, where individuals are called upon to reconstruct their lives in "limbo" (Brun, 2015; Brun & Fábos, 2015), aspirations may serve to facilitate processes of integration. They may be a motivating force driving the individual to engage as an active agent in their integration into the new sociocultural context. The motivation to learn the Greek language, for example, may be substantially driven by aspirations of integrating into Greek society—both socially and economically. Paradoxically, however, the reverse may also be true. Aspirations may serve to impede integration. Stuck in limbo, aspirations are inherently linked to processes of imagination (Zittoun & Cerchia, 2013; Zittoun & Gillespie, 2015), processes which remove the individual from their current "here-and-now" material reality in order that they may dream of a better life "ahead"—elsewhere. To continue with the same example, many feeling trapped in Greece aspire to a better life in Western Europe, and will not find the motivation to learn the Greek language.

Migration is an ongoing process within which past, present and future are folded together in the emergence of migrant lives and subjectivities. The actualisation of migration articulates this complex interplay between these expressions of desire, between strategic planning and opportunism that manifest in movements to achieve or avoid certain kinds of futures. In this respect, it is never singular in its temporality, but rather is an ongoing process where past, present and future are folded together in the emergence of migrant lives (McCormack & Schwanen, 2011). Analysing mobilities as sociocultural constructs therefore contributes to the understanding of forced migrants' mobility choices as well as their individual integration trajectories—providing insight into how the emotionality of subjective experiences, as well as the sociocultural context, are fundamentally involved in people's plans to migrate, the development of their ever-changing aspirations and the process of adapting (or not) to life in a new homeland.

References

Adams, M., & Fleer, M. (2017). International transitions: Generating subjective sense and subjective configuration in relation to the development of identity. *Mind Culture and Activity, 24*(4), 1–15.
Appadurai, A. (2004). The capacity to aspire. *Culture and Public Action, 1,* 59–84.

Bakhtin, M. (1978). *Esthétique et théorie du roman [traduit du russe par Daria Olivier, préface de Michel Aucouturier]*. Paris, France: Gallimard.

Bakhtin, M. (1981). *The DIALOGIC IMAGInation (translated by Caryl Emerson and Michael Holquist)*. Austin, TX: University of Texas Press.

Bakhtin, M. (1986). The Bildungsroman and its significance in the history of realism. In C. Emerson & M. Holquist (Eds.), *Speech genres and other late essays* (pp. 21). Austin, TX: University of Texas Press.

Brun, C. (2015). Active waiting and changing hopes: Toward a time perspective on protracted displacement. *Social Analysis, 59*(1), 19–37.

Brun, C., & Fábos, A. (2015). Making homes in limbo? A conceptual framework. *Refuge: Canada's Journal on Refugees, 31*(1), 5–17.

Bruner, J. (1990). *Acts of meaning: Four lectures on mind and culture (Jerusalem-Harvard Lectures)*. Cambridge, MA: Harvard University Press.

Carling, J. (2002). Migration in the age of involuntary immobility: Theoretical reflections and cape verdean experiences. *Journal of Ethnic and Migration Studies, 28*(1), 5–42.

Carling, J., & Collins, F. (2017). Aspiration, desire and drivers of migration. *Journal of Ethnic and Migration Studies, 44*(6), 909–926.

Carling, J., & Schewel, K. (2017). Revisiting aspiration and ability in international migration. *Journal of Ethnic and Migration Studies, 1,* 1–19.

Cole, M. (1998). *Cultural psychology: A once and future discipline*. Harvard: Harvard University Press.

Collins, F. L. (2018). Keeping bodies moving: Hope, disruption and the possibilities of youth migration. *Journal of Intercultural Studies, 39*(6), 626–641.

González Rey, F. (2008). Subject, subjectivity, and development in cultural-historical psychology. In B. van Oers, W. Wardekker, E. Elbers, & R. Van der Veer (Eds.), *The transformation of learning: Advances in cultural-historical activity theory* (pp. 137–156). Cambridge: Cambridge University Press.

González Rey, F. (2016). Advancing the topics of social reality culture and subjectivity from a cultural–historical standpoint: Moments paths and contradictions. *Journal of Theoretical and Philosophical Psychology, 36*(3), 175.

Goulart, D. M. (2017). The psychiatrization of human practices worldwide: Discussing new chains and cages. *Pedagogy Culture and Society, 25*(1), 151–156.

Goulart, D. M., & González Rey, F. (2016). Mental health care and educational actions: From institutional exclusion to subjective development. *European Journal of Psychotherapy and Counselling, 18*(4), 367–383.

Howden, D. (2017). Greece: Between deterrence and integration. *Newsdeeply*. Retrieved from https://issues.newsdeeply.com/greece-between-deterrence-and-integration?utm_source=rd on the 11 February 2020

Hviid, P. (2008). "Next year we are small, right?" Different times in children's development. *European Journal of Psychology of Education, 23*(2), 183.

Kadianaki, I., & Zittoun, T. (2014). Catalysts and regulators of psychological change in the context of immigration ruptures. In K. R. Cabell & J. Valsiner (Eds.), *The catalyzing mind* (pp. 191–207). New York, NY: Springer.

McCormack, D. P., & Schwanen, T. (2011). Guest editorial: The space—Times of decision making. *Environment and Planning a, 43*(12), 2801–2818.

Kirmayer, L. J., & Ramstead, M. J. (2016). Embodiment and Enactment in Cultural Psychiatry. In C. Durt, T. Fuchs, & C. Tewes (Eds.), Embodiment, Enaction, and Culture: Investigating the Constitution of the Shared World (pp. 397–422). Cambridge, MA: MIT Press

Métraux, J.-C. (2017). L'impact du vécu des réfugiés sur leur apprentissage de la langue d'acceuil. *Tema Babylonia, 1*(2017), 19–22.

Meyer, F. (2017). Navigating aspirations and expectations: Adolescents' considerations of outmigration from rural eastern Germany. *Journal of Ethnic and Migration Studies, 44*(6), 1032–1049.

Salazar, N. B. (2010). Towards an anthropology of cultural mobilities. *Crossings: Journal of Migration & Culture, 1*(1), 53–68.
Salazar, N. B., & Smart, A. (2011). Anthropological takes on (im) mobility. *Identities, 18*(6), 1–9.
Silvey, R. (2004). Power, difference and mobility: Feminist advances in migration studies. *Progress in Human Geography, 28*(4), 490–506.
Valsiner, J. (2007). *Culture in minds and societies: Foundations of cultural psychology*. India: Sage.
Valsiner, J., & Rosa, A. (2007). *The Cambridge handbook of sociocultural psychology*. Cambridge: Cambridge University Press.
Vygotsky, L. S. (1980). *Mind in society: The development of higher psychological processes*. Cambridge, MA: Harvard University Press.
Vygotsky, L. (1987). Speech and thinking. *LS Vygotsky, Collected Works, 1*(3), 39–45.
Wagoner, B., Gillespie, A., Valsiner, J., Zittoun, T., Salgado, J., & Simao, L. (2011). *Repairing ruptures: Multivocality of analyses*. New York: Nova Press.
Wagoner, B., Chaudhary, N., & Hviid, P. (2014). *Cultural psychology and its future: Complementarity in a new key*: Charlotte: IAP.
Zepke, N., & Leach, L. (2002). Contextualised Meaning Making: One way of rethinking experiential learning and self-directed learning? *Studies in Continuing Education, 24*(2), 205–217.
Zittoun, T. (2012a). Life-course: A socio-cultural perspective. In Vaalsiner. J (Ed.), *Oxford library of psychology: The Oxford handbook of culture and psychology* (Vol. 60, pp. 513–535). Oxford: Oxford University Press.
Zittoun, T. (2012b). On the emergence of the subject. *Integrative Psychological and Behavioral Science, 46*(3), 259–273.
Zittoun, T. (2017). Modalities of generalization through single case studies. *Integrative Psychological and Behavioral Science, 51*(2), 171–194.
Zittoun, T., & Cerchia, F. (2013). Imagination as expansion of experience. *Integrative Psychological and Behavioral Science, 47*(3), 305–324.
Zittoun, T., & Gillespie, A. (2015). *Imagination in human and cultural development*. London: Routledge.
Zittoun, T., & Sato, T. (2018). Imagination in adults and the aged person. In T. Zittoun & V. P. Glăveanu (Eds.), *Handbook of imagination and culture* (pp. 187–208). New York, NY: Oxford University Press.

Chapter 9
Working with Shame and Trauma

Not only does the literature attest to the high levels of trauma among displaced populations, research in the past decade has increasingly revealed the hidden yet pervasive role that shame may play in posttraumatic symptomatology. As defined by Wilson and colleagues, "in the posttraumatic self, shame develops from traumatic experiences that render the victim fearful, powerless, helpless, and unable to act congruently with moral values" (Wilson et al., 2006, p. 127). In the context of forced migration in particular, both trauma and shame are ubiquitous, pervasive, and contagious.

Despite its omnipresence, shame is ashamed of itself. Shame activates shame. The mystifying dualism of shame is that it is at once an isolating, intimately intra-psychic phenomenon seeking concealment, yet remains deeply embedded in a visual and public interpersonal space where the self is violently and unexpectedly exposed to the critical gaze of the Other (Womersley et al., 2011). Unlike guilt (typically related to a particular action or behaviour), shame taints the entire landscape of the individual—colouring the very sense of self. Shame is therefore considered to be a more complex intra-psychic process than guilt because it involves processes concerning attributes about the core dimensions of the self, identity, ego processes, and personality (Wilson et al., 2006). Inasmuch as it lies within the interactional space between self and other, at the divide between the intimate and the public, the individual and society—it tries to hide itself by its very nature. As such, it often remains unnoticed. Its powerful yet seemingly invisible impact may be hidden behind a myriad of emotional cloaks—anger, dissociation, blame, resentment... even more so in the context of clinicians working with migrant populations, where a plethora of differently nuanced cultural cloaks may further obfuscate this noxious affect. However, ethically, clinically, professionally, humanly, we cannot ignore it. This is particularly true of work within multicultural contexts, where relations are so typically marked by power differentials in terms of race, class, nationality and socio-economic status. It is here, in this matrix of identities, that shame is located. Therefore, new approaches are needed for clinicians (both researchers and academics) which

G. Theisen-Womersley, *Trauma and Resilience Among Displaced Populations*,
https://doi.org/10.1007/978-3-030-67712-1_9

consider the interactive effects of shame and trauma within sociocultural context among such vulnerable populations.

Migration and Post-traumatic Shame

Shame significantly shapes the migration experience, linked particularly to extreme feelings of powerlessness, degradation and humiliation. It may emerge as a result of the many forms of torture, sexual violence and other atrocities experienced in the country of origin, yet is equally exacerbated by degrading and humiliating asylum procedures, having to accept a new and often devalued social identity of being an asylum seeker, and the embarrassment of not meeting culturally-informed expectations to financially support the family. Shame pervades the experience of no longer being "at home" at home, of being cast out of one's country, of having to metaphorically knock on the door of a potential host country and beg to be accepted, only to be met by significant social discrimination, scrutiny and disbelief at one's claim to asylum.

The process of migration may therefore be in and of itself a shameful experience, wherein individual and social identities risk being negated through the systemic trauma associated with legal and social practices of exclusion (Goldsmith et al., 2014). The bureaucratic systems and procedures with which migrants are faced upon arrival in a host-country may echo feelings of powerlessness and helplessness experienced throughout the migration journey. Indeed, the very status of "victim," of "asylum seeker" may be inherently shameful to some. The outright expulsion of many migrants, the deterioration of living conditions, the uncertainty regarding legal status, the deprivation of rights and the implementation of mechanisms designed to prevent the construction of social links has arguably lead to a shameful "construction of invisibility" (Sanchez-Mazas et al., 2011). Administrative provisions may often make the very presence of migrants as subjects within a State no longer accepted and "this translates all too quickly in the fact that the person as such is no longer accepted" (Torre, 2016). The physical, social and political isolation so typically experienced upon arrival to host countries serves only to feed monstrous feelings of invisibility and disconnectedness (Bhimji, 2015).

Furthermore, the stressful experiences that many asylum seekers and refugees are exposed to during forced migration, and during the resettlement process, make them vulnerable to mental health conditions. As a consequence, the prevalence of psychological distress and mental disorders in asylum seekers and refugees as reported in the literature appears to be generally high, with significantly elevated rates of PTSD being found among this population (Li et al., 2016; Turrini et al., 2017). Traumatology research over the past decade has seen the development of the concept of "posttraumatic shame," with key authors stressing the importance of shame as a social emotion that impacts the severity and course of PTSD symptoms (Hecker et al., 2015; Maercker & Hecker, 2016; Wilson et al., 2006). Indeed, the experience of shame has even been revealed to potentially hold the same properties as traumatic events involving intrusions, flashbacks, strong emotional avoidance, hyper arousal, fragmented states of mind and dissociation (Matos & Pinto-Gouveia, 2010). Shame and trauma are inextricably linked.

Torture in particular represents an extraordinary exception in the psychopathology field—with significant implications for the shame-trauma nexus. The particularity of torture as pathogenic is linked to the fact that the act itself is taught, organized, elaborated, and perpetrated by humans against other humans (Sironi, 1999; Viñar, 2005a). Arguably, the aim of the perpetrator is to shame, to disrupt the connection to all that makes us human (Viñar, 2005a). As such, torture is not an individual act, but a social one. It is an inherently shameful experience, damaging different spheres of an individual including body, personality, hope, aspirations for life, identity, integrity, belief systems, the sense of being grounded and attached to a family and society, autonomy, community relationships, and a sense of safety (Womersley et al., 2018). Humiliation thus arises from torture experiences where the survivor is abused, dehumanized, and made an exhibition for others, essentially representing a profound loss of dignity and power (Wilson & Drožđek, 2004; Wilson et al., 2006). In particular, the dual shame inherent in being both a victim of torture as well a refugee is related to a myriad of losses, human rights violations, shifting power dynamics and other dimensions of suffering linked not only to torture experienced pre-migration, but to different forms of violence experienced during and after migration as well (Hodges-Wu & Zajicek-Farber, 2017).

Cultural Manifestations of Shame and Implications for Clinicians

The source of shame can never be completely in the self or in the Other, but is a rupture of what Kaufman (Kaufman, 1989) calls the "interpersonal bridge" binding the two. In thus theorizing shame as being located at this bridge, we understand the important role it plays in community life through promoting socially acceptable or desirable behaviour. It exerts a force that inclines individuals to adapt to socially sanctioned values, rules and beliefs—an integral component of the promotion of cultural ideals (Swartz, 1988). A significant source of shame is the loss of continuity in upholding culturally defined values, norms and respected patterns of behaviour—and the self-consciousness over disappointing others within one's social network and embedded within one's culture (Wilson et al., 2006). We may therefore understand the importance of the sociocultural context in determining its various manifestations. This has been highlighted in the plethora of cross-cultural and anthropological literature paying attention attesting to the variety of culturally diverse forms of shame (Wong & Tsai, 2007).

This has significant implications for professionals—both clinicians and researchers—working with populations from a variety of cultural backgrounds. A large potential for misunderstandings between clinicians and traumatized individuals is not only because of a language barrier; very little is known about the concepts of illness and treatment expectations in these patients (Maier & Straub, 2011). Furthermore, shame-related cultural codes of behaviour might prevent migrants from directly reporting earlier traumatic experiences, from trusting the professional or from even attending appointments. As noted by Wilson et al. (2006), "the powerful emotions of posttraumatic shame are associated with a broad range of avoidance behaviours: isolation, detachment, withdrawal, hiding, nonappearance, self- imposed exile, cancellation of appointments, surrender of responsibilities, emotional constriction, psychic numbing, emotional flatness, and non-confrontation with others" (p. 138). These signs are easily misread.

The interpersonal dynamics of this clinical encounter may not be so different from the context of research interviews, similarly marked by power asymmetries (Salazar-Orvig & Grossen, 2008). Here, the individual migrant is placed in the role of a patient-participant object, in the face of an arguably more socially powerful professional subject aiming to scrutinize the most intimate details of their life history. It risks being an inherently shameful encounter, exacerbating extreme feelings of powerlessness, degradation, and humiliation. However, as noted by Wilson and colleagues (Wilson et al., 2006), shame is a two-way street; it can exist in the patient and therapist at the same time in different intra-psychic configurations. Working with the complexities of shame in the posttraumatic self, both patient and therapist (and arguably, participant and researcher) share a common ground of human vulnerability whose management likely determines the quality of outcome. As we have illustrated elsewhere in the case of research among survivors of sexual abuse (Gail Womersley et al., 2011), shame pervades the entirety of the relationship. It is contagious. All are affected. As much as the identity of a victim, an asylum seeker, an oppressed ethnic minority may be shaming for the migrant, the identity of the oppressor, the colonizer, the privileged ethnic elite, may be shaming for the clinician or researcher.

We need to consider shame in the context of work with vulnerable migrant populations—not only because it may influence our professional work in profound yet often barely perceptible ways, it is our ethical duty as human beings to reflect on these intersubjective encounters. In order to reflect on some concrete case examples of the ways in which shame may manifest in such encounters, and on some applications in dealing with shame constructively, I draw on my work with asylum seekers and refugees in a centre for victims of torture in Athens.

Case Study One: Research Among Displaced Victims of Torture in Athens, Greece

The case study also appears in a chapter entitled "A Sociocultural Exploration of Shame and Trauma Among Refugee Victims of Torture" in a book entitled "The Bright Side of Shame," edited by Claude-Hélène Mayer and Elisabeth Vanderheiden (Womersley, 2019). As the migration "reception crisis" continues unabated, Greece remains one of the first ports of sanctuary. While the country is still gripped by one of the worst financial and societal crises of the past 40 years, little attention or funding is available to provide mental health and psychosocial support to refugees (Gkionakis, 2016). Many torture survivors in Greece, only some of whom having been identified as vulnerable, are still trapped on the islands, a context characterized by a lack of specialised medical care and poor living conditions. Other torture survivors who have moved to the mainland without permission have also found themselves in limbo, unable to proceed with their asylum claim. The complex asylum system and the many barriers in accessing basic services in Athens and across the country have only increased their hardship (Kotsioni, 2016). Furthermore, according to Mentinis (2013), Greece itself has been diagnosed as being in a never ending crisis of identity; a conflict between two traditions, a hovering between the East and the West. For many Greeks, the major influx of immigrants brings even further challenges to their national identity, because until recently Greece was a very homogeneous society, inhabited by an overwhelming majority of ethnic Greeks who speak Greek and who belong to the Greek Orthodox Church (Voulgaridou et al., 2006). The sources of shame within this context are many: from the Greek citizens themselves who may be ashamed of the poor reception conditions, of not being able to do more to help, of the inadequate institutional structures and hostile reactions to foreigners on the part of their compatriots, of not being up to "civilised" Western European standards; to the asylum seekers suddenly finding themselves in an incredibly precarious and vulnerable position, having lost many aspects of their valued social identity linked to their country of origin.

In this particular context, I conducted participative research in a centre for victims of torture in Athens. This involved three months of participative observation with the medical team of the centre: participating in the team's daily morning meetings and group therapy activities, facilitating psycho-education sessions for the beneficiaries of the project, and teaching English in the centre twice a week. My research also involved conducting qualitative interviews with beneficiaries, the health professionals themselves as well as "community representatives"—leaders of the various refugee communities around Athens. It was thus a complex mixture of being both a clinician and a researcher, requiring an on-going negotiation of these multiple identities.

The beneficiaries of this particular project were identified as "vulnerable"—victims of torture in their countries of origin and in particular need of multidisciplinary care. They came from all over the world, notably regions affected by conflict. The team, offering mental health support, physiotherapy, and medical care, worked in collaboration with social workers and lawyers who were assisting the beneficiaries in their request for asylum. The needs were many, varied yet interrelated. An accompanying team of cultural mediators was required—not only for translation but as mediators of this new and complex medico-legal system with which people were confronted.

The use of the term "beneficiaries" to refer to the individuals coming to the clinic, as opposed to others such as "patients" or "asylum seekers" or "victims of torture" was a deliberate one. When the project opened, all individuals would all be presented with a "patient" card, that is until one individual refused to take his. It was, he said, not how he chose to identify. The word "patient" evoked a deep sense of shame. He felt that it implied a victimizing and humiliating identity. He was neither, he had insisted, a patient nor a victim—but an individual in his own right.

It became apparent, during the course of my time as a participant researcher in this context, that it was not only trauma, but also shame, which pervaded the space—with significant and potentially destructive implications for the micro-interactions among the various actors. It was present in the daily meetings, where professionals kept expressing a feeling that they were not "good enough," not doing enough to help the beneficiary find work or shelter, not feeling experienced enough to handle the complexity of the needs of the vulnerable population with whom they were working, ashamed of belonging to a country where the structures supposedly in place to assist the migrants where not meeting their needs. The result appeared to be either an increased or decreased commitment to the work, a feeling of anger which incited a call to action, to respond to the need in front of them—or a resignation, a feeling that they had very little power to effect concrete changes in the lives of the beneficiaries.

As for the beneficiaries of the project, the shame was even more apparent. Finding themselves at the clinic, unable to help themselves and at the mercy of the team of professionals there to help them, ashamed of not being able to support their families financially, of not having met their aspirations of "succeeding" in Europe, ashamed of the humiliating and horrific experiences which they had endured, of how they may have compromised their perceived moral integrity in order to survive, of not being able to fully master the language nor the cultural nuances of their new environment … this was the shame in some way linked to the identity of "victim." The result, often, was a need to hide oneself, to not want to be seen entering the clinic for fear of the stigma attached to being a victim of torture, to mask aspects of their narratives, to not want to answer the professional's questions directly for fear of certain aspects of their lives being exposed or not believed. It resulted in different versions of their life story being told to different professionals. It resulted in many not wanting to see the psychologist as a result of the shame of being identified as "crazy." It resulted in quiet waiting rooms, where the silence among the various beneficiaries may have been out of respect for shame—for not wanting to expose each other as victims.

Shame was similarly present within the intersubjective space between myself, the health professionals, and the beneficiaries/participants. As noted above, I came as both a researcher and a clinician, an active participant in the space. I was both part of the team, yet in many ways a detached third party observer. Other aspects of my identity were similarly present, becoming more or less salient within the micro-interactions. I am South African. Therefore, as so often raised by the beneficiaries of African origin, I am "an African sister." One of "us." Yet, unlike the rest of "us"—I have White skin, I am not subject to the same degrading or humiliating micro-instances of racism so many experience when coming to Europe. Unlike them, I am "legitimized" in my right to be there, to pass unnoticed in the streets, to move freely around Europe. I am in the privileged position of the professional—I have the right to observe, to direct, to interrogate, to pose questions. I am also a woman, like some and not others. As we have explored elsewhere in reflecting on working with South African survivors of rape (Womersley et al., 2011)—the shame linked to the similarities and differences across marks of identity, so boldly and unavoidably expressed through our bodies, is a fundamental part of the interaction between researcher and researched in the context of qualitative interviews being conducted, particularly among vulnerable populations and particularly when exploring the sensitive topic of trauma.

To explore the myriad manifestations of shame—not belonging to the Self or Other but in the intersubjective space between all of these actors—I present a case study of one beneficiary with whom I had multiple interviews over the course of a year. I intend this to be an illustrative case study which may allow us to track the manifestations of shame as it arose in the interactions between us. It is representative of many of the interviews conducted during this period, and, hopefully, representative of so many qualitative interviews being conducted by qualitative interviewers in multicultural settings across the world. Reflecting on these micro-instances of shame, being able to first of all track it and second of all, through this awareness, allow this reflexivity to influence the way in which we interact with the participants whom we interview in qualitative research, is an ethical obligation. It is our responsibility as researchers, and as human beings.

Applied Approach to Dealing with Shame: The Case of Sylvain

Sylvain is a 35 year old refugee from the Ivory Coast, a beneficiary of the centre for victims of torture in Athens and a participant in my research with whom I conducted five qualitative interviews over the course of the year. Our work together is presented as a study on the myriad of ways in which shame was both manifested, and subsequently transformed, during this period. To analyse the case, instances of manifestations of shame in our interaction were identified in the transcripts, and subsequently grouped according to emerging overarching themes. Four identified sources of shame are presented, accompanied by some reflections on implications for transformation.

The Shame of Dependence

During our first interview, Sylvain described his situation as the following:

> Often we are confronted with strangers, and they mistreat us... when he can help you today, it is in two or three weeks that he will help you. They like to play with people, come and go... You go there and you are told to come back where you left first. It is not easy. But we understand them, we have to accept them, otherwise, it's dangerous [...] but we have to accept it is life, it hurts, it's stressful, it's hard, but when you're out there, we have to accept.

His shame appeared to have been related to being in the vulnerable position of dependence on the help of others, others who may well "mistreat us." Interestingly enough, the "mistreatment" to which he referred was not related to the many instances of racism he reported, nor to the fact that he was handcuffed by the police and thrown in prison without apparent just cause. Rather, he referred to the people who "play," who "come and go." In other words, the mistreatment he referred to is that which he encountered among those meant to "help"—humanitarian aid workers, state social services, medical professionals etc. This, in turn, evoked in me a sense of shame of being somehow related to those who help "when he can." Despite my role as an independent researcher, I was still connected to the clinic where he came for assistance. I was aware of this throughout my fieldwork in Athens. In 2015 and 2016, it was a context characterised by a plethora of well-meaning humanitarian workers coming to assist refugees for short periods of time. So many of the asylum seekers with whom I spoke referred to this phenomenon of "trauma tourism"—painting a picture of people arriving, asking questions, offering to help, and then leaving without fulfilling promises of further assistance.

Implications for Transformation

Sylvain's words offer a sobering reminder of the way in which the shame associated with being dependant on the assistance of others may be transformed through simply being (a) attentive to and aware of the possible impact of shame and (b) aware of the responsibility to avoid "playing" with vulnerable populations, to not just "come and go." I would argue that part of the transformation of Sylvain's shame, particularly shame related to this experience of being dependant on external aid, came through the consistent relationships he was able to form with staff at the centre over a period of two years. In our own relationship, it was linked to the fact that I kept to our agreed meeting schedule and consistently returned over the period of a year. It lay in simple details, such as allowing him to choose the time and place of our meetings together—a change compared to the treatment he reported encountering in his dealing with bureaucratic state institutions where he was often left to wait for hours, only to have the appointment delayed by months. Such basic signs of respect seem to have had a transformative impact on his own shame.

The Shame of Social Discrimination

Throughout our five meetings together, Sylvain reported feeling ashamed at the way in which as an asylum seeker he way he was treated as a "criminal" by a variety of actors, including the police:

> We start from a good one to frustrate you somewhere, and we fled the violence in Africa, arrived in a country where we say there is the human right, you come to sleep in the things that... I am in Greece I have known handcuffs, it is in Greece I have known handcuffs [...] Because they say I don't have papers. Is an unregistered person a criminal? [...]
>
> it's the things we keep in our hearts, in the prison, the police can hit you...

He also noted facing discrimination by not only local Greek populations, but other migrant communities. In reflecting on this, he highlighted my identity as a white person:

> You're South African, where we are sitting, a lot of people think you're European. So you see, but me seeing myself [...] You go to immigration, they say, you wait and give priority to others.

Despite us both being African, a fundamental difference is the colour of our skin. I am able to pass as European, he is not. His words are testament to the very present psychic consequences of shame and the accompanying feelings of envy seen in the context of deprivation and powerlessness as well as in the ubiquitous (and often unspeakable) presence of racial trauma (Harris, 2000).

Implications for Transformation

In outlining his experiences of racism and discrimination encountered in Europe, Sylvain stated the following:

> He [a European] does not distinguish you, he says, "The immigrants." But it's not just immigrants.

His words hint at the shame of a loss of individual identity in favour of being seen as "an immigrant." He contested this notion of being "just immigrants," in favour of being "distinguished"—in other words, of being seen and recognised as a complete and complex individual self. I would argue that the implications for transforming shame related to such social discrimination lie in the need for individual aspects of identity to be made visible, recognised, and valued. In exploring this, we similarly cannot ignore our own sense of shame related to being in a position of social privilege. Here, what seemed to have had a transformative impact on Sylvain's shame was my recognition of it. I needed both to be aware of my own shame linked to social privilege, and to recognise and respect his shame related to social discrimination.

The Shame of Being Unemployed

Throughout the year in which we met, Sylvain referred multiple times to the shame he felt at not being able to provide for his family back home who where waiting for his financial assistance. The shame he felt at not being able to meet their expectations eventually got to the point where he stopped answering their phone calls. He did miss them, he explained to me, but he couldn't face the shame of being unemployed and unable to help:

> Tomorrow when you succeed, you will be the pride of the family: the family and the whole village. But when you become a delinquent, it's [a shame for] the father and mother. These are things you don't really want to talk about.

He reported feeling frozen in time, unable to move on with his life and contribute as a productive member of society. Jobless, he felt "worthless," a delinquent who eventually turned to illegal activities in order to make money:

> The situation in Greece here, if you're not morally strong, it can make you do some bad things. It is not easy. We live like we never existed [...] I'm starting to do bad things. When you become envious, you're exposed to everything. And the easiest thing in Greece is selling drugs.

The shame of being unemployed was therefore double-edged: not only was there shame around being "useless" to society, in other words a "delinquent" family member unable to provide—the situation as an inexistent *persona non grata* lead him to conduct himself in "shameful" ways which previously would have been unthinkable. The behaviour seems to have been judged as immoral not only by others but by himself, a deep source of shame at the interpersonal bridge between himself and his social world. He was led further and further into the metaphorical shadows of society.

Implications for Transformation

Sylvain eventually did find legal work, and the transformative effect on his mental health was remarkable. Not only had his material conditions improved, he felt somehow more legitimate in his environment. He had become an active contributor to society, able to take the bus in the morning along with others heading to work, able to share the little that he had with friends and family, able to "show his face" in public. The fact of being employed seemed to lessen his sense of shame more than any other factor. As concisely and poignantly stated by Buggenhagen (2012), "money takes care of shame."

The shame surrounding Sylvain's unemployment serves as important reminder of the embeddedness of this emotion within a socioeconomic context. In my role as researcher, my primary focus was evidently on his psychological state of mind. However, it became abundantly apparent in interviews, with him and other asylum seekers, that this was significantly dependant on his social and economic environment. His sense of self-worth, relationship with family, socioeconomic status and the material conditions in which he found himself, all mutually reinforced the sense of shame about which he spoke so openly. We may not always have the capacity to effect changes in the socioeconomic lives of the people with whom we interact as clinicians and researchers. We can, however, reflect on this shame in our interactions. This could mean, for example, breaking our professional/ethical codes of conduct to accept gifts which we know individuals can ill-afford but for whom it is a point of pride. It means having the courage to address the sensitive topic of money when raised. Practitioners and researchers working with this population cannot ignore this incredibly salient aspect of shame. To do so risks, in many ways, reinforcing a social silence that so often fosters shame.

Case Study Two: Female Survivors of Sexual Violence in Cape Town, South Africa

The case study also appears in a scientific article published in *Qualitative Inquiry* (Womersley et al., 2011). Shame lies at the heart of the traumatic experience of rape—it is the experience of the body being exposed as inherently damaged or defiled and the consequent disconnection of the self from society. While descriptions of rape commonly identify "shame" as something with which abused women often wrestle, the form of the affect may depend on the value systems of particular communities (Bennett, 2000; Gavey, 2013). Much of the South African literature regarding the stigmatising and shaming effects of rape emphasises how the damage, devaluation and deviance of rape survivors is shaped by underlying contextually-specific patriarchal structures which position African women as moral guardians for their respective cultural values and traditions (Dawes & Donald, 1994; Kiguwa & Hook, 2004). As a result, the attitudes of the police, the medical establishment and the criminal justice system continue to reflect a deeply shaming undercurrent to reactions to rape survivors, contributing to what is referred to in the literature as "secondary traumatisation" (Artz, 1999; Artz & Smythe, 2008; Koss, 2000;Posel, 2005; Steyn & Steyn, 2008).

The pervasive threat of contracting HIV after a sexual encounter adds a further dimension to the shame of the South African rape survivor. The South African context is characterised by an unrivalled rape pandemic as well as having one of the highest HIV infection rates in the world. It is therefore unsurprising that there have been attempts to link the two pandemics conceptually, mediated by the myths and traditional beliefs surrounding female sexuality and its relationship to the virus (Chisala, 2008; Motsei, 2007). Thus, the rape survivor's profound shame lies not only in her experience of the humiliating and degrading event itself, but in the subsequent appraisal processes undertaken by herself and others in an attempt to make sense of the event.

Next to children, black women in South Africa are most vulnerable to ongoing traumatisation on a number of economic, physical and psychological levels, and are also the victims of the majority of rapes reported in the country (Maw et al., 2008). Within this context, it is impossible to consider the shame of the gendered, sexual body without linking it to the shame inherent in racialised identities, which themselves are deeply enmeshed in a complex matrix binding gender, class and socio-economic status (Harris, 2000). Butler (2003), for example, has marked the body as the stage on which traumatic disconnection unfolds. She constitutes the body as a public phenomenon situated squarely in the social sphere, the site of abuse and political oppression reflecting our social identities:

> Each of us is constituted politically in part by virtue of the social vulnerability of our bodies – as a site of desire and of physical vulnerability, as a site of a publicity at once assertive and exposed. Loss and vulnerability seem to follow from our being socially constituted bodies, attached to others, at risk of losing those attachments, exposed to others, at risk of violence by virtue of that exposure…the body implies mortality, vulnerability, agency: the skin and flesh expose us to the gaze of others, and also to touch and to violence (p. 10).

Butler here is not referring directly to the affect of shame. However, her allusion to the exposure of the self to the Other, manifested in the body, speaks directly to processes underlying the shame following violence and bodily abuse. In the context of white women researching gender-based violence among black women in South Africa, there is an added dimension of shame which carries a particularly racialised and politicised dimension. As Burman and Chantler (2005) argue, any investigation of violence or abuse within oppressed communities "faces charges of fuelling racism by perpetuating widespread cultural stereotypes that these groups are more oppressive to women than the dominant culture" (p. 71). This dimension is further highlighted by Mama's (2007) understanding of the role of psychological research in the "construction of African subjects as the objectified Other of the European imagination" (p. 18).

Shame is manifest on the micro-level of our daily interactions and cannot be separated from the complex matrix of gender, ethnicity and socio-economic class informing our public identities, which are so boldly reflected through our bodies. In order to further explore what shame DOES on the micro-level of our daily encounters, the analysis below tracks the affect of shame within the context of a qualitative research interview as a demonstration of how significantly the interview was shaped by the affect.

Presented below is a case study of a particular researcher-researched relationship within the context of qualitative, feminist research in South Africa. It is an analysis of the dialogue between Maria and me, which formed part of a study conducted in order to research the psychological impact of rape in survivors within 72 h of the event. Maria was interviewed at the Thuthuzela Care Centre in the Western Cape, which provides forensic, clinical and counselling support for survivors of rape—the site of the research. A semi-structured interview schedule was used and the conversation was therefore guided by broad, open-ended questions aimed at eliciting a narrative of her experience of the event, including the details of the rape itself, her emotional reaction and her feelings towards the institutions who were dealing with the rape.

The transcript of this dialogue has been analysed as part of this original research, with the focus being on an analysis of the dominant discourses which shaped the narratives of the survivors I interviewed. However, I have subsequently become aware of the pivotal role of shame, which profoundly coloured the exchange between us.

This interaction is therefore presented as a case study in order to delineate the various manifestations of shame which arose in the intersubjective space between us.

In order to track the development of shame as it was co-constructed within this intersubjective field, the analysis follows the interaction from the beginning of the interview to the end. However, specific pieces of dialogue are highlighted as marking particularly salient moments where shame was activated and passed between the two of us. Following the example of Miller (Miller, 2013), who demonstrates an inferential identification of shame themes in interview data, the selection of such moments was based on a triangulated model of data analysis dictating the tracking of the affect—namely based on the form of the conversation, the content of our dialogue as well as my own emotional memory of the event.

Analysis

The analysis offered here illustrates the various manifestations of shame which arose in the interaction between myself and a research participant, Maria. The case illustrates the effects of shame as it is mediated by my identity as a 22 year old, Jewish, middle-class female researcher and Maria's identity as a 32 year old female Coloured rape survivor living in the socially and economically oppressed Cape Flats. Our dialogue is testament to the very present psychic consequences of shame and the accompanying feelings of envy seen in the context of deprivation and powerlessness, as well as in the ubiquitous (and often unspeakable) presence of racial and gendered trauma (Harris, 2000).

The first contact I had with Maria was in the waiting room of the Thuthuzela Care Centre, which forms part of G. F. Jooste Hospital in Mannenberg, Cape Town. She had been brought in by the police, had been seen by a doctor, and was sitting in the waiting room. I approached her to ask whether she would be interested in taking part in my research by speaking to me about her feelings surrounding her experience of having been raped. From the very start of our meeting, our interaction was bound by a potentially shame-inducing social structure. The interview began with Maria expressing her anger and confusion at being raped:

> Now I'm feeling very angry. I feel so confused. I feel that there's no hope. It's almost like I'm trapped. I can't get out. I feel like no one understands, nobody cares. I can't trust even myself. Or even cry…I can't even cry. I don't know what to do. And the most important thing of all that I feel is that I don't feel anything. I feel like nobody cares … I won't even be able to look at myself and I've lost everything.

Maria's sense of "not being able to look at myself" speaks immediately and directly to the shame felt as a result of being raped by her husband, and the subsequent severance of her own sense of self from her social environment, a rupture of what Kaufman (1989, p. 22) terms the "interpersonal bridge" binding self and Other. Her words communicated a sense that the rape has taken away an acceptable form of self from her, and in its place stood a self which even she could not tolerate. At this stage of the interview, her feelings of rage dominated her narrative. She went on to tell me that she was so angry that she could "kill someone, really hurt someone." She outlined the thoughts she had of pouring boiling water over her husband's feet: "he would have gotten so much pain. And all his skins, all his bones would have hanged on him. But most of all he would have had pain…and I wanted him to feel that pain."

Maria then began expressing her sense of helplessness and confusion at the time of the rape: "You can beg, you can scream but they will still hurt you. Nobody will help you. No person…but when I really wanted to, I couldn't end it. But I have to get up from the floor and show no emotions, no feelings." The assumption implicit in her statement is that any display of emotion is strongly equated with a feeling of vulnerability and of being situated in a lower social position ("on the floor"). The rape has tainted her body as spoilt, compromising her social position in the eyes of the Other (Paul Gilbert, 1997; Paul Gilbert & Andrews, 1998; Paul Gilbert & Miles, 2014) and has taken away her own sense of personal agency by placing her in a situation which rendered her powerless to act. Morrison (Morrison, 2014) suggests that the "searing" (p. 113) quality associated with descriptions of shameful experiences reflects a sense of helplessness in the face of an inability to alter the state of the compromised self.

This feeling of unworthiness, of social undesirability, of helplessness leads to a shattering of the core self of the survivor (Herman, 1992), which may lead to a paralysing self-hatred, as illustrated in Maria's subsequent words:

> I know I'm beautiful, I know myself. I'm someone who likes to look in people's faces when I talk to them. I like to look in their eyes. But now I could never look in someone's eyes. I could never look into my own eyes because I'm just lying to myself. I will never see that part of me again. Ever. I will never look another person in the eyes again.

Maria's words suggest that the rape has disconfirmed her previously held positive self-beliefs in her own beauty (Lee et al., 2001), and has replaced this with a shame so paralysing that she is unable to look people in the eyes. As Morrison (Morrison, 1998) notes, "to feel shame, we do not need the presence of an actual shamer or a viewing audience; we need only those internal figures who have become part of who we are" (p. 16).

She went on to say, "I'm in a corner, I can't move. I don't know how to get my life back in order again. I'm a cripple." As Morrison (1998), suggests, "a lack of acceptance by self and others is…a central narcissistic quandary, related to the deeply felt shame of the narcissist" (p. 82). This quandary places the shamed self outside of known relational and contextual structures in the interpersonal field (Broucek, 1991), a significantly disabling position.

She thus described her experience of rape placing her in a lowly social position, her words serving to highlight my relatively high social position as researcher in contrast—a position wherein I could construct my own interpretation of her experience and pass judgement by subjecting her to the scrutiny of my own disciplinary surveillance. My own shame at this juncture in our interaction was significantly informed by a feeling of having forced Maria into this vulnerable position against her will, purely to cater for my own academic needs, or what is referred to in the literature as Guimaraes (Guimaraes, 2007) refers to as "holidaying on someone's misery." In response, I remained silent in order to distance myself from "other" authoritarian figures (in this case not only the police and the medical staff at the hospital, but the numerous white researchers attempting to represent the experiences of black women) who I imagined may have pushed her to expose her experience of being raped.

Maria went on to tell me the story of her first born child, who died on her third day of school at the age of six years old. She told me of how she has come to terms with this death, and how she has been blessed with another child: "Now God gave me another child, He gave me a second child. A Barbie child. That child is so perfect that when I cry, she wipes the tears away." Here there is a striking association of perfection with Barbie—an icon which arguably celebrates the feminine ideal, both in terms of her (white) bodily perfection as well as the middle-class lifestyle she represents. The image of the perfect child reverberates with the projective phantasies of perfection and omnipotence seen as the underside of shame (Hollway, 1989), a defensive identification with the admired Other (Morrison, 2014).

When she uttered these words, I couldn't help but consider the significance of it being this "Barbie child" who was able to alleviate her pain. The allusion resonated with images of the many attempts by powerful white supremacists propelled by humanitarian ideals to "fix" Black and Coloured people (Cushman, 2000). As Maria continued to recount this distressing narrative, she began to cry. She went on to say, "I don't want to be a cry-baby. Growing up, I was told, "Don't you cry, Grown-ups don't cry." At this stage I was made acutely aware of her inability to look me in the eyes. Her head hung low and she avoided my gaze, an indication as to her degree of shame at crying, at being so exposed and placed in such a vulnerable position (Exline & Winters, 1965).

Maria continued by saying, "because what happens if you cry, people slam your face against walls. They take away your dignity, they take away your pride." Her use of the ruthless metaphor of having one's face slammed against a wall, exemplifies her feelings of anger towards the people in her life who have shamed her. The metaphor served as a vivid, concrete example of what such severe feelings of shame might have felt like for her, particularly when one considers its violent depiction of the fragmentation of self.

Maria continued by asking me, "How can someone sleep with you without asking? How can someone just do that to you?" The fact that Maria chose to engage in the use of the second person participle "you" as opposed to the first person singular "I" seems significant on various levels. It was firstly indicative of her desire to remove herself as the subject of the narrative, or indeed as the shamed object of scrutiny. Secondly, it highlighted the salience of our shared gendered identity and thirdly served as an invitation to me to place myself in her position, of imagining myself having been raped by someone who has slept with *me* without asking.

Maria's questions elicited in me a feeling of shame related to my own internal thoughts of immunity to rape, a narcissistically imagined invincibility due to the fact of my own whiteness. Rape doesn't happen in my neighbourhood, specifically not to nice Jewish girls. What rose in the space between us was a recognition of these thoughts, which Maria was able later to expose in a way with her comments that having a nice car will not necessarily prevent me from experiencing similar trauma.

Maria's need for similarity and identification on the basis of a common gendered identity was fighting for space with my own defensive need for distance and difference. I was ashamed that my own silent belief in immunity had been revealed, and was therefore unable to answer her question. Here, my silence acted as an admission of defeat, of acknowledging the shame that I carried which was so deeply connected to notions of my whiteness having marked me as being immune to domestic abuse. Thus, shame in this particular instance served to create blocks in the interaction, potentially obscuring a more natural and spontaneous engagement.

Maria went on to tell me that there was no one else to be trusted "because people talk behind your back. But I do know that there are people out there who care about me." She recounted the ways in which she had been ostracised by many members of her community for being in an abusive relationship, marking her as inferior, unruly and deficient (Ussher, 2006). She told me of the many ways in which she was "not herself," "not the same person I used to be." The experience of being raped, and the subsequent severation of herself from her community had tainted her identity irrevocably, the shame serving to obstruct certain pathways to her social world. She began to cry, turning to me and saying:

> I used to be like…when I look at you, as a young person, we're about the same age and I think, I hope…I hope that you don't have to go through so much pain. It really hurts. I hope you don't have to. I hope nobody kicks you around. Because there's no mercy, no mercy for a poor woman. You can have the car, you can have nice clothes, but don't let anyone take that away from you…don't let anyone do it.

Her words marked a turning point in the interaction between us. I felt as though Maria had turned the tables in a way, positioning herself as the advice-dispensing expert holding significant power and authority, and myself in the position of the shamed and abused. I felt pinned down, trapped, "in a corner" in Maria's words. Her marking my nice clothes and my nice car spoke directly to the reality of my socio-political background, "responsible for the material disadvantage of the majority of South Africans" (Kometsi, 2001, p. 15).

Maria said that were she to go home, that she would not let her husband know that she had been at Thuthuzela, "I would say that I've been at someone else." This provided me with insight into the shame felt by herself, and presumably many other women who came to Thuthuzela Care Centre, at having to come to a hospital centre to receive medical and psychological help. I was only able to imagine the response of Maria's husband, and other important people in their lives, in discovering that she had been there. The sense of silence and secrecy surrounding the space in which we were located mirrored the shame, silence and secrecy which so commonly shroud women's experiences of abuse. Maria told me of how she had waited at the police station for hours the day before in order to get an interdict against her husband:

> And when I came home, I left all those papers at my friend's house because I know that he will take that away from me. They can take my clothes away so that I can't go anywhere. They did take my clothes away, I can't go anywhere. And sometimes they take my stuff,

> my money, my clothes…he always has his brother helping him. And he gave his brother a smile: 'Listen, take my wife's clothes' Take my personal stuff. And anyway, ummm…I went home.

As she said this, Maria pointed to the hair on her head, indicating how her husband had grabbed her hair whilst chasing her. I was immediately filled with a sense of rage at the cruelty of her husband's actions, unable to fully conceive of the sense of utter helplessness and humiliation I assumed must have arisen out of being so mercilessly objectified (Broucek, 1991). It would be possible to suggest that the shame evoked in Maria by such an encounter was significantly informed by a sense of having been objectified by her husband, that her literal nakedness spoke to a much deeper sense of being mercilessly exposed and publicly shamed. At this point in the interview, I was aware of the fact that Maria was not looking me in the eye, and that I too was feeling somewhat disabled by her narrative. My own shame resonated with hers. I was led by a strong desire not to put her any more into a corner, not to appear as yet another judging critic. I felt unable to respond to her shame in a way which was deservedly respectful and thus remained silent whilst she continued to recount her experiences:

> And then he pushed me down on the floor. That is why I had this bump here. It's almost like he forced me down. And he held a screwdriver, an orange screwdriver, against my throat and he said that the more I screamed he would just stab me in the throat. Because I was already so tired and mixed up. I couldn't push him away or anything. And he just forced himself on top of me….and then he had sex with me.

She relayed the narrative with her head down low, avoiding eye contact and evidently distressed. Her shame was palpable. My own silence at this point in the encounter was due in part to a feeling of being overwhelmed with the depth of her pain and feeling a need to limit my identification with her distress and vulnerability. This resonates with the observations of Burman and Chantler (2005) who, upon reflecting on their work researching domestic violence, noted that researchers themselves "might have often felt "shamed" because of their lack of engagement, and/or knowledge, or feelings of being overwhelmed both with issues of abuse and specifically in relation to minoritised women" (p. 390).

Maria then looked up, turned to me with some pride in her voice and said,

> And then I feel, for a second, that I wasn't going to have it. And then I said to myself, "No Maria, remember you have your interdict. You did something" And then, "Don't stop." I wanted to stop, I wanted to get out…This morning I just got up and I just left. I just said to him, 'You will never touch me again' And I left.

Horney (1991) relates pride directly to shame, "pride and self-hate belong inseparably together, they are two expressions of one process" (p. 109). From this perspective, Maria's pride in leaving her husband was an attempt to regain a sense of autonomy and control, a way in which she could reclaim the situation and alleviate her shame.

Maria went on to say:

> Thank you for listening, and I hope that you keep up with what you're doing. I know myself, I know that I can do it. God is all I have because God has put me here. I'm here for a special reason. And I hope that you will make something of your life. That's the kind of person I used to be, talking to people. I can't take your confidence away, I can never put you down.

Maria went on to explain that "because I'm Muslim, I don't have any rights towards the husband," further marking the socio-cultural and religious differences between us. She expressed a sense of powerlessness which she perceived as being inherent to her own identity as a Muslim wife, and all the duties and obligations which that seemed to entail for her. She felt that as a Muslim wife, "they take your money away…because if it's his T.V. it will stay his T.V." Thus, the acknowledgement of religious difference brought with it an acknowledgement of the socio-economic implications of that religious difference, an expression of the meaning which she attributed to her own cultural and religious heritage.

Maria went on to speak about her work as a hairdresser and the sense of autonomy her employment gave her: "I don't depend on him financially to support me. That's the one thing he can't take away from me. I can support myself … I've got my own tools." She explained that being financially independent was of huge significance for her in reclaiming a sense of pride in moments of the most acutely felt shame, because.

> When he hits me, all crumpled up, all hurt, he kicks me, he's injured me, he gives me the … I feel I have no hope. But I pick myself up and I blow someone's hair.

At this stage of our interaction, Maria seemed to have regained a stronger sense of control, as was exemplified in her subsequent comment that "from this point to that point, it's all up to me." She continued by comparing her own physical appearance to mine:

> You look nice with your pink jersey…you like a woman that's in control of her life. That's what I want to look like, not like you, or be you. I can't be you, you are you. I just want to be like you. Just be so confident. Just go somewhere. Just treat people with respect and be like a human being, not like a hoender been [chicken bone]. A hoender been you eat and then you throw it away.

It can be argued that in her construction of me as "confident" and "in control," Maria imbued me with a power which she referred to as having been "stripped away" from her by her husband. Morrison (2014) refers to the interaction between envy and shame, suggesting that "envy leads to the identification (via projective identification) with the powerful object" (p. 108). Seen from this perspective, her words mark me as the powerful object worthy of respect, which sits in stark contrast to Maria's own depiction of herself which positions her as a less-than-human chicken bone. Interestingly, the respect her words mark me as deserving, is intrinsically linked to my "nice pink jersey"—possibly signifying material wealth and thus indicating the link between socio-economic status and immunity from shame.

I replied by acknowledging how difficult it could be for people to talk about their experiences like she had done. The motivation for my words was two-fold. Firstly, in that moment I had become acutely aware my own shame in perceiving myself not to be the caring, ideal Other and of my subsequent desire to detract attention from the uncomfortable feeling of being idealised so overtly by placing her as the subject of our co-constructed narrative, a subject worthy of praise and admiration. Secondly, through the expression of my own admiration for Maria, I was attempting to acknowledge that the potentially shaming experience she may have been going through in having to recount the rape to me, thereby attempting to provide some alleviation from the shame pervading the intersubjective space we had created in order to replace it with a sense of pride and of accomplishment. This lead Maria to reflect on how ashamed she had initially felt in the beginning of our interaction:

> At the beginning you feel like, how can you cry to a stranger? I mean, I don't know you. I don't know where you come from. So I don't know if I can trust you. I don't know if I hate you! I expected you to chase me away, but you didn't….so I can just lift up my eyes.

This acknowledgement of the strangeness of the situation (and allusion to associated shame) served to further emphasise the marked differences in our identities, "where we came from." It is evident that Maria's sense of shame for having cried was significantly compounded by our distinct differences in identity—"how can you cry to a stranger?" A reflection on the degree of devaluation which occurred as a result of the abuse can be seen in Maria's following words:

> I don't know if I can ever look at people again but after the crying and tears, I can look up and I can say, 'You don't deserve it.' Nobody does, but when I look down I can't face a person. I feel that I can chase you and hurt you the way that I am hurt.

It is striking that the alleviation of such shame, expressed by Maria as a feeling of being able to look someone in the eye again, was only made possible "after the crying and the tears." Despite the fact that this was not the aim of our meeting, her words indicate that the journey which we had taken together had been a psychologically beneficial one for her. At this moment the shame resonated between us, facilitating a deeper level of engagement through trust. It is evident that to unpack the impact of shame is a complex process. Shame indeed served thus far in our meeting to hide, obscure and prevent, yet also to facilitate. The sense of hopefulness which dominated the tone of the narrative in that instance may indeed have served to metabolise and remediate some of the shame within the space which we had created, a way for both of us to have constructed a psychologically more coherent and bearable space in which to part.

Shame was certainly making itself felt, both in my own silence and in what Maria was chosing to share and to hide. In retrospect, my comparative silence throughout the interview may be attributed to both my own shame regarding my relatively privileged position in relation to Maria, but equally to a sense of the silence as an appropriate indication of respect for her in making space for her voice to be heard. Ironically, it is her voice which dominated the dialogue throughout our interaction, yet her story remains spoken through my own strong interpretive voice as author.

Our parting was strongly informed by a tension between the various manifestations of shame which had arisen in the space between us, and a need to counteract it through reclaiming a sense of pride and hopefulness for the future. This was reflected in

Maria's parting words, which spoke to a self which had been shattered by shame, and a presumably deeply-felt desire to reclaim a socially acceptable, coherent self:

> In my community, I am not a person that's weak. I'm a person that people look up to. If they could see me now, they'd never believe it. They would just shake their head. And I want that back. I want me back. The way I used to be.

Conclusion

Shame is an individualistic, subjective response to a uniquely constructed experience. However, certain categories of experience may predictably lead to acute feelings of shame connected to both its public and private triggers (Morrison, 1998). Rape is one such category. The shame which attaches itself so strongly to rape, framed the interaction between myself and Maria on numerous levels by opening up a veritable Pandora's box of shameful feelings. However, despite the rape itself having acted as a metaphorical magnifying glass underscoring the shame between us, it only served to highlight a pre-existing shame inevitably framing our interaction.

A consideration of shame is particularly pertinent given the renewed interest in a wider "reflexive turn" in the emotional politics of feminist research which considers the research interview as the point or moment of contact at which subjectivity is formed, negotiated and manoeuvred about (Burns, 2003; Jensen, 2008; Rice, 2009). Given the return of the body and emotions as a site for feminist and psychological inquiry, and a focus on the "emotional geographies" of the research relationship (Burman, 2003, 2006, 2014; Burman & Chantler, 2005), what is called for is a reflexivity that takes into account an acknowledgement of the ways in which we 'affect' the data collected and how our own (powerful) subject positions are implicated in research. As Flax (2004) argues, "content, interpretation, and mechanisms may be partially effects of particular relationships and contexts" (p. 914). From within this paradigm, vigilant ethical practice can be seen a function of the researcher's own self-awareness (Ponterotto, 2010).

I would echo this call to reflexivity by suggesting that qualitative researchers have an ethical responsibility to be aware of the role of shame within the research relationship, both in terms of its potentially traumatizing impact on research participants as well as on the way in which it necessarily impacts data. However, there is similarly a need to challenge discourses of transparency which invite researchers to subject themselves to the scrutiny of others through an incitement to confession. I would argue that such subjugation is, ironically, also motivated by the shame of our limitations as researchers. Indeed, particular perceptions of reflexivity are becoming the index for judgements regarding what is "good" and what is "bad" research (Finlay, 2002; Gray, 2008), leading to a retreat of the privileged researcher into inaccessible and insular "ivory tower angst" (Langhout, 2006, p. 272), "navel-gazing" or an "impasse" of research underlined by fears of (mis)representation (Sultana, 2007, p. 375). Rather, reflexivity should therefore be widened from a self-centred exercise to consider the critical relations which shape academic work (Doucet, 2008).

Shame is a powerfully communicating affect with potentially paralysing effects. Alleviating its noxious effects requires an awareness and acceptance of its ubiquitous presence in our lives, as well as the conditions in which shame plays an important part (Morrison, 1998). We therefore need to reflexively and consciously locate the shame within our racialised, gendered and institutionalised research relationships, and to wrestle with the implications this has for research validity, meaning-making and embodied subjectivity.

Shame is manifest on the micro-level of our daily interactions and cannot be separated from the complex matrix of gender, ethnicity and socio-economic class informing our public identities, which are so boldly reflected through our bodies. What did shame obscure, prevent or facilitate within this space between myself and research participants? What are the implications of this noxious affect for reflexive research, particularly with displaced populations? The above reflections intend not only to shed some light on the role of shame in the research relationship which unfolded but to consider the way in which it was intrinsically linked to the representations of our multiple and constantly shifting identities (Burman, 2006; Gray, 2008). It is clear that both the psychologist and the client's individual shame, as well as the shame which they co-construct within the intersubjective space, play an integral part of the therapeutic process. Similarly, reflexive qualitative research should also take into consideration the powerful impact of this affect within the research relationship.

References

Artz, L. (1999). *Violence against women in rural Southern Cape: Exploring access to justice within a feminist jurisprudence framework.* Doctoral dissertation, University of Cape Town,

Artz, L., & Smythe, D. (2008). *Should we consent?: Rape law reform in South Africa.* Cape Town: Juta and Company Ltd.

Bennett, J. (2000). The politics of writing. *Agenda, 16*(46), 3-12.

Bhimji, F. (2015). Collaborations and performative agency in refugee theater in Germany. *Journal of Immigrant and Refugee Studies, 1,* 1–23.

Broucek, F. J. (1991). *Shame and the self*. New York, NY: Guilford Press.

Buggenhagen, B. A. (2012). *Muslim Families in Global Senegal: Money takes care of shame.* Indiana: Indiana University Press.

Burman, E. (2003). From difference to intersectionality: Challenges and resources. *European Journal of Psychotherapy and Counselling, 6*(4), 293–308.

Burman, E. (2006). Emotions and reflexivity in feminised education action research. *Educational Action Research, 14*(3), 315–332.

Burman, E. (2014). Taking Women's voices: The psychological politics of feminisation 36. *The Discursive Turn in Social Psychology,171.*

Burman, E., & Chantler, K. (2005). Domestic violence and minoritisation: Legal and policy barriers facing minoritized women leaving violent relationships. *International Journal of Law and Psychiatry, 28*(1), 59–74.

Burns, M. (2003). I. Interviewing: Embodied communication. *Feminism and Psychology, 13*(2), 229–236.

Butler, J. (2003). Violence mourning politics. *Studies in Gender and Sexuality, 4*(1), 9–37.

Chisala, S. (2008). Rape and HIV/AIDS: Who's Protecting Whom? In L. Artz & D. Smythe (Eds.), *Should we consent* (pp. 52–71). Cape Town: Juta.

Cushman, P. (2000). White guilt, political activity, and the analyst: Commentary on paper by Neil Altman. *Psychoanalytic Dialogues, 10*(4), 607–618.

Dawes, A. E., & Donald, D. E. (1994). *Childhood and adversity: Psychological perspectives from South African research.* Cape Town: David Philip Publishers.

Doucet, A. (2008). "From her side of the gossamer wall (s)": Reflexivity and relational knowing. *Qualitative Sociology, 31*(1), 73–87.

Exline, R. V., & Winters, L. C. (1965). Affective relations and mutual glances in dyads In S. Tomkins & C. Izard (Eds.), *Affect cognition and personality* (pp. 319–351). New York: Springer.

Finlay, L. (2002). "Outing" the researcher: The provenance, process, and practice of reflexivity. *Qualitative Health Research, 12*(4), 531–545.

Flax, J. (2004). What is the subject? Review essay on psychoanalysis and feminism in postcolonial time. *Signs: Journal of Women in Culture and Society, 29*(3), 905–923.

Gavey, N. (2013). *Just sex?: The cultural scaffolding of rape.* London: Routledge.

Gilbert, P. (1997). The evolution of social attractiveness and its role in shame humiliation guilt and therapy. *British Journal of Medical Psychology, 70*(2), 113-14

Gilbert, P., & Andrews, B. (1998). *Shame: Interpersonal behavior psychopathology and culture.* London: Oxford University Press

Gilbert, P., & Miles, J. (2014). In *Body shame: Conceptualisation, research and treatment.* London: Routledge

Gkionakis, N. (2016). The refugee crisis in Greece: Training border security, police, volunteers and aid workers in psychological first aid. *Intervention, 14*(1), 73–79.

Goldsmith, R. E., Martin, C. G., & Smith, C. P. (2014). Systemic trauma. *Journal of Trauma and Dissociation, 15*(2), 117–132.

Gray, B. (2008). Putting emotion and reflexivity to work in researching migration. *Sociology, 42*(5), 935–952.

Guimaraes, E. (2007). I. Feminist research practice: Using conversation analysis to explore the researcher's interaction with participants. *Feminism Psychology, 17*(2), 149–161.

Harris, A. (2000). Haunted talk, healing action: Commentary on paper by Kimberlyn Leary. *Psychoanalytic Dialogues, 10*(4), 655–662.

Hecker, T., Braitmayer, L., & van Duijl, M. (2015). Global mental health and trauma exposure: The current evidence for the relationship between traumatic experiences and spirit possession. *European Journal of Psychotraumatology, 6*(1), 29126.

Herman, J. (1992). Complex PTSD: A syndrome in survivors of prolonged and repeated trauma. *Journal of Traumatic Stress, 5*(3), 377–391.

Hodges-Wu, J., & Zajicek-Farber, M. (2017). Addressing the Needs of Survivors of Torture: A Pilot Test of the Psychosocial Well-Being Index. *Journal of Immigrant and Refugee Studies, 15*(1), 71-89

Hollway, W. (1989). *Subjectivity and method in psychology: Gender meaning and science (gender and psychology).* Thousand Oaks, CA: Sage.

Horney, K. (1991). In *Neurosis and human growth: The struggle toward self-realization.* New York, NY: WW Norton and Company

Jensen, T. (2008). I. Speaking as a Mother': Notes on Becoming a Researcher and Not Getting onto Supernanny. *Feminism and Psychology, 18*(3), 384–388.

Kaufman, G. (1989). In *The psychology of shame: Theory and treatment of shame-based syndromes.* New York: Springer.

Kiguwa, P., & Hook, D. (2004). Feminist critical psychology in South Africa. *Self Community and Psychology, 7,* 1–38.

Kometsi, K. (2001). Multi-racial clinical settings and the counter-transferential feelings of a black trainee psychologist. *Psycho-Analytic Psychotherapy in South Africa, 9*(1), 11–21.

Koss, M. P. (2000). Blame, shame, and community: Justice responses to violence against women. *American Psychologist, 55*(11), 1332.

Kotsioni, I. (2016). *Rehabilitation for survivors of torture and other forms of ill-treatment in Athens, Greece—Responding to a protracted refugee crisis.* Paper presented at the 4th MSF Workshop on the thematic of torture : caring for the human beyond the torture Rome, Italy

Langhout, R. D. (2006). Where am I? Locating myself and its implications for collaborative research. *American Journal of Community Psychology, 37*(3–4), 267–274.

Lee, D. A., Scragg, P., & Turner, S. (2001). The role of shame and guilt in traumatic events: A clinical model of shame-based and guilt-based PTSD. *British Journal of Medical Psychology, 74*(4), 451–466.

Li, S. S., Liddell, B. J., & Nickerson, A. (2016). The relationship between post-migration stress and psychological disorders in refugees and asylum seekers. *Current Psychiatry Reports, 18*(9), 82.

Maercker, A., & Hecker, T. (2016). Broadening perspectives on trauma and recovery: A socio-interpersonal view of PTSD. *European Journal of Psychotraumatology, 7*, 293033

Maier, T., & Straub, M. (2011). "My head is like a bag full of rubbish": Concepts of illness and treatment expectations in traumatized migrants. *Qualitative Health Research, 21*(2), 233–248.

Mama, A. (2007). Is it ethical to study Africa? Preliminary thoughts on scholarship and freedom. *African Studies Review, 50*(1), 1–26.

Matos, M., & Pinto-Gouveia, J. (2010). Shame as a traumatic memory. *Clinical Psychology and Psychotherapy, 17*(4), 299–312.

Maw, A., Womersley, G., & O' Sullivan, M. . (2008). The psycho-social impact of rape and its implications for expert evidence in rape trials. In L. Artz & D. Smythe (Eds.), *Should we consent?: Rape law reform in South Africa* (pp. 121–143). Cape Town: Juta.

Mentinis, M. (2013). The entrepreneurial ethic and the spirit of psychotherapy: Depoliticisation, atomisation and social selection in the therapeutic culture of the 'crisis.' *European Journal of Psychotherapy and Counselling, 15*(4), 361–374.

Miller, S. (2013). In *The shame experience.* London: Routledge

Morrison, A. P. (1998). *The culture of shame.* New York, NY: Jason Aronson Incorporated.

Morrison, A. P. (2014). *Shame: The underside of narcissism.* London: Routledge.

Motsei, M. (2007). *The kanga and the kangaroo court: Reflections on the rape trial of Jacob Zuma.* Johannesburg: Spinifex Press.

Ponterotto, J. G. (2010). Qualitative research in multicultural psychology: Philosophical underpinnings, popular approaches, and ethical considerations. *Cultural Diversity and Ethnic Minority Psychology, 16*(4), 581.

Posel, D. (2005). The scandal of manhood:'Baby rape'and the politicization of sexual violence in post-apartheid South Africa. *Culture Health Sexuality, 7*(3), 239-252

Rice, C. (2009). Imagining the other? Ethical challenges of researching and writing women's embodied lives. *Feminism and Psychology, 19*(2), 245–266.

Salazar-Orvig, A., & Grossen, M. (2008). Le dialogisme dans l'entretien clinique. *Langage Et Société, 1*, 37–52.

Sanchez-Mazas, M., Efionayi-Mäder, D., Maggi, J., Achermann, C., Schaer, M., Escoda, R. I., & Coumou-Stants, F. (2011). *La Construction de l'Invisibilité: Suppression de l'Aide Sociale dans le Domaine de l'Asile.* Geneva: IES.

Sironi, F. (1999). *Bourreaux et victimes: psychologie de la torture*: Paris: Odile Jacob.

Steyn, E., & Steyn, J. (2008). Revictimisation of rape victims by the South African Police Service. J Acta Criminologica: African Journal of Criminology Victimology, 2008(Special Edition 1), 41-60.

Sultana, F. (2007). Reflexivity, positionality and participatory ethics: Negotiating fieldwork dilemmas in international research. *ACME: An international E-journal for Critical Geographies, 6*(3), 374–385.

Swartz, M. J. (1988). Shame culture and status among the Swahili of Mombasa. *Ethos, 16*(1), 21–51.

Torre, L. D. (2016). The Sans-Papiers. Blog writtein for the *National Centre of Competence in Research - The migration-mobility nexus* (Vol. 2016). Retrieved from https://blog.nccr-onthemove.ch/the-sans-papiers/?lang=fr on the 13 February 2020.

Turrini, G., Purgato, M., Ballette, F., Nosè, M., Ostuzzi, G., & Barbui, C. (2017). Common mental disorders in asylum seekers and refugees: Umbrella review of prevalence and intervention studies. *International Journal of Mental Health Systems, 11*(1), 51.

Ussher, J. M. (2006). *Managing the monstrous feminine: Regulating the reproductive body*. London: Psychology Press.

Viñar, M. N. (2005). La spécificité de la torture comme source de trauma. *Revue Française De Psychanalyse, 69*(4), 1205–1224.

Voulgaridou, M. G., Papadopoulos, R. K., & Tomaras, V. (2006). Working with refugee families in Greece: Systemic considerations. *Journal of Family Therapy, 28*(2), 200–220.

Wilson, J. P., & Drožđek, B. (2004). Broken spirits: The treatment of traumatized asylum seekers, refugees and war and torture victims. London: Routledge

Wilson, J. P., Droždek, B., & Turkovic, S. (2006). Posttraumatic shame and guilt. *Trauma Violence and Abuse, 7*(2), 122–141.

Womersley, G., & Arikut-Treece, Y. (2019). Collective trauma among displaced populations in Northern Iraq: A case study evaluating the therapeutic interventions of the free Yezidi foundation. *Intervention, 17*(1), 3.

Womersley, G., Maw, A., & Swartz, S. (2011). The construction of shame in Feminist reflexive practice and its manifestations in a research relationship. *Qualitative Inquiry, 17*(9), 876–886.

Womersley, G., Shroufi , A., Severy, N., & van Cutsem, G. (2018). Post-traumatic stress disorder among refugees following xenophobic attacks in Durban, South Africa. In Psychology Applications & Developments III (pp. 3-12). Lisbon: in Science Press.

Womersley, G., Kloetzer, L., Van den Bergh, R., Venables, E., Severy, N., Gkionakis, N., Popontopoulou, C., Kokkiniotis, M., & Zamatto, F. (2018). "My mind is not like before": Psychosocial rehabilitation of victims of torture and other forms of ill-treatment in Athens. *Torture Journal, 28*(2), 72-84.

Wong, Y., & Tsai, J. (2007). Cultural models of shame and guilt. In J. Tracy, R. Robins, & J. P. Tangney (Eds.), *The self-conscious emotions: Theory and research* (pp. 209–223). New York, NY: Guilford.

Chapter 10
Working with Cultural Mediators

While Western mental health professionals are working to provide assistance to displaced populations around the world, it is important to take a step back and consider the unique contexts in which this work is done (Nicolas et al., 2015). The collaboration between mental health professionals, and the refugees frequently faces language barriers, thereby rendering communication difficult during consultations, and increasing the risk of misunderstanding, misdiagnosis and errors in treatment (Gard, 2015; Hecker et al., 2015; IASC, 2015; Karageorge et al., 2016; Maier, 2006; Maier et al., 2010; Maier & Straub, 2011; Rechtman, 2000; Wang, 2012, 2016). In clinical contexts, the use of everyday expressions and proverbs or metaphors to express distress may be misunderstood as "resistance" to direct communication, or even misinterpreted as psychotic symptoms (Hassan et al., 2015). This is especially true in the context of trauma. Often, there are simply no words to describe the horror. For those affected by this trauma, "their problem is not the limits of memory but of language—the inadequacy of ordinary words to express all they have witnessed" (Kirmayer, 1996).

Trauma begets trauma. Exposure to trauma, itself connected to a breakdown in social connection, risks the individual being caught up in a vicious cycle where no addressee may be found, no language exists to form a coherent narrative whereby the event may itself be collectively represented and made sense of. Indeed, many authors highlight that trauma remains simply inaccessible to verbal recollection (Brewin, 2001; Brewin et al., 1996; Brewin et al., 2009), paradoxically the very recollection itself necessary for healing. Returning to the specific context of migration in particular, itself characterized by a rupture in connection to "home" (and all the social, cultural and linguistic connections that this implies)—the physical, social and political isolation so typically experienced by displaced populations serves only to feed monstrous feelings of invisibility and disconnectedness (Bhimji, 2015). In such a state, there is no coherently constituted individual: no memory, no clear defining of the Self and of the world in the safe confines of time—only speaking in embodied signs. Disaffiliation, de-culturation and de-linking both in terms of family and social ties similarly affects the internal capacity to make links between different events and

G. Theisen-Womersley, *Trauma and Resilience Among Displaced Populations*,
https://doi.org/10.1007/978-3-030-67712-1_10

moments in life. Without the container of home-as-it-was, there is little membrane to hold the symbolic (Goguikian Ratcliff, 2012).

According to Kirmayer (1996):

> Traumatic experience is not a story but a cascade of experiences, eruptions, crevasses, a sliding of tectonic plates that undergird the self. These disruptions then give rise to an effort to interpret and so to smooth, stabilize and recalibrate. The effect of these processes is to create a specific narrative landscape. This landscape must fit with (and so is governed by) folk models of memory" (p. 14)

Narratives of trauma, then, may be understood then as cultural constructions of personal and historical memory: What is registered is highly selective and thoroughly transformed by interpretation and semantic encoding at the moment of experience (Kirmayer, 1996). Particularly in cases where trauma has been prolonged, "the survivor may be left with large chunks of endured experience with no meaning, creating disquieting gaps and discontinuities in the experience of one's life history" (Sucharov et al., 2007).

For displaced populations—particularly asylum seekers and refugees who have arguably been exposed to a plethora of traumatic events both before, during and after migration – what is potentially lost is the ability to draw on meaningful socio-cultural symbolic resources to make sense of these events as well as the ear of a listening Other to whom and with whom the process of sense-making of traumatic experiences may be addressed. In order to illustrate the importance of social recognition as a "powerful element for healing in the aftermath of trauma," Larrabee and colleagues (2003) refer to the works of Agger (1994) wherein she details her journey through the narratives of forty refugee women. In documenting the healing process among these woman, Agger writes: "in this space they begin to experience the necessary turning point between the wordless nothing dominated by chaotic anxiety and the wordless fellowship given form and expression in the symbol of the circle and its healing ritual" (p. 126). What is interesting to note in her words is the particular value given to "fellowship" as crucial to the healing process of giving "form and expression" to a coherent narrative of trauma.

Telling a story of trauma or reliving it necessarily occurs in a larger dialogical matrix of narrative and social praxis (Kirmayer, 1996). The communicative function of language as a tool, concrete semiotic and symbolic devices provide the connections to an Other and to one's Self (Daiute & Lucić, 2010). As such, symbolic elements in socio-cultural practices are resources for repairing ruptures in intersubjectivity. Indeed, they are lenses through which experiences may be collectively and individually reflected upon. Within this paradigm, cultural representations are considered in their function not only as shared symbols but also as subjectively appropriated and emotionally invested representations (Sturm et al., 2010). It is therefore through language that one is able to constitute and actualize a coherent sense of Self. Furthermore, this can only take place in the context of 'interlocution' or 'addressivity'—towards and with an Other; there is evidently a continual dialogue between the person's inner world and the socio-cultural context in which internalized configurations or representations of traumatic events are processed (Lemma & Levy, 2004).

The critical issue here is that of the notion of reciprocity (Van Der Kolk, 2015) inherent to social recognition (Marková, 2016). For the transformation of traumatic memories into semiotic forms which connects it through language to its rightful place in time, the elaboration needs to be socially situated and intersubjectively acknowledged (Zittoun, 2014). This is because social resources provide a time orientation, and, consequently, a self-continuity between past and future (Kadianaki & Zittoun, 2014) necessary for the construction of a coherent narrative, and, ultimately, the Self.

The importance of culturally contextualised understanding of trauma when working with refugee populations in particular has been explored, among others, by cultural psychiatrists (Greene et al., 2017; Hassan et al., 2015; Kirmayer, 2001; Rousseau et al., 2014; Silove et al., 2017). In cultural psychiatry, cultural idioms of distress refer to common modes of expressing distress within a culture or community that may be used for a wide variety of problems, conditions, or concerns. Explanatory models refer to the ways that people explain and make sense of their symptoms or illness, in particular how they view causes, course and potential outcomes of their problem, including how their condition affects them and their social environment, and what they believe is appropriate treatment. These cultural psychologists therefore argue that what they refer to as culturally shaped or collective representations of trauma may provide a frame for the construction of narrations which informs the processing of traumatic experiences and the way in which the individual may be able to convey their distress in socially understandable and acceptable ways. This includes, for example, theories about the origins of pain and the possibilities of healing, conceptions of family and social bounds, religious or metaphysical conceptions of the world, ideologies, or positions in a field of political conflicts.

Various linguistically- and culturally-specific examples of different "idioms of distress" and "culture-bound syndromes" in response to trauma have been documented in the literature (Afana et al., 2010; Hinton & Lewis-Fernández, 2010; Jayawickreme et al., 2012; Lewis-Fernández & Kirmayer, 2019; Nicolas et al., 2015; Summerfield, 1996; Ventevogel et al., 2018). Ventevogel and colleagues (2018) for example, highlight the rise the rise of exorcistic healing in Burundi, whereby afflicted persons are assisted to enter into a peaceful and accepting relation with the possessing spirit. Cultural psychiatrists use these examples to show how such distinctive, historically-bound idioms illustrate communal reflections on the meaning behind experiences of violence, forced displacement, social exclusion, and humiliation. Behind all of the various idioms of distress found across the world, they argue, lie the social representations of trauma and ways in which it is defined and processed on a socio-cultural level:

> The idioms we have described borrow from everyday language to make sense of the impact of violence in a situation of protracted conflict. They do not represent discrete syndromes or sharply delimited categories. Rather, they are familiar ways of speaking about traumatic events that invoke specific networks of meaning. They serve to communicate to others within the community about the dimensions of suffering through language that references collective experience and that conveys assumptions about the expected bounds of behaviour, the likely course of distress, and outcome of clinical or social intervention. Generally, these cultural idioms of trauma are not diagnostic entities that require treatment but a vocabulary through which distress is expressed and social support mobilized (Afana et al., 2010)

This literature has emphasized the diversity of experiences of interventions for traumatized members of displaced populations across the globe (Goguikian Ratcliff, 2010; Goguikian Ratcliff & Suardi, 2006; Harvey, 2007; Diallo et al., 2009). Drožđek and Wilson (2007) offer examples: among Cambodian refugees who had suffered multiple life-threatening trauma during the Khmer Rouge regime, many who suffered from PTSD and depression understood their symptoms in light of their Buddhist beliefs in karma as a station in life, an incarnate level of being and fate where personal suffering is considered from a particular religious-cosmological perspective on the meaning of life. Among the Native American people, illness is thought to result from imbalance, loss of harmony and being dispirited with oneself due to a loss of vital connectedness. A common explanation for the 1988 Yuannan earthquake in China was that a "great dragon" was moving below the earth because he was angry with the people… these are all striking examples of how cultural variations in ways of life and social contexts shape experiences of trauma (Kirmayer & Ramstead, 2016).

In the specific context of migration in particular, itself characterized by disruptions in connection to "home" (and all the social, cultural and linguistic connections that this implies)—the physical, social and political isolation so typically experienced by asylum seekers upon arrival to host countries and often imposed by the state through legal requirements, serves only to feed monstrous feelings of invisibility and disconnectedness (Bhimji, 2015). In such a state, disaffiliation, de-culturation and de-linking both in terms of family and social ties similarly affects the internal capacity to make links between different events and moments in life through the use of words. Without the container of home-as-it-was, with no interlocutor to whom to address the distress (Womersley & Kloetzer, 2018), there is little membrane to hold the symbolic (Goguikian Ratcliff, 2012). In this context, the role of cultural interpretation and mediation, defined as a "negotiation process" (Wang, 2016, p. 141), is necessary in the healing process.

As the number of refugee mental health programs has increased in recent years, so has the use of cultural mediators, without whom clinical services for refugees could not be provided (Miller et al., 2005). Here, the term "cultural mediator" is purposefully used instead of "interpreter" in order to reflect the dynamic and complex nature of their work which often extends far beyond that of simple translation; they are often the mediators between the world of the health professional and that of the refugee. Wang (2012, 2016) points out the complex "subjectivity" of the cultural mediator: "he or she has to be interested in both the content and the form of the discussion, and gives attention to interpersonal relationships" (Wang, 2016, p.141). As noted by Resera and colleagues (2015), this comes with challenges surrounding the need to be precise, emotionally detached, firm, to know how to behave in relation to a specific culture, and being neutral and impartial.

This is particularly true in the context of mental health were words are the tools of the professional. Indeed, the literature highlights mental health as being the most demanding context for cultural mediators compared to their work with other professionals. Here, cultural mediators have been shown to have to negotiate multiple positions including that of a cultural broker, community organizer and even a directly implicated co-therapist (Goguikian Ratcliff et al., 2017; Miller et al., 2005; Mitschke et al., 2017; Pestre & Benslama, 2011; Resera et al., 2015; Wang, 2012, 2016). Miller and colleagues (2005) go even further in arguing that not only is mental health a unique context for cultural mediation among refugee populations, but that this is particularly true for victims of torture and other political refugees. They identify two factors: (1) the prevalence of exposure to extreme violence and deprivation and the subsequent development of severe and persistent psychological trauma and (2) the experience of multiple losses—of social networks, personal possessions, valued social roles, and environmental mastery. In these traumatic contexts in particular, the challenge of translation goes beyond a literal transcription from one language to another (Pestre & Benslama, 2011). As stated by Maqueda (2005):

> the presence of an interpreter enables to calm fantasies of infringement and involvement of one culture by another. The interpreter is a transitional space both to the migrant and the caregiver. He or she symbolizes the comparable and different to both of them. He or she occupies the position of cultural mediator clarifying the understatements, implicit information in any culture. He or she uses singular words, embodying the particular story of the individual in a background group. The interpreter symbolizes the possible development between both contexts: cultural but also temporal, between a before and an after. He or she represents the cultural weaving, thereby enabling to adapt oneself without quite being another (p. 3)

So how are the different representations and understandings of trauma managed in this space? How are they negotiated among the various actors (refugees, psychologists, cultural mediators) in the complex context of psychotherapy in humanitarian settings? To explore this question, I present the case study of cultural mediators working in a centre for refugee victims of torture in Athens, Greece.

Case Study: Cultural Mediation Among Victims of Torture in Athens

Since the height of the migration reception crisis that shook the continent in 2015–2016, Greece remains one of first sanctuary ports in Europe. In a country exposed to a serious financial crisis, fewer resources are available to ensure quality mental health services to refugees (Gkionakis, 2016). Several refugees who enter Greece through the Aegean Sea remain blocked on Greek islands, far from the adequate medical care they could receive in Athens. Others continue their way illegally through the Balkan route and find themselves trapped in limbo, unable to make their asylum application. The asylum system is often long and opaque, and the numerous obstacles to the access of basic services in Athens, and throughout the country add to the day-to-day difficulties (Kotsioni, 2016).

In order to explore this diversity of perspectives on trauma, I present the analyses of 12 months of fieldwork in an NGO-run centre for refugee victims of torture in Athens, Greece. Ten refugee victims of torture (9 men and 1 woman) treated in the clinic were identified by the medical staff to participate in this research. Participation was entirely voluntary. Exclusion criteria included psychosis, serious dissociative symptoms, and acute suicidality. The over-representation of male participants reflects to some extent the demography of the beneficiaries of the centre, of whom 80% are men. I carried out five in-depth qualitative interviews with each of them throughout this one-year period. Interviews with refugees were focused on symptoms of PTSD, subjective experiences and explanatory models of trauma, and the integration process within Greece. Interviews were conducted in English or French without a translator.

To further a sociocultural understanding of trauma within this particular context, I conducted 36 interviews with health professionals working with refugees victims of torture in various humanitarian organizations across Athens, as well as with seven cultural mediators,[1] speaking French, Arab and Farsi, and working with patients diagnosed with the PTSD These seven cultural mediators were all full-time employees of the project who had been recruited on the basis of their language skills, and work experience with NGOs. They consisted of 3 French-speaking women, and 4 Arab/Farsi men respectively, aged 22 to 65. Like several other humanitarian actors, the centre officially uses the term "cultural mediator" instead of "translator"—in order to highlight the importance of their work as mediating between cultural norms—a job which goes far beyond a simple translation *verbatim.* The other two French-speaking mediators were retired Greeks locals, and the third was a young Congolese of 23 years living in Athens for three years on a student visa. One of the Arab mediators was an Egyptian migrant of 40 years living in Greece for four years, while the three others were themselves refugees recently arrived in the country. No mediator had a translation or cultural mediation certificate or diploma.

Qualitative in-depth interviews were also carried out with 21 community representatives and leaders of various refugee associations around Athens in order better to understand the perspectives, and explanatory models that exist in their respective communities at a sociocultural level. Furthermore, I engaged in three-months of participant observation, which included attending daily staff meetings as well as facilitating sessions and workshops with beneficiaries of the project.

In this case study, I particularly focus on the accounts of cultural mediators, by taking into account their work as revealing existing tensions between representations of trauma among health professionals and those of their patients. The analysis will focus on three themes: (1) the negotiation of the cultural mediators' complex roles, (2) alliances with health professionals, and (3) working with "culturally inexperienced" health professionals.

Through analyzing cultural mediation in this context, I explore the role of culture in the care of refugees diagnosed as having mental disorders, and the implications of these diagnoses for treatment, issues that pose significant challenges to health professionals regarding the relationship between trauma, culture, and subjectivity (Rechtman, 2000).

---

[1] We are using the term "cultural mediator" and "community interpreter' in order to respect the official title used in this project.

Cultural Mediators as Negotiating Different Interpretations of Trauma

Interviews with cultural mediators highlight three main themes: (a) the difficulty of positioning their translation between *verbatim* accuracy and interpretation; (b) the complexity of the alliance process between emotional proximity with refugees, and allegiance to a professional mental health approach; (c) the challenge of working with "culturally incompetent" health professionals.

Translation: Accuracy Versus Interpretation

In regards to experiences with the PTSD diagnosis in particular, none of the cultural mediators referred spontaneously to the diagnosis of trauma. At the request of the researcher, all seven expressed doubts in regard to (i) the exact meaning of the diagnosis, as well as (ii) the usefulness of this diagnosis to the refugee population. For instance, one cultural mediator explains:

> KI28: they don't have such stress because they were used to the joy of living. We can have it but they don't. They knew how to hustle on a daily basis. These are habits and traditions. You cannot find this kind of depression there.

It should be noted that the individual life history of each cultural mediator has a substantial impact on their position. This particular cultural mediator is Greek—as alluded to in her distinction between "we" (culturally the same, we can experience with the PTSD), and "them" (others, culturally different, they cannot). The fact that no cultural mediator had previous training in the fields of medicine or psychology may explain, to an extent, their doubts regarding the use and exact meaning of the PTSD Many of them seem to prefer referring questions of PTSD to the medical doctor or psychologist, even during our interviews with them.

Several cultural mediators are confronted to the following dilemma: on the one hand, they are asked simply to provide a literal translation of what is said, and in the other hand, they have to play the role of a more implicated and nuanced mediator. As one participant states:

> KI4 : My role consist of just translating words or images, the message they want to transmit to the psychologist in regard to their trauma, uh, in the past. I try to do my best to use the interpretation and not words.

Despite his initial affirmation that his role is "just to translate words," it is clear that he sees the need to broaden this function by offering something more complex than a simple translation ("interpretation and not only words"). This ambiguity is also reflected in the opinion of another cultural mediator:

> KI39: You try to transmit the same messages as the psychologist [...] but at the same time, you also do the mediation of terms.

Most often, discussions in this area focus on accuracy (where cultural mediators who are considered to be the most professional are those who can translate the words with technical precision) versus mediation (where cultural mediators who are considered to be more professionals are those who manage better to grasp the cultural nuances). To be understood by both parties, the cultural mediator is supposed to adapt his position and translation to a situation with flexibility, and in a dynamic way. As one participant states, "we are facilitating an appointment, you switch your role in a continuous way to adapt yourself to millions of cultural barriers." As another one underscored, "I cannot behave like a machine, a Google translation." Indeed, a complex system of interpersonal dynamics seems to play out in the triad between psychologist, cultural mediator and refugee where the cultural mediators are tasked with taking on an active role—that of a co-therapist:

> KI5 : It's not easy, translating for psychology because the person have many mental problems, many psychological problems. First, I want that he feels safe with me, the interpreter, not with the psychologist. Because he has to trust me. When I feel that he doesn't trust me, I can't work. I can't make an appointment with the person. Because for me, especially if he shares, he wants to talk with the person, he's not scared to talk. First of all, with this way I create the, the, trust between the interpreter and the patient to not feel uncomfortable.

This active role of co-therapist similarly involved an emotional investment in the well-being of the refugee beneficiaries:

> KI26: I'm touched, I really like it because I think that I'm offering something to these people. I think I'm helping them in this way to externalize their feelings, to be able to express themselves, and mostly what they have in themselves And obviously, I'm touched, and I get attached. I don't show it, but during the consultation I want to know what happened in their life, about their experiences

What is noteworthy in the above statement is the clear active voice, and use of the first person "I." There is no mention of the role of the therapist themselves, it is the cultural mediator who sees herself as being the one to facilitate the psychotherapeutic process. Indeed, all of the cultural mediators interviewed referred to the idea that they felt closer to the refugee beneficiaries than the health professionals:

> KI4: Always, the interpreter is the person who he is understanding more deeply the patient who has any kind of problem because the interpreter is the person that he is native of this language and maybe he's more closer because he's closest with, ah, things that happened to the country. Ah, but, ummm, I try even to explain even when we finish the session to explain why, why we say that, just to have message. Because the patient has in his mind always the message that 'you don't understand me, the doctor don't understand what's going on'
>
> KI5: You have to see every person in the room, the psychologist, the interpreter and the person. Many times, the person will not see the psychologist, many times. Because they all see me, talk with me. Every time they say, 'I don't see, I want to see you, the interpreter.' They never want to see the psychologist. You'll ask something and he'll say this one, « you understand what happened ». You see, you ask about something that happened, they say, « N [cultural mediator], N, I have this problem. »
>
> KI39: I will see [the sessions in] exactly the same way as a psychologist.

For some cultural mediators, this active role was not of their own choosing but which they felt was imposed upon by refugee beneficiaries seeking assistance who turned to the cultural mediators, rather than the health professionals, as their primary source of aid:

> KI29: A lot of people from our country, when they come here, when I'm the cultural mediator, the interpreter, they think I am the best one who decide about everything. A lot of people, they are thinking, I am the first one, I am the manager, I am the psychologist, I am the doctor, and I am everyone here.

To defend against being placed in this often unwanted position of being an active co-therapist and, furthermore, even having to assume the role of "everyone here" with the responsibility for "everything," many explained the need to clarify their roles and keep within the limits of their job descriptions:

> KI29: We have to explain them, « this is not my decision to give you ». Because I am cultural mediator, [I cannot] give her money, pharmacy, medicine, accommodation, everything. We must be clear for the first time [...] they are thinking that 'R [himself, the cultural mediator] is here, and he will decide about everything.

> KI39: The major thing for me is to keep neutrality. My primary role is just to facilitate appointments I'm not a psychologist. I am not a medical doctor or a physiotherapist to put things in my own way.

The strategy of maintaining neutrality and clarifying the limitations of their role implies deferring to the expert position of the health professional. Straddled between two worlds, that of the health professional and that of the refugee beneficiary, many drew on a "us" versus "them!" discourse—whereby as cultural mediators, they were positioned as a member of the health professional team, in other words in alliance with the health professionals and not the refugee beneficiary.

A Game of Alliances Between Refugees and Health Professionals

Alliances done in the triadic interaction are complex. Cultural mediators are by definition in both "camps"—at times, they themselves are often from the same migrant population, as well as being members of the professional team. These alliances can influence the quality of the collaboration. As cultural mediators adapt intelligently to the context, the quality of their interventions are often most visible in field of mental health (Goguikian Ratcliff et al., 2017).

Working as an intermediary between health professionals (especially mental health professionals), refugees who may have never met a psychologist has its challenges. Sometimes, being identified as "agents of the medical system" (Leanza, 2011), cultural mediators are often employed to serve as "defenders" of mental health services, explaining for instance, the role of the psychologist, and the advantages that the refugee may have from psychotherapeutic sessions:

> KI25: Furthermore, they explain to them that the work of the psychologist is to discuss with someone who is in danger. And someone who is going through tough moments, they advise

him of her to talk with the psychologist. When you talk to the psychologist, he or she listens to you, he or she liberates you, and you tell your story and what hurts you. When you are talking, it is just as if you are narrating a normal story. It won't hurt you anymore. It is a story that won't affect your health anymore.

One cultural mediator, for example, describes being proud of assisting the psychologist in convincing refugee beneficiaries to attend psychotherapeutic sessions. This was because, according to her,

KI26: With sessions, [...] the psychologist succeeds in achieving what she or he wants

Her words imply that the therapeutic sessions are what the psychologist wanted and is searching to obtain. It is their goal, not necessarily that of the refugee beneficiary. She further continued to give a specific case as an example:

KI28: We succeeded to convince her to see a psychologist. She didn't want because she was ashamed. You can quite understand because the mentality is different. This is a lady who is not educated. She grew in a very strict and closed society. On one hand, her only worry was not to remain pregnant and to keep to herself. Finally, we succeeded because she started to see a psychologist in the evening, and she had a four-month baby with her. It was really successful […]. When we convinced her to go and see a psychologist, it was really a party for us.

In this example, the words "it was really a party for us" allude to the fact that managing to convince a refugee to see the psychologist was a cause for celebration, a party for the whole team including the cultural mediator herself. As such, it is part of the role of the cultural mediators to convince the refugee population about the "truth" of western psychiatric knowledge and the benefits of seeing a psychologist, as similarly reflected in the words of one cultural mediator who gave another example of such a case:

KI4 I understand the guy, that he was not having knowledge before and when he get understanding and the peadopsychiatrist explained his problem or his story or his trauma with another way, of explaining, by drawing, by feelings, then he understand that, 'yeah,this is the truth.'

There is an implicit acceptance of the "truth" in what says the psychologist, and through an explanatory process, the professionals manage to convince the refugee of this truth as well. It is also noteworthy that, despite the apparent alliance with health professionals regarding the "truth" of western psychiatric knowledge, the words below also underscore the complexity of the position: the sentence "I understand the guy" may indicate the fact that cultural mediators are seeing both the perspective of the refugee and that of the medical doctor. Such an understanding of these different perspectives is not without challenges, and is often a source of responsibility for cultural mediators who, according to Wang (2016), defines their work as a "negotiation process, eased by a third party not exercising the power of decision, whose purpose is to allow the parties concerned to solve a conflict situation or a relationship" (p. 141).

Working with Health Professionals Perceived as "Culturally Inexperienced"

In negotiating the variety of complex roles, including that of an active co-therapist in alliance with the health professionals, many cultural mediators also alluded to the challenges of working with health professionals who they perceived as lacking a certain cultural proficiency. This was a specific challenge manifesting within the therapeutic triad between refugee beneficiary, health professionals and the cultural mediators who found themselves between the two.

In some cases, the cultural mediators took on a more "experienced" role as a "cultural *passeur*" (Leanza, 2011) in relation to the health professional, who needed to be "taught" by the cultural mediator, in a manner of speaking, of the cultural norms relating to specific refugee populations:

> KI4: For me, as an experience, the psychologist, okay especially the psychologist, I see that they have difficulties to, in communication between the patients. This is, I think, especially for somebody who doesn't know about the cultural, where does this guy from, what his culture, how he think, how he look at you, how he look at things, of course this is not like as we look, as we think, so, I try to a little bit to give some tips to colleagues that you can use it or you can try some things that will, where he comes from, some words or some things, okay try, that helps the person to feel comfortable and that this guy, he knows about me and my culture and I can trust him, I can be comfortable.
>
> KI23: For the psychologist this is a little bit hard, because this culture doesn't understand psychology.
>
> KI29: I saw in my experience life, many psychologists who are not experienced. And she says, she asks the patient, it was too directly, it was too directly. And he was afraid to say correct. But this is my job, this is my job like interpreter. I cannot say other words. For example, you are psychologist and you ask her if she had in her country sexual violence, yeah? You cannot ask her like directly. But you find a way.

As such, the cultural misunderstandings were perceived as emanating not only from the side of the refugee beneficiary, possibly unused to seeing a psychologist, but also from the health professionals, possibly unused to working with refugee populations:

> KI39: Sometimes there are cultural barriers - not only from the client's side but also from the professional side.

This discrepancy in cultural knowledge and *savoir-faire* seemed to inverse an expected hierarchy within the power dynamics. It is often the cultural mediators, not the health professionals, who position themselves in the role of the expert:

> KI39: If a psychologist is trying to help them to understand their problems then [...] some of them culturally is not appropriate to the patients and some of their suggestions. Even describing things in a particular way that is not appropriate. If I just come with this message exactly as it is to the patient then it harms the trust in the therapeutic relationship that wasn't there with. It would decrease the efficiency and quality of the session.

Therefore, there appears to be a significant sense of responsibility felt by the cultural mediators to assume the role of "expert" in relation to cultural knowledge of refugee populations. This lead them to assume an active role in facilitating sessions, in mediating between the health professional and the refugee beneficiary, when they felt it was necessary to do so. Thus, mediating between refugees and western medical professionals, psychologist and traumatized patient, it is clear that the role of cultural mediators extend far beyond that of a simple translation. It is a complex task requiring a myriad of subtle negotiations of power. A professional dilemma exists between the fact of wanting more responsibilities in sessions with professionals who are often culturally inexperienced, and on the contrary, refusing this responsibility which is not supposed to be theirs. This research work reveals the complex challenges and tensions surrounding the diagnosis and the implementation of mental health interventions.

Conclusion

Many refugees have lived through horrors beyond description, indeed beyond words in any language. In this context, humanitarian organisations are engaging in the important work of implementing mental health interventions for communities whose lives have been devastated by a multitude of traumas. Here, the role of cultural mediators is an essential one. Indeed, as stated by Summerfield (2006), the challenges they face are "not…of translation between languages but of translation between worlds" (p. 255). Within this context, they are active co-therapists, advocates of mental health and experts assisting health professionals to explore the culturally-informed psychic worlds of traumatized refugees.

What further characterizes the position of the cultural mediator is the emotional investment in the relationship on the part of refugees. Working in a neutral and impartial way in this context necessites taking a detached professional and inter-professional position (in their work in and of itself as well as in the collaboration between health professionals and cultural mediators) which takes into account the substantial emotional impact of the work, rather than denying it. The construction of this position a significant, collective and ongoing task. To ignore these factors runs the risk of ignoring (or worse, denigrating) local support systems, pathologizing and stigmatizing individuals, and usurping resources from social and structural interventions (Nicolas et al., 2015). In the face of extreme adversity, people often turn to collective cultural systems of knowledge, values and coping strategies to make meaning in the face of adversity. In this context, providing culturally safe environments, including competent cultural mediators and culturally adapted tools for respectful dialogue and collaborative work, is essential to assist displaced populations in constructing meaning from suffering and finding adaptive strategies to cope with their situation (Hassan et al., 2015).

References

Afana, A.-H., Pedersen, D., Rønsbo, H., & Kirmayer, L. J. (2010). Endurance is to be shown at the first blow: Social representations and reactions to traumatic experiences in the Gaza Strip. *Traumatology: An International Journal, 16*(4), 73–84.

Agger, I. (1994). The Blue room. Trauma and testimony among refugee women. A psycho-social exploration. *Resources for Feminist Research, 24*(1/2), 40.

Bhimji, F. (2015). Collaborations and performative agency in refugee theater in Germany. *Journal of Immigrant & Refugee Studies, 1,* 1–23.

Brewin, C. R. (2001). A cognitive neuroscience account of posttraumatic stress disorder and its treatment. *Behaviour Research and Therapy, 39*(4), 373–393.

Brewin, C. R., Dalgleish, T., & Joseph, S. (1996). A dual representation theory of posttraumatic stress disorder. *Psychological Review, 103*(4), 670–686.

Brewin, C. R., Lanius, R. A., Novac, A., Schnyder, U., & Galea, S. (2009). Reformulating PTSD for DSM-V: Life after criterion A. *Journal of Traumatic Stress, 22*(5), 366–373.

Daiute, C., & Lucić, L. (2010). Situated cultural development among youth separated by war. *International Journal of Intercultural Relations, 34*(6), 615–628.

Drožđek, B., & Wilson, J. P. (2007). *Voices of trauma: Treating psychological trauma across cultures.* New York, NY: Springer.

Gard, C. (2015). Migration et santé mentale: Quelques enjeux politiques et cliniques de la psychiatrie contemporaine. *L'information Psychiatrique, 91,* 111–117.

IASC. (2015). *Inter-Agency Standing Committee (IASC) reference group for mental health and psychosocial support in emergency settings: Guidelines on mental health and psychosocial support in emergency settings.* Geneva: Inter-Agency Standing Committee.

Gkionakis, N. (2016). The refugee crisis in Greece: Training border security, police, volunteers and aid workers in psychological first aid. *Intervention, 14*(1), 73–79.

Goguikian Ratcliff, B. (2010). Différences culturelles et exercice de la psychothérapie avec un interprète. In G. Thésée, N. Carignan, & P. Carr (Eds.), *Les faces cachées de l'interculturel: De la Rencontre des Porteurs de Cultures* (pp. 78–96). Paris, France: L'Harmattan.

Goguikian Ratcliff, B. (2012). Repenser les liens entre migration, exil et traumatisme. *(Re)penser l'Exil, 1,* 1–8.

Goguikian Ratcliff, B., & Suardi, F. (2006). L'interprète dans une consultation thérapeutique: Conceptions de son rôle et difficultés éprouvées. *Psychothérapies, 26*(1), 37–49.

Goguikian Ratcliff, B., Pereira Kraft, C., & Fierro, I. (2017). L'évaluation de la collaboration entre interprètes et intervenants primaires dans différents services publics. *Dragoman, Journal of Translation Studies, 5*(7), 164–189.

Greene, M. C., Jordans, M. J., Kohrt, B. A., Ventevogel, P., Kirmayer, L. J., Hassan, G., et al. (2017). Addressing culture and context in humanitarian response: Preparing desk reviews to inform mental health and psychosocial support. *Conflict and Health, 11*(1), 21.

Harvey, M. R. (2007). Towards an ecological understanding of resilience in trauma survivors: Implications for theory, research, and practice. *Journal of Aggression, Maltreatment and Trauma, 14*(1–2), 9–32.

Hassan, G., Kirmayer, L. J., Mekki-Berrada, A., Quosh, C., El Chammay, R., Deville-Stoetzel, J., & Coutts, A. (2015). *Culture, context and the mental health and psychosocial wellbeing of Syrians: A review for mental health and psychosocial support staff working with Syrians affected by armed conflict* (pp. 14–15). Geneva: UNHCR.

Hecker, T., Braitmayer, L., & van Duijl, M. (2015). Global mental health and trauma exposure: The current evidence for the relationship between traumatic experiences and spirit possession. *European Journal of Psychotraumatology, 6*(1), 29126.

Hinton, D. E., & Lewis-Fernández, R. (2010). Idioms of distress among trauma survivors: Subtypes and clinical utility. *Culture, Medicine, and Psychiatry, 34*(2), 209–218.

Jayawickreme, N., Jayawickreme, E., Atanasov, P., Goonasekera, M. A., & Foa, E. B. (2012). Are culturally specific measures of trauma-related anxiety and depression needed? The case of Sri Lanka. *Psychological Assessment, 24*(4), 791.

Kadianaki, I., & Zittoun, T. (2014). Catalysts and regulators of psychological change in the context of immigration ruptures. In K. R. Cabell & J. Valsiner (Eds.), *The Catalyzing Mind* (pp. 191–207). New York, NY: Springer.

Karageorge, A., Rhodes, P., Gray, R., & Papadopoulos, R. (2016). Refugee and staff experiences of psychotherapeutic services: A qualitative systematic review. *Intervention, 15*(1), 51–69.

Kirmayer, L. J. (1996). Landscapes of memory: Trauma, narrative and dissociation. In P. Antze & M. Lambek (Eds.), *Tense past: Cultural essays on memory and trauma* (pp. 173–198). London: Routledge.

Kirmayer, L. J. (2001). Cultural variations in the clinical presentation of depression and anxiety: Implications for diagnosis and treatment. *Journal of Clinical Psychiatry, 62,* 22–30.

Kirmayer, L. J., & Ramstead, M. J. (2016). Embodiment and Enactment in Cultural Psychiatry. In C. Durt, T. Fuchs, & C. Tewes (Eds.), *Embodiment, enaction, and culture: Investigating the constitution of the shared world* (pp. 397–422). Cambridge, MA: MIT.

Kotsioni, I. (2016). *Rehabilitation for survivors of torture and other forms of ill-treatment in Athens, Greece—Responding to a protracted refugee crisis.* Paper presented at the 4th MSF Workshop on the thematic of torture: Caring for the human beyond the torture.

Larrabee, M. J., Weine, S., & Woolcott, P. (2003). "The wordless nothing": Narratives of trauma and extremity. *Human Studies, 26*(3), 353-382.

Leanza, Y. R. (2011). *Exercer la pédiatrie en contexte multiculturel: Une approche complémentariste du rapport institutionnalisé à l'autre.* Georg éditeur.

Lemma, A., & Levy, S. (2004). *The impact of trauma on the psyche: Internal and external processes.* London: Whurr Publishers.

Lewis-Fernández, R., & Kirmayer, L. J. (2019). Cultural concepts of distress and psychiatric disorders: Understanding symptom experience and expression in context. *Transcultural Psychiatry, 56*(4), 786–803.

Maier, T. (2006). Procédure d'asile et rapports médicaux. *Bulletin des médecins suisses| Schweizerische Ärztezeitung| Bollettino dei medici svizzeri, 87,* 25.

Maier, T., & Straub, M. (2011). "My head is like a bag full of rubbish": Concepts of illness and treatment expectations in traumatized migrants. *Qualitative Health Research, 21*(2), 233–248.

Maier, T., Schmidt, M., & Mueller, J. (2010). Mental health and healthcare utilization in adult asylum seekers. *Swiss Medical Weekly, 140,* w13110.

Maqueda, F. (2005). L'accès aux soins psychiques pour les demandeurs d'asile: Position soignante, position citoyenne. *L'Autre, 6*(1), 111–123.

Marková, I. (2016). *The dialogical mind: Common sense and ethics.* Cambridge: Cambridge University Press.

Miller, K. E., Martell, Z. L., Pazdirek, L., Caruth, M., & Lopez, D. (2005). The role of interpreters in psychotherapy with refugees: An exploratory study. *American Journal of Orthopsychiatry, 75*(1), 27.

Mitschke, D. B., Praetorius, R. T., Kelly, D. R., Small, E., & Kim, Y. K. (2017). Listening to refugees: How traditional mental health interventions may miss the mark. *International Social Work, 60*(3), 588–600.

Nicolas, G., Wheatley, A., & Guillaume, C. (2015). Does one trauma fit all? Exploring the relevance of PTSD across cultures. *International Journal of Culture and Mental Health, 8*(1), 34–45.

Pestre, E., & Benslama, F. (2011). Traduction et traumatisme. *Recherches En Psychanalyse, 1,* 18–28.

Rechtman, R. (2000). Stories of trauma and idioms of distress: From cultural narratives to clinical assessment. *Transcultural Psychiatry, 37*(3), 403–415.

Resera, E., Tribe, R., & Lane, P. (2015). Interpreting in mental health, roles and dynamics in practice. *International Journal of Culture and Mental Health, 8*(2), 192–206.

Rousseau, C., Guzder, J., Santhanam-Martin, R., & de la Aldea, E. (2014). Trauma, culture, and clinical work: The "House of Stories" as a pedagogical approach to transcultural training. *Traumatology: An International Journal, 20*(3), 191–198.

Silove, D., Ventevogel, P., & Rees, S. (2017). The contemporary refugee crisis: An overview of mental health challenges. *World Psychiatry, 16*(2), 130–139.

Sturm, G., Baubet, T., & Moro, M. R. (2010). Culture, trauma, and subjectivity: The French ethnopsychoanalytic approach. *Traumatology, 16*(4), 27–38.

Sucharov, M. S., Buirski, P., & Kottler, A. (2007). Kafka's window and Kohut's mirror: A dialogic journey to the center of traumatic worlds. In P. Buirski & A. Kottler (Eds.), *New developments in self psychology practice* (pp. 193–206). Lanham: Jason Aranson.

Summerfield, D. (1996). *L'impact de la Guerre et des Atrocités sur les Populations Civiles: Principes Fondamentaux pour les Interventions des ONG et une Analyse Critique des Projets sur le Traumatisme Psychosocial.* London: Overseas Development Institute.

Summerfield, D. (2006). Survivors of the tsunami: Dealing with disaster. *Psychiatry, 5*(7), 255–256.

Sylla Diallo, T., Dembele, D. S., Ndiaye, S. M., & Konare, K. (2009). Femmes d'émigrés et conjugopathie au Senegal: Une souffrance banalisée. *Psychopathologie Africaine, 35*(1), 25–36.

Van Der Kolk, B. (2015). *The body keeps the score: Brain, mind, and body in the healing of trauma.* Penguin Books.

Ventevogel, P., Niyonkuru, J., Ndayisaba, A., Reis, R., & de Jong, J. T. (2018). Change and continuity in Burundian divinatory healing. *Journal of Eastern African Studies, 12*(1), 22–43.

Wang, S. (2012). Analyses sociologiques des pratiques de l'interprétariat-médiation en pédopsychiatrie: l'exemple des familles d'origine chinoise à Paris. *Enfances & Psy, 3,* 136–145.

Wang, S. (2016). Aidez-nous à comprendre vos Chinois! *Genèses, 4,* 141–156.

Womersley, G., & Kloetzer, L. (2018). Being through doing: The self-immolation of an Asylum seeker in Switzerland. *Frontiers in Psychiatry, 9,* 110.

Zittoun, T. (2014). Three dimensions of dialogical movement. *New Ideas in Psychology, 32,* 99–106.

Chapter 11
Working with PTSD in the Asylum Procedure

Europe is living through a refugee crisis of historic proportions, with subsequent evolving responses having now become one of the continent's defining challenges of the early twenty-first century (Médécins Sans Frontières, 2016; UNHCR, 2015). Assessing the thousands of applications of asylum claims on a case-by-case basis remains one of the most significant challenges for host countries. In the face of significant anti-migration sentiment, procedures for testing refugee claims continue to be applied by most countries of the West in order to manage and restrict the flow of displaced persons by drawing on increasingly harsh policies to justify "humane deterrence" (Silove & Mares, 2018; Steel et al., 2004). Therein lies the many contradictions between the emerging human right discourse and the appalling reality of asylum (Wenzel & Drožđek, 2018). Within this "adverserial" (Crumlish & Bracken, 2011, p. 57) context, the burden of proof of refugee status rests upon the individual asylum seeker. Refugees may feel pressured not only to prove persecution, but also that they've also been damaged by it (Joles, 2018).

In terms of Article 1, Chapter 1 of the Geneva Convention of 1951, a refugee is defined as being someone with a 'well-founded fear of being persecuted for reasons of race, religion, nationality, membership of a particular social group or political opinion.' The word 'fear' here is of particular interest as it implies that a refugee is defined to some extent by his or her psychological response to events, not only by the events themselves. Therefore, when persecuted individuals seeking asylum cannot give evidence of marks on their body, they have the alternate possibility of proving the violence to which they have been exposed through what is sometimes designated as the "wounds of the soul," notably a diagnosis of post-traumatic stress disorder (PTSD) (Fassin, 2011). As noted by Steel and colleagues (2004), the refugee determination process therefore represents a point of intersection between the domains of psychology and administrative law, a setting in which these frameworks may well collide. Such a setting, it is argued, "starkly demonstrates the ineluctable intersection of mental health, human rights, ethics and social policy" (Silove & Mares, 2018). d'Halluin (2009, 2016) similarly demonstrates the dangers inherent in this contentious relationship between immigrant, psychiatry and social security, arguing

G. Theisen-Womersley, *Trauma and Resilience Among Displaced Populations*,
https://doi.org/10.1007/978-3-030-67712-1_11

that a diagnosis of PTSD risks ultimately becoming a 'pre-requisite' for validating the experiences of migrants, thereby reifying and reducing these experiences by placing them within an exclusively psychiatric paradigm. Furthermore, she contests, by pathologizing asylum seekers, mental health damages inherent to this population have been used in anti-immigration public discourse to highlight security issues related to refugees as a damaged, diseased "other."

As such, PTSD as a political tool historically has limited and controlled the influx of migrants. For this reason, as recently stated in an article by Peter Ventevogel, senior mental health officer for the UNHCR, trauma is not part of how the agency evaluates asylum or settlement claims: "a resettlement interview is not meant as a therapy session, the goal is to get as much information is as needed to prepare a good, credible resettlement case" (Joles, 2018). However, it is nation states which have the primary responsibility for determining the status of asylum-seekers, and around the world, a diagnosis of PTSD continues to feature in the refugee determination process. In the Greek context in particular, Eleftherakos and colleagues (2018) have recently argued that "a vulnerability status can potentially help in accelerating the asylum procedures, the transfer to a better accommodation or to the mainland through the lift of geographical restrictions. The identification of vulnerability however is subject to constant modification and prolonged delays, and therefore migrants become obsessed with the pursuit of (potentially) necessary documents" (p. 6). Being diagnosed with PTSD is one such marker of vulnerability.

In this chapter, I explore the multiple and often contradictory role PTSD plays as a psychiatric diagnostic category in the refugee determination process. Firstly, I review the literature related to PTSD among refugee populations and the criticisms levelled against PTSD in this context, then turn to the role it may play as a specific legal category in the refugee determination process and the implications for professionals working within the asylum system. By drawing on case studies of victims of torture claiming asylum in Greece, I highlight the ways in which PTSD is understood by the various actors concerned throughout the asylum procedure—including among lawyers, health professionals as well as asylum seekers themselves. I argue that PTSD is a cultural tool, serving to narrate the lives of asylum seekers during the refugee determination process and how, as a cultural tool, it "embeds institutional values, power relations, circumstances of the physical environment and individual motivations" (Dauite, 2013, p. 7).

PTSD Among Refugee Populations

Despite the popularity of PTSD as a "sexy diagnosis" (Struwe, 1994) and its dominance in Western cultural discourse as an integral part of humanitarian interventions for refugee populations, various criticisms levelled against the diagnosis have long been documented in the literature ever since the period leading up to its codification as a disorder in the DSM-III (Bracken, 2001; Bracken et al., 2016; Steel, 2001; Summerfield, 1999, 2001; Young, 1995). Questions remain about the common elements underlying the diverse experiences of people across the world exposed to trauma. The work of anthropologists (Young, 1995), psychiatrists (Bracken, 2001; Bracken et al., 2016, 1997; Summerfield, 2001) and sociologists (Fassin & Rechtman, 2009), among others, have long criticised PTSD as a heavily politicized and westernised social construct. This is in light of the plethora of research indicating that sociocultural and linguistic heritage influences what experiences are interpreted as 'traumatic,' the manifestations and expressions of post-traumatic symptomatology, the interpretation of symptoms, narratives of distress as well as culturally-informed healing models (Droždek, 2015; Janoff-Bulman, 1985; Kirmayer et al., 2010; Kleinman & Good, 2004; Luno et al. 2013; Marsella, 2010). As a diagnostic construct developed for use in Western contexts, PTSD has been criticized for ignoring this significant variability among symptoms evident in different cultural settings across the world (Hinton & Lewis-Fernández, 2011; Kirmayer et al., 2010; Momartin et al., 2003; Steel et al., 2009; Tummala-Narra, 2007). Further criticism is based on the fact that one cannot always link post-traumatic symptoms directly and uncritically to a single event in the life of an individual—a pre-requisite of a PTSD diagnosis by its very definition.

As noted by Young (2016), this research calls into question the validity of using the current version of the DSM for legal purposes without modification. The literature attests to the risk of PTSD reifying and minimizing the trauma experienced by refugee populations by within an exclusively psychiatric paradigm in order to render narrative accounts of asylum seekers believable in the refugee determination procedure (Fassin & d'Halluin, 2005; Maier, 2006; McFarlane, 1995; Rogers et al., 2015; Wilson-Shaw et al., 2012; Young, 1995). According to Summerfield (1996) such a politically loaded use of PTSD may lead to "absurd" (p. 14) situations whereby victims of torture and other atrocities fear not being believed unless they can 'check off the tick list of symptoms' required by PTSD.

Despite these criticisms, as Young (2016) concludes:

> Despite what some might contend in their narratives about PTSD, it is not a mental disorder that has no validity and, if it is diagnosed, it is not often reflective of malingering. Unlike the opposite point of view, it is valid, it can be validly diagnosed, and malingering does not confound it to any great degree. This opposition in views on PTSD illustrates that there is much work to do forensically to improve assessment and diagnostic procedures (p. 239).

In other words, we cannot disregard the diagnosis entirely and throw the metaphorical baby out with the bathwater. Rather, this literature emphasises the necessity of deepening our understanding of trauma as it affects refugee populations.

The Importance of Correctly Identifying Trauma in the Refugee Determination Process

There is an increasing body of scientific evidence looking at the assumptions recorded by authorities in their asylum decisions and the psychological processes at play during the court proceeding. This literature suggests not only that there may be marked uncertainty in how to reach the correct determination, but also that there is often the potential for bias against the person genuinely fleeing from trauma and persecution. This is because trauma negatively impacts the credibility and consistency of verbal accounts. PTSD has been shown to impair memory and capacity for coherent verbal recollection. It may even itself be seen as a disorder of memory: traumatic stress overwhelms the brain's ability to store autobiographical memories in the normal way, and fragmented memories of traumatic experiences are typical (Crumlish & Bracken, 2011). As noted by Linton (2015), "ironically, the fraudulent applicant is better situated to relate a detailed story with appropriate demeanour than the genuine applicant" (p. 1085).

Furthermore, the varied responses to traumatic events (including dissociation or emotional numbing, for example) may fall outside of given cultural norms surrounding expectations of how a traumatised individual "should" act (Bögner et al., 2010; Linton, 2015; Mueller et al., 2011; Rogers et al., 2015; Schock et al., 2015; Silove & Mares, 2018; Turner, 1992, 2015). Among the factors that require sensitive consideration are risk of cultural and linguistic misunderstandings and the effect of posttraumatic stress disorder and depressive symptoms on the capacity to provide a coherent narrative (Silove & Mares, 2018). Such a consideration is particularly pertinent when seen in light of the literature which demonstrates that the refugee determination process risks being a traumatic event in and of itself (Rogers et al., 2015; Schock et al., 2016, 2015; Turner, 1992, 2015).

Within the asylum seeking procedure itself, a culturally sensitive recognition of trauma may assist judges and other decision makers in recognizing and being more attentive to the difficulties asylum seekers may have in verbalising and constructing their case as a result of a compromised mental state which "may impede the applicant's ability to testify in a manner that appears direct, specific, and emotionally appropriate" (Linton, 2015, p. 1085). Thus, identifying the impact of trauma—and accounting for cultural and linguistic barriers—may avoid discrepant accounts being seen as evidence of fabrication (Crumlish & Bracken, 2011). This recognition of impairment is critical to assist the comprehensive assessment of refugee claims—as it limits the risk of erroneous decision making based on testimonies distorted by psychological trauma (Silove & Mares, 2018).

There is therefore a need to explore these tensions surrounding the controversial use of PTSD as evidence in court, as well as to deepen the way in which the impact of trauma among refugee populations is understood. Nowhere is this more pertinent than in the refugee determination procedure, where questions of legitimacy are central.

PTSD and the Question of Legal Causality

According to Young (2017) causality (or causation) is central to every legal case, yet its underlying philosophical, legal, and psychological definitions and conceptions vary. Based on the five-point scale he outlines regarding causation in psychological inquiry, drawing on a diagnosis of PTSD as proof of refugee status would fall in the level 1 explanation, defined as the following:

> The index event is the "sole cause" of the resulting psychological condition (disorder(s) and/or functional effect(s)). There are neither overt nor latent psychological conditions evident in the pre-event state, that is, there are no pre-existing psychological vulnerabilities or risk factors. The psychological condition at issue would not have occurred, either in the present or later on, had the subject event not occurred. (pg. 12)

Indeed, it could be argued that PTSD is the only psychiatric diagnosis that tells a story. By its very definition, it is based on the following premises:

(i) There were no pre-existing psychological vulnerabilities or risk factors
(ii) An event occurred (criteria A according to the DSM V, (Association, 2013))
(iii) This event was experienced by the individual as being traumatic
(iv) As a result, the individual responded with a specific set of thoughts, feelings and behaviors as outlined in the criteria of the diagnosis of PTSD
(v) The traumatic event was the sole cause of this response

In order for a PTSD diagnosis to be made, a traumatic event needs to have occurred by definition and this denotes an implied level of believe in the asylum seekers' narrative—thus fulfilling a legal requirement that it be *credible* (Maier, 2006). Conversely, "if rape/torture/persecution happened to someone then they would have psychological difficulties" is prey to the counter-argument "we don't believe it did happen, so we don't accept that the difficulties are genuine," as frequently seen in responses to medico-legal reports themselves" (Good, 2007, p. 203–204). The political implications for asylum procedures are clear. For example, PTSD may serve as evidence of the trauma which they experienced in their country of origin, their subsequent "well-founded fear" of being persecuted if forced to return, and therefore, ultimately, as a justification of their claim to refugee status.

The premises outlined above are based on a universalist model of trauma situated in western psychiatric discourse and developed only after the second World War. As highlighted by Bracken and colleagues (2016), this universalist model—the dominant paradigm in psychiatry—is technological. With it's origins in the European asylums of the nineteenth century, it responds to the technical challenges of the refugee determination procedure requiring a scientific response: to classify accurately, to identify universal causal factors and pathways, and to seek efficient forms of interventions. However, this universalist model of trauma rejects a priori any notion of singularity, or of ethnic or cultural differences (d'Halluin, 2009, 2016). Understanding trauma in the context of the refugee determination procedure should necessarily recognise the social-cultural context in which it occurs, in relation to the activity of which it is a part and within a broader systems of relations in which it has meaning (Van der Riet, 2009, 2012). I therefore explore the refugee determination procedure as a system of activity—arguing that such a systemic analysis allows for a broad contextualisation of practices around PTSD, revealing and exposing tensions and contradictions in how various actors involved in the asylum seeking process understand trauma among refugee populations and the implications for the refugee determination process.

The Refugee Determination Procedure as a System of Activity

I explore the refugee determination procedure is an activity system (Kloetzer et al., 2015; Roth & Lee, 2007; Toomela, 2014; van der Riet, 2012), defined according to Vygotskian cultural-historical psychology as a system of settings, institutions, physical environments, formal and informal, social relations, and events wherein a multitude of actors intersects. This includes, for example, the lawyers, doctors, psychologists, bureaucrats, and asylum seekers themselves, for whom PTSD has a different meaning. Here, the activity of individuals are considered as inherently embedded in social context and mediated by cultural tools (Kloetzer et al., 2015). I draw on Dauite's (2014) definition of a cultural tool as "symbolic process developed in human relations for interacting purposefully in the world" (p. 23). From a Vygotskian perspective, therefore, cultural tools act on others and on the world, coordinating actions. In other words, by examining PTSD within the asylum activity system, it is considered as a cultural tool purposefully aimed at "conduct[ing] human influence on the object of activity" (Vygotsky, 1980, p. 55), circulating at the crossroads where asylum seekers' narratives meet a 'centered' bureaucratic language system (Maryns & Blommaert, 2001).

To examine the use of PTSD as a cultural tool used both in a medical and legal sense in the treatment of asylum seekers, I propose to take a narrative approach to examining how a human story is translated into legal one (Di Donato, 2014). Such a narrative approach, significantly developed by the likes of Jerome Brunner (Amsterdam & Bruner, 2000; Bruner, 1990, 1991, 2003) and others, examines how "the client's story gets recast into plights and prospects, plots and pilgrimages into possible worlds…this endless telling and retelling, casting and recasting is essential to the conduct of the law…stories construct the facts that comprise them. For this reason, much of human reality and its 'facts' are not merely recounted by narrative but constituted by it. To the extent that law is fact-contingent, it is inescapably rooted in narrative" (Amsterdam & Bruner, 2000, p. 110). In other words, cultural tools used in a court of law shape the world not according to how it is but according to its very own categories. Such categories are, according to Bruner (Amsterdam & Bruner, 2000) "the badges of our socio-political allegiances, the tools of our mental life, the organization of our perception" (p. 19). They produce theories and about causes and connections in the natural world (for example, that experiencing a single traumatic event in the past would logically lead one to display symptoms of PTSD). As such, cultural tools may be regulative, overtly normative and potential instruments of power in that they institutionalize customs and traditions. To categorize an asylum seeker with PTSD is therefore "an act of meaning making" (p. 29) which may become entrenched in the habits of medical and legal institutions with very concrete social, material and legal consequences.

There are inherent power imbalances found within the activity system of the refugee determination process. Cultural tools, such as PTSD, are embedded in systems of resources hierarchized in terms of functional adequacy (Blommaert,

2001a). Blommaert and colleagues (Blommaert, 2001a, b; Maryns & Blommaert, 2001), for example, argue how asylum seekers narrating their experiences in the context of the asylum procedure are confronted with a complex set of administrative procedures which presuppose access to various codes (for example, psychiatric or legal codes) requiring a very specific set of westernized narrative resources which may not be available to migrants. Added to this is the power imbalance inherent in the process of diagnosing asylum seekers, as outlined above, which privileges western above local knowledge. Here, as chillingly noted by Blommaert (2001b), "Foucault's image of subjects being transformed into knowable objects of clinical observation by means of a multilayered complex of discursive and material practices is looming large" (p. 31). I would argue that PTSD as a cultural tool may represent just such practices.

According to Blommaert (2001a), "the resources controlled by the narrators and their interlocutors are part and parcel of the interpretations given to their stories, and given the central role of the stories in the asylum procedure, matters of resources may influence the outcome of their asylum application" (p. 23). Medical certificates stating PTSD among asylum seekers therefore "come with a history of use and abuse; they also come with a history of assessment and evaluation… put into a legal/procedural framework, in sum, that every step in the systematically and uniformly performed process involves not replication but far-reaching transformations of the 'original' story" (Blommaert, 2001a). The story of trauma, then, is also replicated and transformed into the form of a medical certificate attesting to PTSD, a "narrative shaping of individualized experience through contextualization processes [which] entails a shaping of linguistic and narrative tools that operate as contextualization cues" (Maryns & Blommaert, 2001, p. 62). These "contextualization cues" permit the very concept of PTSD to circulate as a "boundary object" (Star & Griesemer, 1989) understood differently by various actors. The messy story of trauma then is decoded and converted into a "depersonalized case" (Maryns & Blommaert, 2001, p. 65) based on "overly tidy stories" (Bruner, 1990, 1991, 2003) and thus easily convertible into established legal categories.

To explore this further, I propose to usefully shift to dynamic storytelling from the perspectives of those involved (Daiute, 2017) and to investigate the roles of those actors in constructing the legal facts (Di Donato, 2011). The investigation is based on the results of a yearlong research projects among asylum seekers diagnosed with PTSD as well as their treating health professionals (including doctors, psychologists and psychiatrists) in a center for victims of torture in Athens, Greece. I explore how PTSD circulates as a cultural tool among the various actors within the asylum activity system, specifically in relation to social structures, power relations and each actor's diverse activities and objectives.

Case Study

I conducted 12 months of research among asylum seekers and refugees in a center for victims of torture in Athens, Greece run by *Médecins Sans Frontières* and their local partner, Babel. This longitudinal study involved participant observation as well as qualitative, in-depth interviews with 74 various actors. This included a year-long follow up of 10 victims of torture seeking asylum (interviewed an average of five times)—as well as in-depth interviews with 43 health professionals working with refugee victims of torture from a variety of humanitarian organizations, including cultural mediators working in psychosocial interventions for individuals diagnosed with PTSD Furthermore, I conducted qualitative, in-depth interviews with 21 community representatives and leaders of diverse refugee associations around Athens in order to explore culturally determined narratives of trauma.

Framework analysis.

To analyse the data, I specifically draw on a systemic framework analysis to examine the refugee determination process as an activity system—particularly the various and often contradicting ways in which PTSD serves as a cultural tool drawn upon by the different actors within this activity system. This enables an exploration of the activity of the various actors concerned, in order to identify the various narratives they draw upon to understand trauma and highlight the various dilemmas with which they are faced in the refugee determination process.

The five stages to conducting this framework that I followed, based on the method as outlined by Pickup and colleagues (2014), were:

(1) Familiarising myself with the data
(2) Delineating overall narratives concerning trauma and/or PTSD in relation to the refugee determination process
(3) Identifying the various actors within the refugee determination process to determine a framework of themes and subthemes
(4) Indexing specific responses by copying relevant participant quotes from interview transcripts into this framework
(5) Iteratively reviewing and revising the initial framework
(6) Mapping and interpreting the subthemes with a summary of the main descriptive comments
(7) Selecting representative quotes and individual cases for each subtheme

Results.

Asylum seeker	Tell his or her story to be granted refugee status	Used to testify (to fear/suffering), reinforces the story	Culturally informed	To tell the "trauma story" (risking retraumatization) or not, how to tell the story in a credible way

(continued)

(continued)

Medical professional	Treat	Used to determine course of treatment	Psychiatric/medical	To diagnose PTSD or not, to write the medical certificate or not
Bureaucrat in asylum procedure	Assess	Used as evidence to assess the case	Legal, institutional	To grant refugee status or not, to believe the asylum seeker or not

As indicated by the framework analysis above, the results highlight the various ways in which trauma is seen and understood by various actors in the refugee determination process. For asylum seekers, the activity is narrating their story, their objective is to be believed, and the diagnosis of PTSD is used to this end as testament to their suffering. PTSD is coloured by culturally informed narratives of trauma, and they are the victim in need of assistance. For health professionals, their activity is diagnosing, their objective is to treat the patient, as well as to attest to their psychological state of mind and the diagnosis of PTSD is used as a tool to this end. PTSD is informed by a medicalized discourse of psychiatric categories and the asylum seeker is the patient. For judges and other officials in the asylum tribunal, their activity is to assess the legal case, their objective is to determine the refugee status of the individual in front of them and PTSD serves as evidence to this end. PTSD is colored by a technical, legal discourse and the asylum seeker is the defendant whose case is being assessed.

Asylum Seeker Perspectives

An analysis of the asylum seekers' narratives highlight the following:

(i) Discrepancies exist among the various narratives of trauma in the refugee determination process
(ii) Existing power imbalances underlie these discrepancies, privileging westernized narratives of trauma above others
(iii) Asylum seekers sometimes deliberately drew on specifically "westernized" narratives of trauma in order to best present their case, and
(iv) Many asylum seekers appeared to be retraumatized by the refugee determination process.

I explore these themes through representative case studies and quotes from participants.

Discrepancies in Narratives of Trauma

Discrepancies in how narratives of trauma circulated among various actors were reflected in seven out of 10 participants. One stated that "here, we don't speak like in Africa." Another said "because there *[in their country of origin]*, there are many people who, when they have something, don't write. They keep it [in their head]. When they have a problem, they just forget about it....here, they note it." In the context of seeking asylum, the medical certificate was seen as a reflection of western values, knowledge, and ways of being, where the written word is privileged. This finding echoes the words of Blommaert (2001b) who argues that the "process of (re)structuring talk into institutionally sanctioned text involves a dynamic of entextualization that is based on power asymmetries" (p. 3). Differences were evident in individual asylum seeker's experience of the asylum tribunal itself: "here, it's a new world. I don't know how things are done."

Many felt at a loss as to how to narrate their trauma narrative in the face of these asymmetries:

> What is happening to your country? how you can come here?" ... these are not questions you can answer.
>
> I don't know what to tell them. I don't have words to explain the things.
>
> What happened in Africa, it's not easy to explain.
>
> I have a fear that I don't know how to explain.

According to one participant: "the people asking you questions, it's like you're sitting across from a psychologist. They're professionals who know their work." The professionalism of the bureaucrats in the asylum tribunal is highlighted—and, by extension, their superior position. An interesting comparison is made between the bureaucrats of the asylum tribunal and the psychologist: asking questions, probing, evaluating, judging from a superior position. In the words of one asylum seeker, it's a situation "where one doesn't understand anything." Another participant drew a similar parallel: "The psychologist, it's a game. It's a toy. He asks you questions, and bases his deductions on your response—and the asylum [procedure] itself, it's the same." The metaphor of a game is an interesting one: on the one hand, it arguably denotes the power imbalance between those who are tasked with assessing their case—who take it as lightly as though it was just a game to be played, nothing more—and those whose lives are dependent on the outcome. On the other hand, the fact that asylum seekers recognized the procedure as a game may also be indicative of the fact that it is a situation to be played: a knowledge of the rules is needed in order to strategize and, ultimately, to win.

Asymmetries in Trauma Narratives, Asymmetries of Power: The Case of Dilraj

Dilraj is a 30-year-old Indian asylum seeker of Sikh religion. As a university student in India in 2007, he was arrested and tortured on numerous occasions due to his involvement as a Sikh political activist. The detainment and torture often lasted months at a time, and involved other members of his family as well is himself. According to him, his father was allegedly killed by the Indian Secret Services in 2009. He himself managed to escape from prison with the help of an uncle, and arrived, alone, in Athens to seek asylum in September 2015. He was referred to the centre for victims of torture in June 2016, where his treating doctor describes "a clear case of post-traumatic stress disorder," including symptoms of flashbacks and nightmares, at the first consultation. Dilraj himself stated that:

> Mr. Psychologist doctor, he gave me the report. In that report, he has written that I'm in very big depression. Actually, I don't know I'm in depression or not. I know only one thing, that my world is just only this room. If I'm going out, if I'm having any appointment with my social worker, or with doctor, then only I'm going out from this room... What I do all day long, I just go through all the papers. This is my life.

Firstly, Dilraj begins by addressing the doctor as "Mr Psychologist doctor." On the one hand, it could be argued that the "Mr" and "Dr" is intended as a sign of respect, positioning the health professional as a respected and superior authority. On the other, it indicates some confusion as to the exact role or title of the professional. What is striking is that he refers to the report as stating that he has "depression"—despite the diagnosis being that of PTSD The report is seen as something "given" to him, as a passive recipient. He displays an element of doubt as to the veracity of the report: "I don't know if I'm in depression or not." Given this element of doubt, he relies instead to his own subjective experience that defies any psychiatric labelling. Despite his uncertainty as to whether or not what it says is true, the "papers," seem to hold significance for him. The medical certificate is a cultural tool that has become an integral part of "his life" now. As such, his words imply an assumed respect and value for the papers. However, their inevitable role in his life appears to be met with ambivalence. He notes, "every time I go to the people they only write and they don't really listen to me." Here, the activity of noting is seen as a communicative barrier between himself and the unnamed "they."

His doctor noted:

> He doesn't seem to understand it as an illness. He says that he feels abnormal, he feels wrecked; he says that he's not dangerous; that he is not crazy. Every time I say to him, "These voices is just a symptom of a disease that will go away eventually," he doesn't seem to listen.

Again, there is a substantial difference in the way in which the symptoms are interpreted. Neither feels listened to by the other. Dilraj again does not seem to understand his state as fitting into a western, psychiatric narrative. For him, it is "not an illness." Furthermore, the assumed superior authority of the health professional is implicit in his words "he doesn't seem to listen" to the fact that it is "a disease." Dilraj is positioned as a patient who simply needs to listen to the doctor. His illness is presented as an irrefutable fact to be understood. Western knowledge trumps local.

Adapting the Trauma Narrative: The Case of Jules

Arguably aware of the evident power asymmetries inherent in the way in which narratives of trauma are presented and perceived in the tribunal, many participants described successfully drawing on a specifically western narrative of trauma (as exemplified by the diagnosis of PTSD) in order to best present their case during the refugee determination process. In the words of one participant, "crying makes your story more believable." To explore this, I present the case of Jules.

Jules is a Congolese 35 year old male who was arrested and tortured as a result of his political activism. He arrived in Greece in 2015 to claim asylum. Upon preparing for his appearance in front of the asylum tribunal, he was told by his lawyer to remove his earrings when he went in front of the asylum tribunal. He explained that the "flashy" jewellery reflected "joy" and that his narrative, to the contrary, needed to be one of trauma:

> Between a made-up story and the story of what happened, it's not the same...I can tell the story 1500 times, even 15000 times, without fault, because it's what I experienced. It's different to the story that they gave me. That's another person. It's different. It's what you experienced but the way in which you tell it must necessarily change. Some people know how to talk – 'they'll believe this and believe that' but it's no longer the story, the real story. It's the real story that they've complicated. It's the lawyer who will say things and take out certain dirty things to be clean… All people who tell stories can tell made-up stories. You need to show people that this story really is your true story, so that they can accept that 'no, he's telling the truth.' You can tell a good story, but you can also tell it without emotion.

To be granted asylum, he needs to be believed. To be believed, he needs to tell "a good story." To tell a good story, it needs to be "clean." Indeed, the literature shows the importance of the "emotional congruence" afforded by a PTSD diagnosis as a critical factor used to judge the credibility of asylum seeker's narratives (Rogers et al., 2015). It could be argued that the "clean" story (or, an emotionally congruent narrative) required by the tribunal is reflected in the medical certificate stating that he has PTSD and which Jules insisted on using as evidence in the court. Using his trauma narrative as a cultural tool in order to be believed, he draws upon what Hymes (1998) refers to as "fully formed narratives" - narratives which display growing tightness and structure due to repeating instances of narrating. In other words, he rehearses. According to Jules, the difference between the "real" story and the rehearsed one is the fact that his real story is far more emotionally nuanced: throughout the course of our interviews with him, he constantly referred to his childhood and early adulthood where he represents himself as a strong and active member of the community. In the rehearsed story, he draws on what Amsterdam and Bruner (2000) refer to as a "script." They define such a script as "stories that provide walk-through models of a culture's canonical expectations" (p. 45). Jules realises that in order to "play the game" and be granted refugee status, he needs to construct a narrative of himself as a traumatized refugee. This leaves little space for a more complex picture of multiple aspects of his identity to emerge. He is, in essence, an actor rehearsing his script.

As noted by Blommaert (2001b), such rehearsals involve "an acute awareness of the categories and interpretive resources of the hearer" (p. 22). This awareness is reflected in Jules' words, "you need to show people that this story really is your story." He does this by drawing on a specific "clean" trauma narrative. This is a narrative that "they" (an unnamed yet present Other) gave him and which is based on specific socially, culturally, politically, and historically informed constructions of what it means to be a traumatized refugee. It has been circulating among various actors and passed onto Jules. Such fully formed narratives "testif[y] to the gradual and discursive practice-based construction of such refugee identities" (Blommaert, 2001b, p. 20). When Jules constructs such an identity, he notes that it is not his "real story," it is a "made-up" self.

Following the script is not without difficulty. As with many other participants, Jules was confronted with the dilemma of how much to tell. He realises that to increase credibility, the narrative needs to be emotionally congruent, despite the significant potential of sharing the trauma narrative in the asylum tribunal for re-traumatisation (Rogers et al., 2015; Turner, 1992; S. Turner, 2015). Jules' insistence on the importance of rehearsals is clear. However, he continued the interview by saying.

> But it hurts to have to tell it…yes, it hurts. Even during the interview, it hurts you … but they're looking for sadness, during the interview …

The dilemma centres on the emotional difficulty associated with sharing the trauma narrative, and the intended objective of being granted asylum status. Jules' words indicate an acknowledgement that, despite the fact that sharing the trauma narrative "hurts," it is a necessary and required condition for being granted refugee status. Even the "sadness" is used to validate his experience, addressed to his intended audience in the tribunal who are "looking for it."

Jules walks a tightrope—the narrative is required to be formal (without being too formatted or rehearsed) but also emotional (without being too emotional), this optimal balance assumed to enhance credibility (Montagut, 2016). All of this comes at an emotional cost: having to follow the script may also run the risk of re-traumatization.

As was the case for Jules, six out of 10 participants referred to the emotional distress they experienced as a result of having to speak about potentially traumatic events in the asylum tribunal. Despite the risk of retraumatization, most appeared to face this psychological challenge with a resilient acceptance. As neatly expressed by one participant, Sylvain:

> We are obliged to do it. You say that you want a paper, you're obliged to explain why you left your country. We're at a point where you're obliged to say everything. You want the papers, you speak, you don't want the papers, you don't speak.

Health Professionals' Perspectives

The health professionals similarly highlighted tensions around the use of medical certificates for the asylum tribunal. Many strategically and purposefully weighed up the risks and benefits of using a PTSD diagnosis across various settings and among various actors, recognising the activity of diagnosing as one loaded with political significance:

> A certified traumatic experience opens many advantages, ummm, the doors to, ummm, asylum and added to the facts, it's a way of saying that the, the health professional has more relevance to his words when he certifies the existence of trauma, more than the person him- or herself
>
> In this case, the clinician has a certain power

Implicit power dynamics are highlighted in the above words, where the health professionals are placed in a superior position, their own medicalised narratives valued above the words of the asylum seekers themselves. Given this power, many alluded to the purposeful and strategic use of providing a PTSD diagnosis to help the asylum-seeker within the asylum seeking process:

> [PTSD] is something that we can try to drag the process on for a while if we're getting a negative response.
>
> They [the commission] can understand if you provide PTSD
>
> It's about all the only ammunition that we have.
>
> It was a way to protect them during the commission.
>
> I guess [PTSD] is a construct which we have to work because um, that's the way we communicate about what trauma is and as for the asylum process we have to often say that somebody has PTSD because that's going to be important to sort of validate what they're saying happened to them.

Words such as "protect" and "ammunition" connote war narratives, with asylum seekers positioned as soldiers going into battle, the medical certificate the "ammunition" provided by their superiors (in this metaphor, the health professionals). We can infer that health professionals are not naïve to the legal weight given to PTSD They position themselves as one of the actors who influence the asylum process. "We" or "us" refers to either the group of health professionals ("the only ammunition that *we* have") or to the health professional and the asylum seeker ("if *we're* getting a negative response"); "they" or "them" referring to the commission or the asylum seeker ("a way to protect *them*"). Within these shifting alliances, the health professionals are not politically neutral actors. They described purposefully using PTSD as "ammunition" in cases where, in the words of one participant, the asylum seekers' narratives are "not as psychiatric and not as theoretical and psychological as ours is." The use of the word "construct" implies a recognition of the diagnosis as being socially constructed and relevant in certain situations, a cultural tool used to "communicate" about what trauma is—in this case to communicate to the actors of the asylum tribunal.

Like the individual asylum seekers themselves, the necessity of having a "coherent" and "linear story" was widely recognised:

> They need something very sure to evaluate a demand, whether they will give asylum or not, which is the simplest way to have a coherent, and very linear story. The more linear and straightforward it is, the best [sic] it is for them.

The "clean story" narrative is one permeating the activity system, passed around among actors. One participant stated, "a very, very coherent and linear story is a story prepared with a lawyer." What is implied in these words is the fact that (a) it is impossible for any individual to have a very, very coherent and linear story, (b) the asylum seeking process may require it and (c) professionals may purposefully reconstruct the narrative to fit into pre-established legal categories. As an interesting aside, this particular participant seems to imply that, as much as it would be impossible for the "genuine" story to be coherent and linear, it would be impossible for the asylum seeker him- or herself to have reconstructed it.

The health professionals, therefore, allude to an implicit knowledge that their position is a powerful one. By virtue of the fact that they are able to diagnose an asylum seeker with PTSD, they are in a position to construct the narrative of the individual. The use of a clean and coherent (linear) narrative, however, was not perceived as being without complications. Many health professionals raised doubts about fitting the trauma narrative into such a "clean" story:

> I'm afraid that it victimizes the person. I mean, I tell him, "Okay, you have PTSD and for this reason you can claim that." … And so, it becomes that he or she becomes passive, waiting for others to do things for him. Because he's vulnerable. Because he suffers with PTSD This doesn't have to do with PTSD This has to do with how the policy concerning refugees is formed and is applied.
>
> It has to do with identity if it's totally stripped off, what he was before. He's like just an object. He's treated like an object from everyone.
>
> They are very, they are basing all of their work on PTSD diagnosis, they completely medicalise and victimise people

The concerns of the health professionals centred on the fact that to have a "clean narrative" (as seems to be implied by a PTSD diagnosis) is to reduce the asylum seeker's story. Their unique and individual "identity" is "stripped off" in order to make the story clean. Thus, a trade-off is implicitly recognised. On the one hand, the benefits of being recognised as a "victim" of PTSD (and by extension, having one's story believed and being recognised as a refugee) are many. On the other hand, the very mechanism of reconstructing the trauma narrative in order to fit into, in the words of one participant, "a perfect victim template" risks reducing the individual to an "object" without identity. As a result, the use of the diagnosis is met with some ambivalence:

> They want to victimize the patient. It's already a mistake from me that I talk about the patient. Sorry, I'm medical. I'm referring to people as the patient and very often people will not be a patient, neither psychiatrically or physically.

The above participant engages in a narrative (re)positioning. Firstly, like others, he refers to "they" (presumably the actors of the asylum tribunal) as intentionally looking to "victimize" the "patient." There is an implicit recognition of, and disagreement with, such victimization. He then refers to the asylum seekers with whom he works as "patients." Thereafter, he immediately repositions himself, by taking himself out of the normative, medical narrative within which he acknowledges he has placed himself unintentionally. He self-identifies as "medical," using this as a justification for drawing on medical narratives of the individual asylum seeker as a patient. The reason he gives for it being a "mistake" is that, to be a patient is to imply, in some way or another, that one is a psychiatric or physical victim. There is an implicit acknowledgement of the complexity of individual asylum seekers' narratives which extends beyond the medical narrative.

Furthermore, an attempt to reduce these complex narratives to a medical one paradoxically denies those whose narrative is not "clean" (linear, coherent, "medicalisable") access to certain rights, recognitions, and privileges:

> I think [PTSD is] being used to filter rights, to filter certain rights and access to certain services, which could be open to everybody.
>
> This is extremely dangerous, because being a refugee doesn't mean that you have obvious consequences, even psychological. I'm very, very skeptical that people that they don't have symptoms, they might be considered liars. What should we do then?
>
> I think there is a disconnection between what you see in the clinical setting and the evaluation process, there's a, there's a break in the system. And, it's very traumatizing also for the professionals working in such a setting, because you feel helpless. You see the case, and you see that, yes, this person is in need of support and help and is really traumatized, but his claim doesn't fit the official, what do you say, profile...

Implicit in the above words of the participants is an understanding of PTSD as a cultural tool with political significance, and furthermore that the narratives of many asylum seekers "don't fit the official" narrative required. This clear "break in the system," arguably resulting from conflicting narratives, places the health professionals in a "traumatizing" and "helpless" position. Referring to the conflicting narratives around trauma, another participant similarly stated that "we need a common knowledge to share with the commission." The words of one participants reflects the strategies developed to negotiate this complex position:

> for me the diagnosis is something that if you use it, you should know for what reason you use it. You use it because you want to understand better the patient, you use it because you want to help him with the asylum process and you know that if there is a diagnosis that this person will be helped, you use it because it's a great way to communicate with other professionals, so if I say "PTSD" the other will understand, but for me it's very important if you use a diagnosis to explain exactly what's happening with this person, not only to say "okay, he has PTSD" and it's not clear.

Her strategy includes an implicit understanding of the multiple ways in which PTSD is understood by the various actors. For herself as a professional, it is a way of better understanding the patient. For other professionals, it is a way to communicate this understanding clearly and efficiently. For the asylum seeker in front of her, it is a way to help him or her in the asylum procedure. Given the various ways in which PTSD is understood by the various actors, she highlights the importance of addressing medical reports to match the understanding of the intended audience being addressed.

Conflicting Narratives Across the Activity System

The health professionals found themselves having to negotiate a variety of conflicting discourses of trauma within the refugee determination process. Here, their activity of diagnosing patients similarly includes needing to address a variety of different actors, including bureaucrats of the asylum tribunal, lawyers, as well as the asylum seekers—themselves occupying multiple positions associated with being a patient, a client and an asylum seeker. The complexity of this is highlighted in the words of one participant:

> Then you sit down, the interpreter, the professional, and the patient. The professional is reading the report with the interpreter and on the spot they explain to the patient what everything means. Then the patient receives the report. Very often he will say that, "This is wrong. With that what you write, you say that I'm crazy, I'm not crazy." Then, of course, you have to try to explain to the patient that, "I don't understand what you meant by crazy, I never said that you are crazy. I say that you are suffering from post-traumatic stress disorder.

What is noteworthy is the multiple actors involved in the above-mentioned exchange. Present in the moment described are three actors: the professional, the interpreter and the patient (asylum seeker). Furthermore, there are a myriad of actors not physically present but implicitly addressed, including, for example, the lawyer or the bureaucrats of the tribunal. For the asylum seeker, having PTSD is equivalent to being seen as "crazy." It is not evident, but we could suppose that this narrative is associated with a certain social stigma for the asylum seeker, who rejects the psychiatric labelling. For the health professional, PTSD is a familiar cultural tool of the profession. The word "crazy" does not enter into this medical narrative. It is also interesting to note the implicit power dynamics inherent in this exchange, as illustrated by the words "you have to try to explain," indicative of the value given to his expert medical knowledge above that of the patient's. This is similarly reflected in the words of other health professionals:

> We will give the report to the patient who will read it and translate it to him and explain to him exactly what he has.
>
> They don't understand that they have it.

PTSD is implicitly acknowledged as fact, something that the asylum seeker "has." Rather absurdly, despite the fact that it concerns the psychological condition of the individual, there is an implicit assumption that his own thoughts, feelings and behaviors need to be explained to him—in other words, fitted within a pre-established medical narrative. Conflicting narratives circulated among the actors, but appeared to create specific tension when it came to the written reports of PTSD:

> Very often he will not accept it. Very often the beneficiary will tell you, "I don't want you to write that.

Health professionals reported a variety of reactions of asylum seekers to the medical certificate stating PTSD:

> Some patients, they will insist to write something worse, exactly because they know that this thing I will use it like a leverage for my asylum… For someone it's very important to know what they have: "I feel better to know that I have this so I can do that to be better" but for someone else, they don't accept diagnosis. They don't like diagnosis because they think that they are crazy or you are saying to them "you are not okay, something wrong is happening.
>
> You see when they ask the report, that they expect to [see written in the report is] this vulnerable identity is that deep inside. They speak of vulnerability. They speak about, "I have to prove to them that I'm vulnerable because they didn't believe.

The above quote raises some key considerations (i) PTSD is used by some (but not all) of asylum seekers in a purposeful and strategic manner in their asylum seeking procedure as "proof" of vulnerability (ii) it is also used within a therapeutic setting as a helpful clinical diagnosis used to understand symptoms being experienced and receive appropriate psychosocial treatment (iii) many asylum seekers disagree with the diagnosis, due to a belief that it suggests something "wrong"—an indication of resistance to their symptoms fitting into a medical narrative of deficiency. The above-mentioned reactions also seem to be related to whom the diagnosis is addressed (for example, positively regarded when shared with the bureaucrats of the tribunal and with the treating health professional of the consultation room as compared to being negatively regarded within the asylum seekers' community space where the diagnosis may carry a social stigma). As such, its use is highly context dependant and continually negotiated across activity systems.

Discussion: An Overview of the Various Critiques of PTSD Within the Asylum Process

For asylum seekers and their lawyers, the medical certificate, including evidence of PTSD, is an "open sesame" (Fassin & d'Halluin, 2005, p. 600); for officials and judges it is a piece of evidence among others; and for both it is an innovation in governmentality. This labelling of asylum seekers is supported by a system in which tabulation of numbers with psychiatric labels forms a crucial basis for the mobilisation of broader social supports (Watters, 2001) and a new form of the transnational administration of people (Fassin & d'Halluin, 2005). It risks tearing individuals away from the potential protection of their own resilience as well as from their community's traditional means of coping with trauma (Losi, 2002). As Papadopoulos (2002b) argues, in our efforts to express our justified condemnation of the individuals, groups and policies that lead to political oppression and crimes against humanity, we offer as "proof" the fact that people have been "traumatized" by these despicable actions. In doing so, we ignore all psychological considerations of how people process traumatic experiences and, unwittingly, we end up doing violence to the very people we want to help through psychologizing the political dimensions of human suffering.

As noted by Daiute and Lucic (2010) 'the almost-exclusive focus on psychopathology as a response to war defines traumatic reactions and recoveries in terms of the direct exposure of individuals to violence and reactions to these events as automatic emotional responses' (p. 615). This medical narrative of trauma, linked to fixed 'traumatic' events in the past, risks rendering us blind to other ongoing aspects of interpersonal, political and social violence on a more global scale (Maier & Straub, 2011; Silove et al., 1998, 2000). Furthermore, "although there is evidence that some …people experience trauma and others interpret violence in terms of cultural values and practices, we know little about the broader range of strategies … people use to understand the myriad material and symbolic circumstances they encounter in their daily lives" (Dauite & Lucić, 2010, p. 616). By placing human suffering within this medical narrative, a thin description of the individual is created where other important socio-cultural and political considerations are easily lost or hidden (Marlowe, 2010). Such a shift away from a wider understanding of the political context from which asylum seekers may be fleeing, towards this medical narrative may equally lead to the moral disqualification and criminalization of unsuccessful asylum seekers who are not found to be "traumatized" (Sturm et al., 2010).

Deconstructing the "Traumatized Refugee" Narrative

An obvious but often neglected point is that not all refugees are traumatized. This assumption, Summerfield (2001) argues, reflects "a globalization of western cultural trends towards the medicalization of distress" (p. 1449). A narrative of refugees as invariably damaged, weak or scarred, manifest (as indicated by the diagnosis of PTSD), may have unintended negative consequences for refugee populations by minimizing strengths and positive adaptation mechanisms (Afana et al., 2010; Losi, 2002; Marlowe, 2010; Papadopoulos, 2002b; Sturm et al., 2010). The "traumatized refugee" narrative ignores systematic complexities such as the relational nature of the event's impact among family, community and ethnic group members, as well as the effects of the wider societal discourses which colour the meaning, emphasis and quality of events and experiences (Papadopoulos, 2002b). It also neglects to consider the fact that different reactions or non-reactions to trauma—not matching those prescribed by PTSD—may indeed serve as a defensive and adaptive survival mechanism for individuals who may not have the "luxury" of allowing the experience of psychological distress to impede the urgent and daily task of surviving.

As such, the "traumatized refugee" narrative risks placing asylum seekers in the role of passive victims, their own choices, traditions, survival strategies and competencies ignored, and the role of Western "experts" and their technology in the field of mental health exaggerated (Summerfield, 1996). It may thus represent a form of western cultural imperialism (Steel, 2001) which denies the resilience of survivors (Marlowe, 2010) and serves to reinforce existing imbalances of power between Western "expert" and "victim-patient" (Summerfield, 1996). As stated by Pupavac (2002):

> Internationalization and professionalization of adversity, indigenous coping strategies are thus not merely demeaned and disempowered. The community itself is pathologized as dysfunctional and politically delegitimized (p. 493).

The narrative further serves to detract attention away from the structural violence inherent in the asylum seeking procedure of host countries to which many asylum seekers are exposed - a "colonization of intimate psychic spaces" (d'Halluin, 2009).

Implications for Health Professionals Working with Asylum Seekers

Losi (Losi, 2002), an ardent critic of humanitarian interventions focused on PTSD, argues that the use of PTSD by professionals working with asylum seekers leads to a reductive assessment of their plight, victimization and a shift in the interpretation (and understanding) of the refugees' experiences, where the reasons for their exile are no longer socio-political but belong to a more neutral, "technical" dimensions; a de-contextualization of the lived experience of refugees leads to languages and concepts being lost and replaced by medical jargon and obscure terms.

In practice, many health professionals are increasingly called upon to provide medical information in order for the state to distinguish between "true" and "fake" refugees. However, a number of criticisms have been raised regarding the potential subjectivity and partiality of health professionals providing a PTSD diagnosis as evidence in asylum procedures. Such criticisms perceive the diagnosis provided by the professionals to be less based on objective medical "expert" information and more on "therapeutic" clinical intuition (Dromer & Grandmaison; Hauswirth, Canellini, & Bennoun, 2004; Lechenne, 2012; Maier, 2006; Montagut, 2016). Such criticisms may pose a dilemma for the professionals themselves, who are often faced with their own doubts regarding the diagnosis and their attempts to be as objective as possible (Joksimovic, Schröder, & van Keuk, 2015; Maier, 2006). They may in fact be seen as agents of de-culturalisation and de-politicisation in that they transfigure the refugees' accounts of atrocities into individualised pathology—a process refugees themselves may not be averse to as it may be the only avenue available to secure wider legal and welfare benefits. The resulting ethical dilemmas faced by health professionals is aptly described by Steel et al. (2004):

> The life-and-death struggle implicit in the refugee claim process presents the mental health clinician with additional professional and ethical dilemmas. Clinicians working with asylum applicants often find themselves in a position where forensic demands—namely, the need to obtain trauma testimonies to support refugee applicants' claims—can be of such a pressing nature that they outweigh usual clinical caution in delving too quickly into traumatic material that could undermine the emotional well-being of their patients (pg. 512).

Similarly, Fassin and d'Halluin (2005) quote the June 2002 newsletter of the organization Primo Levi which aptly asks, 'does one need a paper to prove torture?' The authors state:

> For immigrants, the poor, and more generally, the dominated – all of whom have to prove their eligibility to certain social rights – [the individual body and mind] has also become the place that displays the evidence of truth...asylum seekers are more and more submitted to the evaluation of their physical sequels and psychic traumas, as if their autobiographical accounts were not sufficient... Medical authority progressively substitutes itself for the asylum seekers' word. In this process of objectification, it is the experience of the victims as political subjects that is progressively erased (p. 597).

They argue that the medical certificate is detached from the lived experience of the victims of persecution, attempting a process of objectification through expert's words and thus desubjectifying individual narratives. A health professional they interviewed is quoted as saying that "by issuing certificates, we're busy judging who's guilty and who's innocent. What situation are we in? We're neither experts nor jurists" (p. 601). Another explains: "it is part of a programme designed to destructure and depersonalize the individual" (p. 602). Elsewhere, Joksimivic and colleagues (2015) similarly quote a professional as saying "I'm not paid to write certificates for authorities, I'm paid to treat my patients" (p. 233). This highlights the multitude of challenges often posed to health professionals, torn between the "moral demand" for PTSD to be diagnosed at the risk of influencing the therapeutic relationship, which by definition is less based on 'truth funding' and more on an exploration of the subjective experience of the individual. For many professionals who find themselves on the horn of this dilemma: "it is their burden and their duty to testify" (p. 604). The other health professionals interviewed by the authors similarly perceived the gap between the meaning that potentially traumatic acts can have for the people who were subjected to them and the "semantic reduction" (p. 603) of the clinical examination and medical report.

However, despite the potential damage caused to the individual by the use of a PTSD diagnosis, it is critical to highlight that there are indeed instances where it can be used in the service of marginalized individuals or groups. A persuasive argument therefore is the co-occurrence with policies, rights, and benefits through providing a foundation for status claims (Daiute, 2017). For example, a PTSD diagnosis is a way of validating the violent acts and traumatic events to which the individual has been subjected—not only are people listened to, it is a recognition that the suffering has been seen. It thus carries a deeply symbolic value.

Conclusion

Making use of the PTSD diagnosis in asylum procedures may present a double-edged sword. On the one hand, it acknowledges the deep pain experienced by asylum seekers and assists them in getting their refugee status recognized. On the other, it risks becoming a trendy "catch-all" diagnosis open to various forms of political abuse or manipulation. In this chapter, I have explored how PTSD may limit and control, yet at the same time how it is a powerful tool for public recognition and political response. It has been examined it as a boundary object (Star & Griesemer,

1989) used differently by health professionals and asylum seekers to facilitate the asylum process yet "glued together by the practices, technologies, and narratives with which it is diagnosed, studied, treated and represented and by the various interests, institutions, and moral arguments that mobilised these efforts and resources" (Young, 1995).

As noted by Dauite (2014), "storytelling shapes public life, and individuals transform public life in their own personal stories. It is through storytelling that societies indicate who belongs and who does not" (p. 7). The asylum procedure is one in which storytelling—rhetorical accomplishments and discursive constructions of reality—are of critical importance; the politics of asylum is a politics of representation in which discursively constructed and disseminated gross categories are crucial political instruments (Blommaert, 2001b). The category of "traumatized refugee," as reflected in a PTSD diagnosis, is one such instrument. It privileges certain events to develop a plausible version of the story in a context where the asylum seeker may be constructed as someone with a fragile memory, a fragmented subject who lies, an actor playing a role to deliver his subjectivity (Demazière, 2007).

The results indicate that neither the health professionals nor the asylum seekers are naïve to the potential benefits of fitting the traumatic events experienced into a narrative framed by PTSD, as a cultural tool, in the refugee determination process. However, there are apparent discrepancies in the way in which it is understood and used across the asylum activity system. Within this activity system, it functions as a "boundary object" (Trompette & Vinck, 2009), circulating among different actors yet with specific meanings within each sub-system. It is used by health professionals in certain activity systems to communicate among each other about the clinical symptoms experienced by the patient, and by the bureaucrats of the tribunal as evidence in court of the individual having survived a traumatic experience. The asylum seekers themselves experience the diagnosis in a myriad of different ways. Positioned as political subjects in the asylum procedure, as patients in the consulting room, as clients with their lawyers, as members of their community at home—PTSD appeared to have different meanings across these spaces. For the health professionals needing to address a variety of different actors outside of their clinical community, PTSD is helpful to explain (both to patients as well as to the bureaucrats of the asylum tribunal), to treat and, in some cases, to attest to the trauma experienced by the asylum seeker.

PTSD represents a refocalisation of the trauma narrative in a way that:

> shifts the epistemic center from the asylum seeker to the administrator processing the application… the story of the applicant is relocated in another space and time frame: that of the administrative procedure and its pace, that of its standard categories, criteria and textual formats…[it shifts] away from the local, away from the experiential, the affective, the emotional, the individual positioning of people in conflicts, towards generalizable categories and space-time frames (Blommaert, 2001b, p. 27)

As such, it is not politically neutral. Despite the many ways in which it can effectively assist asylum seekers who have indeed experienced significant psychological trauma, we cannot neglect the risks inherent to the "psychologization" (Rose, 1998) of persons and identities. In this context, not only are the accounts of the asylum seekers describing the persecutions they have endured and the risks they would incur if they were to return to their home country discredited, but their voice can no longer be heard: lawyers speak in their stead; volunteers help with their application, some even specializing in the so-called preparation of narratives; physicians and psychologists attest to their past experience (Fassin & d'Halluin, 2005; Fassin & Rechtman, 2009). PTSD risks creating narratives in which asylum seekers are seen in terms of deficits and security threats, which risks facilitating ongoing exclusion from human communities: if the asylum seeker is always represented as an individual victim of psychological damage, object of sympathy, scorn, or fear, initiatives for social inclusion are undermined (Daiute, 2017).

Yet despite the risks of victimization, psychological evaluation offers professionals a unique and privileged opportunity to help survivors to address and recover from the devastating consequences of trauma. As argued by Gangsei and Deutsch (2007), such evaluations may significantly increase an understanding of the survivors' background and experiences as well as their manner of self-presentation in the courtroom or interview. A recognition of trauma thus empowers individuals to present experiences more fully and confidently, helps them understand the necessity of telling the story, illuminates the often poorly perceived link between current emotional suffering and past trauma, facilitates the development of cognitive and emotional control, and heals the wounds of mistrust, humiliation, marginalization and fear. Indeed, as noted by Hanewald et al. (2016), in the case of traumatized refugees, the coaction of legal and medical aspects has to be acknowledged seriously by the medical, legal and political parts involved. Professionals—both legal and medical—working with asylum-seeking populations need to incorporate a nuanced and contextually informed understanding of each individual's trauma narrative.

References

Afana, A.-H., Pedersen, D., Rønsbo, H., & Kirmayer, L. J. (2010). Endurance is to be shown at the first blow: Social representations and reactions to traumatic experiences in the Gaza Strip. *Traumatology: An International Journal, 16*(4), 73–84.

Amsterdam, A. G., & Bruner, J. (2000). *Minding the law*. Cambridge, MA: Harvard University Press.

Blommaert, J. (2001a). Context is/as critique. *Critique of Anthropology, 21*(1), 13–32.

Blommaert, J. (2001b). Investigating narrative inequality: African asylum seekers' stories in Belgium. *Discourse and Society, 12*(4), 413–449.

Bögner, D., Brewin, C., & Herlihy, J. (2010). Refugees' experiences of Home Office interviews: A qualitative study on the disclosure of sensitive personal information. *Journal of Ethnic and Migration Studies, 36*(3), 519–535.

Bracken, P. (2001). Post-modernity and post-traumatic stress disorder. *Social Science and Medicine, 53*(6), 733–743.

Bracken, P., Giller, J. E., & Summerfield, D. (1997). Rethinking mental health work with survivors of wartime violence and refugees. *Journal of Refugee Studies, 10*(4), 431–442.

Bracken, P., Giller, J., & Summerfield, D. (2016). Primum non nocere. The case for a critical approach to global mental health. *Epidemiology and Psychiatric Sciences, 25*(6), 506–510.

Bruner, J. (1990). *Acts of meaning: Four lectures on mind and culture (Jerusalem-Harvard Lectures)*. Cambridge, MA: Harvard University Press.

Bruner, J. (1991). The narrative construction of reality. *Critical Inquiry, 18*(1), 1–21.

Bruner, J. (2003). *Making stories: Law, literature, life*. Cambridge, MA: Harvard University Press.

Crumlish, N., & Bracken, P. (2011). Mental health and the asylum process. *Irish Journal of Psychological Medicine, 28*, 57–60.

d'Halluin, E. (2009). La santé mentale des demandeurs d'asile. *Hommes et migrations. Revue française de référence sur les dynamiques migratoires*, (1282), 66–75.

d'Halluin, E. (2016). Le nouveau paradigme des «populations vulnérables» dans les politiques européennes d'asile. *Savoir/Agir*, (2), 21–26.

Daiute, C. (2014). *Narrative inquiry: A dynamic approach*. Los Angeles: Sage Publications.

Daiute, C. (2017). Narrating Refuge. *Europe's Journal of Psychology, 13*(1), 1–15.

Daiute, C., & Lucić, L. (2010). Situated cultural development among youth separated by war. *International Journal of Intercultural Relations, 34*(6), 615–628.

Demazière, D. (2007). À qui peut-on se fier? Les sociologues et la parole des interviewés. *Langage Et Société, 3*, 85–100.

Di Donato, F. (2011). Constructing legal narratives: Client-lawyers' stories. In A. Wagner & L. Cheng (Eds.), *Exploring courtroom discourse: The language of power and control* (pp. 129–146). London: Routledge.

Di Donato, F. (2014). Narratives in cultural contexts: The legal agentivity of the protagonists. Available at SSRN 2469436.

Drožđek, B. (2015). Challenges in treatment of posttraumatic stress disorder in refugees: Towards integration of evidence-based treatments with contextual and culture-sensitive perspectives. *European Journal of Psychotraumatology, 6*, 24750.

Eleftherakos, C., van den Boogaard, W., Barry, D., Severy, N., Kotsioni, I., & Roland-Gosselin, L. (2018). "I prefer dying fast than dying slowly," how institutional abuse worsens the mental health of stranded Syrian, Afghan and Congolese migrants on Lesbos island following the implementation of EU-Turkey deal. *Conflict and Health, 12*(1), 38.

Fassin, D. (2011). The trace: violence, truth, and the politics of the body. *Social Research, 78*(2), 281–298.

Fassin, D., & d'Halluin, E. (2005). The truth from the body: Medical certificates as ultimate evidence for asylum seekers. *American Anthropologist, 107*(4), 597–608.

Fassin, D., & Rechtman, R. (2009). *The empire of trauma: An inquiry into the condition of victimhood*. Princeton, N.J.: Princeton University Press.

Gangsei, D., & Deutsch, A. C. (2007). Psychological evaluation of asylum seekers as a therapeutic process. *Torture Quarterly Journal on Rehabilitation of Torture Victims and Prevention of Torture, 17*(2), 79–87.

UNHCR. (2015). *The sea route to Europe: The Mediterranean passage in the age of refugees*. Geneva: United Nations High Commissioner for Refugees.

Good, A. (2007). *Anthropology and expertise in the asylum courts*. London: Routledge.

Hanewald, B., Gieseking, J., Vogelbusch, O., Markus, I., Gallhofer, B., & Knipper, M. (2016). Asylum law and mental health: An interdisciplinary analysis of the coaction of medical and legal aspects. *Psychiatrische Praxis, 43*(3), 165–171.

Hinton, D. E., & Lewis-Fernández, R. (2011). The cross-cultural validity of posttraumatic stress disorder: Implications for DSM-5. *Depression and Anxiety, 28*(9), 783–801.

Hymes, D. (1998). When is oral narrative poetry? Generative form and its pragmatic conditions. *Pragmatics, 8*, 475–500.

Janoff-Bulman, R. (1985). The aftermath of victimization: Rebuilding shattered assumptions. *Trauma and Its Wake, 1*, 15–35.

Joksimovic, L., Schröder, M., & van Keuk, E. (2015). Psychotherapy with Immigrants and Refugees from Crisis Zones. In M. Schouler-Ocak (Ed.), *Trauma and Migration* (pp. 223–241). Cham: Springer.

Joles, B. (2018). How refugees' trauma became 'currency' in resettlement. *NewsDeeply: Refugees Deeply*. Retrieved from https://www.newsdeeply.com/refugees/articles/2018/08/10/how-refugees-trauma-became-currency-in-resettlement on the 11th of Feb. 2020.

Kirmayer, L. J., Kienzler, H., Afana, A. H., & Pedersen, D. (2010). Trauma and disasters in social and cultural context. *Principles of Social Psychiatry, 2,* 155–177.

Kleinman, A., & Good, B. (2004). Culture and depression. *New England Journal of Medicine, 351,* 951–952.

Kloetzer, L., Clot, Y., & Quillerou-Grivot, E. (2015). Stimulating dialogue at work: The activity clinic approach to learning and development. In L. Filliettaz., & S. Billett (Eds.), *Francophone perspectives of learning through work* (pp. 49–70). Springer.

Lechenne, J. (2012). *Violences sexuelles à l'encontre des femmes en situations de conflit et de post-conflit: La procédure d'asile en Suisse vue sous l'angle d'un continuum de la violence.* Masters' Dissertation, University of Geneva.

Linton, R. (2015). A presumption of disclosure: Towards greater transparency in asylum proceedings. *Seattle University Law Review, 38,* 1069–1139.

Losi, N. (2002). Some assumptions on psychological trauma interventions in post-conflict communities. In R. Papadopoulos (Ed.), *Therapeutic care for refugees: No place like home* (pp. 103–120). London: Karnac.

Luno, J. A., Beck, J. G., & Louwerse, M. (2013). Tell us your story: investigating the linguistic features of trauma narrative. *The Cognitive Science Society, 35,* 2955–2960.

Maier, T. (2006). Procédure d'asile et rapports médicaux. *Bulletin des médecins suisses| Schweizerische Ärztezeitung| Bollettino dei medici svizzeri, 87*, 25.

Maier, T., & Straub, M. (2011). "My head is like a bag full of rubbish": Concepts of illness and treatment expectations in traumatized migrants. *Qualitative Health Research, 21*(2), 233–248.

Marlowe, J. M. (2010). Beyond the discourse of trauma: Shifting the focus on Sudanese refugees. *Journal of Refugee Studies, 23*(2), 183–198.

Marsella, A. J. (2010). Ethnocultural aspects of PTSD: An overview of concepts, issues, and treatments. *Traumatology, 16*(4), 17.

Maryns, K., & Blommaert, J. (2001). Stylistic and thematic shifting as a narrative resource: Assessing asylum seekers' repertoires. *Multilingua, 20,* 61–84.

McFarlane, A. C. (1995). PTSD in the medico-legal setting: Current status and ongoing controversies. *Psychiatry, Psychology and Law, 2*(1), 25–35.

Médecins Sans Frontières (M.S.F.) (2016). *Neglected Trauma - Asylum seekers in Italy: an analysis of mental health distress and access to healthcare.* Rome, Italy. Retrieved from https://www.msf.org/sites/msf.org/files/neglected_trauma_report.pdf on the 12th of Feb. 2020.

Momartin, S., Silove, D., Manicavasagar, V., & Steel, Z. (2003). Dimensions of trauma associated with posttraumatic stress disorder (PTSD) caseness, severity and functional impairment: A study of Bosnian refugees resettled in Australia. *Social Science and Medicine, 57*(5), 775.

Montagut, M. (2016). L'emprise de la torture: Les troubles langagiers des demandeurs d'asile face aux attentes institutionnelles. *Langage Et Société, 4,* 89–105.

Mueller, J., Schmidt, M., Staeheli, A., & Maier, T. (2011). Mental health of failed asylum seekers as compared with pending and temporarily accepted asylum seekers. *The European Journal of Public Health, 21*(2), 184–189.

Papadopoulos, R. (2002b). *Therapeutic care for refugees: No place like home.* Karnac Books.

Pickup, J. C., Holloway, M. F., & Samsi, K. (2014). Real-time continuous glucose monitoring in type 1 diabetes: A qualitative framework analysis of patient narratives. *Diabetes Care, 38*(4), 544–550.

Pupavac, V. (2002). Pathologizing populations and colonizing minds: International psychosocial programs in Kosovo. *Alternatives, 27*(4), 489–511.

Rogers, H., Fox, S., & Herlihy, J. (2015). The importance of looking credible: The impact of the behavioural sequelae of post-traumatic stress disorder on the credibility of asylum seekers. *Psychology, Crime and Law, 21*(2), 139–155.

Rose, N. (1998). *Inventing our selves: Psychology, power, and personhood*. Cambridge: Cambridge University Press.
Roth, W.-M., & Lee, Y.-J. (2007). "Vygotsky's neglected legacy": Cultural-historical activity theory. *Review of Educational Research, 77*(2), 186–232.
Schock, K., Rosner, R., & Knaevelsrud, C. (2015). Impact of asylum interviews on the mental health of traumatized asylum seekers. *European Journal of Psychotraumatology, 6*, 26286.
Schock, K., Böttche, M., Rosner, R., Wenk-Ansohn, M., & Knaevelsrud, C. (2016). Impact of new traumatic or stressful life events on pre-existing PTSD in traumatized refugees: results of a longitudinal study. *7*, 32106.
Silove, D., & Mares, S. (2018). The mental health of asylum seekers in Australia and the role of psychiatrists. *BJPsych International, 15*(3), 65–68.
Silove, D., Steel, Z., McGorry, P., & Mohan, P. (1998). Trauma exposure, postmigration stressors, and symptoms of anxiety, depression and post-traumatic stress in Tamil asylum-seekers: Comparison with refugees and immigrants. *Acta Psychiatrica Scandinavica, 97*(3), 175–181.
Silove, D., Steel, Z., & Watters, C. (2000). Policies of deterrence and the mental health of asylum seekers. *JAMA, 284*(5), 604–611.
Star, S. L., & Griesemer, J. R. (1989). Institutional ecology, translations' and boundary objects: Amateurs and professionals in Berkeley's museum of vertebrate zoology, 1907–39. *Social Studies of Science, 19*(3), 387–420.
Steel, Z. (2001). Beyond PTSD: Towards a more adequate understanding of the multiple effects of complex trauma. In C. Moser & D. Nyfeler (Eds.), *Traumatiserungen von Flüchtlingen und Asyl Schenden: Einflus des politischen, sozialen und medizinischen Kontextes* (pp. 66–84). Zurich: Seismo.
Steel, Z., Frommer, N., & Silove, D. (2004). Part I—The mental health impacts of migration: The law and its effects: Failing to understand: Refugee determination and the traumatized applicant. *International Journal of Law and Psychiatry, 27*(6), 511–528.
Steel, Z., Chey, T., Silove, D., Marnane, C., Bryant, R. A., & Ommeren, M. V. (2009). Association of torture and other potentially traumatic events with mental health outcomes among populations exposed to mass conflict and displacement: A systematic review and meta-analysis. *JAMA, 302*(5), 537–549.
Struwe, G. (1994). Training health and medical professionals to care for refugees: Issues and methods. In A. J. Marsella, T. Bornemann, S. Ekblad, & J. Orley (Eds.), *Amidst peril and pain: The mental health and well-being of the world's refugees* (pp. 311–324). Washington DC: American Psychological Association.
Sturm, G., Baubet, T., & Moro, M. R. (2010). Culture, trauma, and subjectivity: The French ethnopsychoanalytic approach. *Traumatology, 16*(4), 27–38.
Summerfield, D. (1996). *L'impact de la Guerre et des Atrocités sur les Populations Civiles: Principes Fondamentaux pour les Interventions des ONG et une Analyse Critique des Projets sur le Traumatisme Psychosocial*. London: Overseas Development Institute.
Summerfield, D. (1999). A critique of seven assumptions behind psychological trauma programmes in war-affected areas. *Social Science and Medicine, 48*(10), 1449–1462.
Summerfield, D. (2001). The invention of post-traumatic stress disorder and the social usefulness of a psychiatric category. *British Medical Journal, 322*(7278), 95–98.
Toomela, A. (2014). There can be no cultural-historical psychology without neuropsychology. And vice versa. In A. Yasnitsky, R. van der Veer, & M. Ferrari (Eds.), *The Cambridge Handbook of Cultural-Historical Theory* (pp. 315–349). Cambridge University Press.
Trompette, P., & Vinck, D. (2009). Revisiting the notion of boundary object. *Revue D'anthropologie Des Connaissances, 3*(1), 3–25.
Tummala-Narra, P. (2007). Conceptualizing trauma and resilience across diverse contexts. *Journal of Aggression, Maltreatment and Trauma, 14*(1–2), 33–53.
Turner, B. (1992). *Regulating bodies: Essays in medical sociology*. London: Routledge.
Turner, S. (2015). Refugee blues: A UK and European perspective. *Psychotraumatology, 6*(1), 29328.

Van der Riet, M. (2009). *The production of context: using activity theory to understand behaviour change in response to HIV and AIDS (Doctoral dissertation).* (PhD), University of KwaZulu-Natal, Pietermaritzburg. Retrieved from https://www.researchgate.net/profile/Mary_Van_Der_Riet/publication/267259128_The_production_of_context_using_activity_theory_to_understand_behaviour_change_in_response_to_HIV_and_AIDS/links/55d1c66808ae3dc86a4f2eb3.pdf on the 02.06.2020.

van der Riet, M. (2012). Working with historicity: Tracing shifts in contraceptive use in the activity system of sex over time. *Psychology in Society, 43,* 23–39.

Vygotsky, L. S. (1980). *Mind in society: The development of higher psychological processes.* Cambridge, MA: Harvard University Press.

Watters, C. (2001). Emerging paradigms in the mental health care of refugees. *Social Science and Medicine, 52*(11), 1709–1718.

Wenzel, T., & Droždek, B. (2018). *An uncertain safety: Integrative health care for the 21st Century refugees.* New York: Springer.

Wilson-Shaw, L., Pistrang, N., & Herlihy, J. (2012). Non-clinicians' judgments about asylum seekers' mental health: How do legal representatives of asylum seekers decide when to request medico-legal reports? *European Journal of Psychotraumatology, 3*(1), 18406.

Young, A. (1995). *The harmony of illusions.* Princeton: Princeton University Press.

Young, G. (2016). PTSD in court I: Introducing PTSD for court. *International Journal of Law and Psychiatry, 49,* 238–258.

Young, G. (2017). PTSD in Court II: Risk factors, endophenotypes, and biological underpinnings in PTSD. *International Journal of Law and Psychiatry, 51,* 1–21.

Chapter 12
Conclusion

The number of refugees across the globe is growing dramatically—a trend predicted to continue due to a global increase in social and political instability as well as socioeconomic conflicts. In places where violence is seen as a necessary factor in achieving peace, ongoing armed conflict, and displacement will likely contribute to continued psychological impairment and suffering among those affected (Morina et al., 2018). Indeed, research overwhelmingly attests to the alarmingly high rates of PTSD among this population (Schouler-Ocak et al., 2019). This is no surprise. What is surprising, however, is the lack of knowledge concerning refugee experiences of potentially traumatic events from a sociocultural perspective. As recently noted by Zipfel and colleagues (2019):

> we still know very little about how evidence-based concepts of assessing and treating mental health conditions actually work when applied to traumatised refugee populations... Also, the interplay between pre-migration adverse or potentially traumatic experiences, various stressors during the flight, post-migration living difficulties, and mental health is far from being understood (p. 22).

Within humanitarian interventions targeting refugee populations, "trauma" seems to be something taken-for-granted and assumed. It is a ubiquitous buzzword permeating discourse. Yet, there continues to be very little critical reflection—or indeed consensus—on what it *actually* is. Having worked as a clinician in mental health projects with displaced populations—across a variety of cultural contexts—this was a constant source of personal frustration and concern. I would repeatedly be called upon to report on the number of refugees with PTSD Repeatedly, I would sit in front of individual refugees for whom the diagnosis made little sense. It seemed a ludicrous discrepancy. Similarly absurd was the implicit assumption that the mental health of this population had very little to do with their current daily reality. I was working as a psychologist, not a social worker, lawyer, or human rights advocate. Yet the social, legal, and economic needs of the beneficiaries continually found their way into our

G. Theisen-Womersley, *Trauma and Resilience Among Displaced Populations*,
https://doi.org/10.1007/978-3-030-67712-1_12

consultations. From a personal perspective, this compelled me to develop this body of research. Importantly, it is research intended to speak to the concrete reality of the humanitarian field. It is research intended simply to make sense.

Given the ubiquitous nature of the diagnosis in popular discourse in general, and humanitarian discourses centering on "suffering refugees" in particular, what is missing is an understanding of the context in which experiences of potentially traumatic events are embedded. The staggering discrepancy in rates of PTSD noted among refugee populations (Morina et al., 2018) could be seen as a further indication that we need to go *beyond* the diagnosis to see what is happening "in the field." This is not to say that we need to disregard the diagnosis. This book does not intend to position itself as being "for" or "against" its use at such. Rather, the intention is to peek *behind* the metaphorical curtain and explore the stories behind the high prevalence rates of PTSD—and to explore the borders of the diagnosis itself. Echoing the research aims of Shala and colleagues (2020), the intention is thus "to go beyond such labelling to explore participants' assumptions about the causes of their suffering, their implicit concepts of how body and mind interact, how language is used to express psychological distress in a culturally congruent and socially acceptable manner, and what expectations people hold about the course (and relief) of their suffering." (p. 19).

The notion of the "traumatised refugee" is a complex one. It holds symbolic power. There is a complete narrative behind this tragic figure. Many have seen the images flashed across the media: devastated and impoverished communities, sinking ships, abandoned children, fences and barriers and brutal European regimes attempting to control the influx. There is no denying the brutal reality facing refugees arriving in Europe. The suffering is real, and multifaceted. Trauma does not stop at the border.

However, the results of this research have highlighted the existing tensions among conflicting narratives of trauma circulating among the actors involved. They bring to light the discrepancies in the way in which experiences of potentially traumatic events are understood, and in which narratives of trauma are used across legal and medical activity systems. Broadly speaking, the way in which "trauma" is understood by lawyers is different to that of health professionals such as doctors and psychologists, and again to that of refugee populations themselves. Furthermore, the way in which experiences of potentially traumatic events and their sequelae is i) understood or made sense of and ii) (re)presented in narratives, addressed to other actors across settings, changes to adapt to the context, and changes over time. The use of a diagnosis of PTSD in particular seems to be unnervingly context-dependant. A doctor may diagnose PTSD strategically, to inform an individual treatment plan within a medical context, but not to inform the asylum tribunal to assist them in their decision-making process—or vice versa. A lawyer may decide to focus on the "headline" of the potentially traumatic event in representing the narrative to a judge—and encourage a refugee to frame this narrative within a certain way that is most easily understood by the court. Refugees may decide to present the trauma narrative in one way to a psychologist, and in another way to their lawyer. They may go to the psychologist with the explicit intention of receiving a medical certificate attesting to a diagnosis of PTSD for use in the legal system. They may deny being traumatised altogether—the implicit understanding of "trauma" inherent to a PTSD diagnosis seemingly too far from their own subjective understanding of what was happening to them. The results indicate that PTSD as an instrument circulates among the different actors yet with specific meanings and functions within each activity system, and which change over time.

Not only are there multiple tensions associated with such a diversity of narratives of trauma, but there is an inherent hierarchy within medical and legal activity systems which places the knowledge of one group as superior to another. The narratives are not created equal. They are embedded within sociocultural and political structures with very real political, economic, and social consequences for refugees. Within this system, it appears that the medicalized narrative of trauma, as manifested concretely in the diagnosis of PTSD, holds particular political power. Neither the health professionals nor the refugee research participants appeared naïve to the potential benefits of using PTSD as a cultural tool to be used in the asylum seeking procedure in particular. PTSD as a diagnosis appears instead to have been used strategically by the various actors in a way that was explicitly interactive, communicative, and purposeful. It is not a politically neutral tool.

The results also clearly highlight the changing nature of the subjective experiences of exposure to potentially traumatic events by individuals over time. For the individual refugee research participants—negotiating complex legal and medical systems had a substantial impact on their mental health. It confirms what is increasingly being highlighted in the literature: there is very little "post" about the post-traumatic stress being experienced by refugee populations in Europe. It seems absurd to focus on the "headline events" of what happened in the country of origin when individuals are struggling to survive—today and every day. Yet it is not a question of "here or there," "past or present." No such dichotomies exist. Rather, the potentially traumatic experiences of the past echo the current reality. Trauma begets trauma.

Another issue explored in the book concerns that of the use of the diagnosis of PTSD as a cultural tool: for what, by whom, and for whom? None of the refugee participants in the research were familiar with the concept of PTSD before being diagnosed with it themselves. What strikes me is the way in which this diagnosis was appropriated and/or contested by various participants. There were a variety of responses to being confronted with this novel, medicalized notion of suffering. For some participants, it appeared as though the notion was so far from their own conceptualisation of what was happening that very little appropriation took place. The diagnosis was something for western health professionals, from western health professionals, that was of very little direct concern or consequence. As such, it was not so much of a rejection of the diagnosis. It was a rendering it irrelevant. For others, it was a useful tool. In this latter case, it seems that the use of the tool lay in its concrete political, legal, and social relevance. It was a tool for use within various medical and legal activity systems—not a personal usefulness as such, but a practical and concrete usefulness in the sociocultural environment. In such cases as these, there similarly seems to have been very little appropriation of the diagnosis at a personal or subjective level among participants. In other words, PTSD as a cultural tool was used with certain concrete intentions in mind. For example, it was useful to have the diagnosis as evidence of refugee status within the asylum tribunal. The diagnosis was a cultural tool used to act in the world, but not to further a process of psychological rehabilitation, or to make personal sense of suffering. None of the participants seemed to have drawn upon the diagnosis to inform their own personal way of making sense of potentially traumatic events or as a significant factor in their journey to recovery.

It is perhaps understandable that PTSD be used as a tool by various actors attempting to negotiate the complex procedure that is asking for asylum. It may even perhaps be viewed as a question of the survival of certain refugees. We need, on one hand, to be shocked by the potentially traumatic events—and to bear witness the impact of this on their mental health. To recognise this, in the concrete form of the diagnosis, is imperative. The wounds are real. What I find more surprising, however, were results indicating the same power struggles playing out in the court playing out in the consultation room. From a personal perspective, it has lead me to reflect on the implication of this for health professionals working with this population. Might refugee patients be rehearsing their trauma stories for the psychologist, as they do for the court? Might they experience being seated in front of a psychologist in the same way as being seated in front of a judge?

I refer back to the words of one refugee with whom I had a conversation:

> The people asking you questions [in the tribunal], it's like you're sitting across from a psychologist. They're professionals who know their work…for the psychologist, it's a ***game***. It's a ***toy***. He asks you questions, and bases his deductions on your response - and the asylum [procedure] itself, it's the same.

His words suggest a deep distrust in mental health professionals. It also highlights how different the subjective experience of being seated in front of a psychologist may be for refugees to that of what we might imagine it to be. For him, the psychologist is similarly playing a game. He himself is a toy in this context, being manipulated by the medical system as much as the legal system. For many who have experienced torture in particular, it sadly seems to echo the deep sense of powerlessness at the hands of an aggressor experienced in their countries of origin. There are inevitably power imbalances inherent to the relationship. There are inevitably differences in how we make sense of trauma, how we narrate trauma to ourselves and others. As there are multiple traumas, there are multiple stories of trauma, and multiple listeners to the stories.

Trust is central to these dynamics. Within the dialogical approach adopted throughout this book, trust is considered as positional: "social power holders insist upon a positional monologization of trust…we are assumed to trust institutions [and] all that monogolization happens through words -words inserted into specific locations." (Linell & Marková, 2013) p. xi). Yet, "trust is a dialogical feeling in which the person relies on someone else based on expectation of positive ethical reciprocity…thus trusting psychotherapy, in a macro-sense, implies to trust a distributed institution, in which social roles are established, as well as the generic rules that govern the activity that may reach a legal format" (Salgado, 2013) p. 110). In the consultation rom, refugee victims of torture are expected to trust the mental health professional when diagnosed with PTSD They are socially and institutionally in the (inferior?) position as the patient within this dynamic. For some of the refugees I encountered, trust in the mental health professional was a given. For most, however, there was a marked ambivalence around how much the professionals charged with their care could be trusted. In light of the multitude of potentially traumatic events to which this population has been exposed—all along the migration journey—the lack of trust is not surprising. Indeed, for some, the implicit obligation to trust the professional may prove an impossible task. Being in the privileged and arguably hierarchically superior position of health professional in relation to refugee "patient" therefore comes with an ethical responsibility to be aware of the discrepancies in trauma narratives, and the power dynamics inherent to this context of which trust is a core component.

What is further worth highlighting in reflecting upon these results is the notion of agency or the will and ability to extend one's power to act (Clot, 2011; Clot & Béguin, 2004; Clot & Litim, 2008; Kloetzer et al., 2015). None of the research participants–refugees, health professionals, community leaders–were passive in engaging with these legal and medical activity systems. To some degree or another, there was more or less power to act as individual agents. This power extends to the refugee participants themselves. Despite the inevitable imbalances of power characterising these systems, and the multitude of barriers faced, all of the refugee participants found ways to act within the system in order to survive and thrive: rehearsing a speech for the tribunal, disagreeing with a psychologists' interpretation of their symptoms, actively seeking the support of a local community … even within the most ostensibly powerless positions, there is a power to act, there is resistance. Research participants, refugee victims of torture, found the will and ability to exert power over a seemingly hopeless situation.

To summarize, this book highlights.

(i) the way in which a PTSD diagnosis is being used strategically as a cultural tool by various actors within medical and legal activity systems put in place to address the large influx of refugees arriving in Europe
(ii) the changing development of experiences of potentially traumatic events over time. This includes the substantial impact of the current (sociocultural, legal, economic, and political) environment on refugee trauma trajectories
(iii) the culturally diverse narratives of trauma informing refugee mental health, which may compete, contradict, or conform to the narrative of trauma inherent to a diagnosis of PTSD This includes the substantial lack of the use of the PTSD diagnosis as a resource for personal recovery among participants
(iv) the ways in which refugee victims of torture manage to draw on multiple resources in order to exert and extend their power to act as active agents, despite being positioned as "victims".

Towards a Sociocultural Definition of Trauma

I begin these reflections by returning to psychoanalytic conceptualizations of the term "trauma." According to Freudian psychodynamic theory, trauma is defined as a frightful experience which overwhelms the psyche to such an extent that images, words or other memories related to the event are unable to be integrated into the system of representations which structure the experience of the individual (Garland, 2002; Sturm et al., 2007). Within this paradigm, one commonality of trauma experience is the feeling of a chaos of seemingly unutterable experiences collapsing into that "wordless nothing" (Larrabee et al., 2003, p. 354). As eloquently expressed by Lester (2013):

> Pushed to the very precipice of physical and/or psychological annihilation, the bonds that tether a person to the everyday world become stretched, distorted, and even torn; sometimes irreparably so. Such a state of ontological alienation is profoundly distressing. To regain their footing, people often turn to culturally available practices, symbols, and structures to help reorient them to the world (p. 753).

What this research demonstrates is the mediating impact of narrating potentially traumatic experiences to Others, in processes of recovery. This is because telling a story of a potentially traumatic event or reliving it necessarily occurs in a larger dialogical matrix of narrative and social praxis (Kirmayer, 1996). The communicative function of language as a tool, concrete semiotic and symbolic devices provide the connections to an Other and to one's Self (Daiute & Lucić, 2010). As such, symbolic elements in socio-cultural practices are resources for repairing ruptures in intersubjectivity. They are lenses through which experiences may be collectively and individually reflected upon. **Language** is central. Cultural representations, carried through language, are considered in their function not only as shared symbols but also as subjectively appropriated and emotionally invested representations (Sturm et al., 2010). It is therefore through language that one is able to constitute and actualize a coherent sense of Self. Furthermore, this can only take place in the context of "interlocution" or "addressivity" (Bakhtin, 1978, 1981, 1986)—towards and with an Other. There is evidently a continual dialogue between the person's inner world and the socio-cultural context in which internalized configurations or representations of potentially traumatic events are processed (Lemma & Levy, 2004). The critical issue here is that of the notion of reciprocity (Van Der Kolk, 2015) inherent to **social recognition** (Marková, 2016).

Zittoun (2004) argues that:

> The embodied quality of experiences is, in its origin, given as a brutal happening. To be apprehended mentally, these experiences have to be linked to semiotic mediations. Mnemonic traces of previous comparable experiences, in their minimal definition or socially shared signs, either previously internalized, or available in one's environment, have to be attached to them. Semiotic mediation minimally authorizes the grouping of fuzzy embodied impressions and then designate these groups of impressions (by a linguistic term, or also just by attaching

> them to any image), and eventually to include them into an articulated sequence in the flow of thinking. Thus, semiotic mediations can allow experience to become part of, and thus transform, other thoughts. Thanks to semiotic mediation, normal elaboration of experiences allows processes of linking and transformation through which they progressively fade in the flows of memories and thinking. (p. 484).

Reflecting on the process by which semiotic mediation allows for memories of potentially traumatic events to be processed and ultimately stored in the flows of memories and thinking, a traumatic rupture in this very process would lead to the usual semiotic work of making sense, which demands to bind traces of events to other traces, in time and in experience, not taking place. The potentially traumatic events and the actual sphere of experiences are disconnected. Should this prove to be the case, the lack of connection of past and present can also be understood as preventing the emergence of possible futures. From within this dialogical paradigm, this lack of connection to the future is intrinsically linked to a severe disruption of the relational processes by which meaning is dialogically created—the bedrock of which is social recognition. Viewed through the lens of a dialogic systems sensibility, the traumatic world's slipping away from the categories of meaning can be seen as a severe disruption of those relational processes in which meaning is formed (Sucharov et al., 2007).

Within a sociocultural framework than, **trauma may be defined as that which cannot be elaborated through semiotic means.** I would argue that, implicitly contained within this definition, is the idea that the Self is inextricably connected to the Other, and that it is language which acts as the mediating conduit between the two. Trauma has a social and a cultural dimension. For the transformation of memories of potentially traumatic events into semiotic forms which connects it through language to its rightful place in time, the elaboration needs to be socially situated and "intersubjectively acknowledged" (Zittoun, 2014, p. 485). Here, I refer to a Vygotskian conceptualization of language as a system of signs. This does not necessarily mean that the elaboration needs to be conducted verbally. Language is more than words. Many processes of recovery from potentially traumatic events have resulted from making use of alternative ways in which to elaborate upon the experiences. Drawings, puppets, dolls, sandtrays, to cite a few examples, have all been used to facilitate this process of elaboration in creative ways without depending on words.

A sociocultural definition of trauma, sees it first and foremost as **relational, intersubjective** experience. It relates to a **crisis** that is situated, negotiated, and sometimes mended in relationships. From this perspective, mental health comes into view as "a problem of social Ecology, which may involve crises of kinship, of relations of reciprocity and obligation, of maintaining proper relations with ancestors, and, importantly, the therapeutic relationships" (Bemme & Kirmayer, 2020, p. 13). Trauma should be seen as a social phenomenon, viewed at communal and societal levels (Daiute et al., 2006).

Due to the fact that the experience of trauma unfolds within the complex ecology of sociocultural systems, it is **nonlinear and non-dose dependant.** Being exposed to a "dose" of potentially traumatic event(s) will not result in a directly proportional symptomatic response to these events. Rather, the experience is mediated through language, and through our connections to others. The way in which post-traumatic symptoms may manifest is similarly nonlinear: symptoms do not necessarily gradually weaken over time. Furthermore, as explored in **chapter eight**, the suffering is not in direct opposition to aspects of resilience and growth.

A sociocultural understanding of trauma takes into account notions of **temporality**. Social resources provide a time orientation, and, consequently, a self-continuity between past and future (Kadianaki & Zittoun, 2014) necessary for the construction of a coherent narrative, and, ultimately, the Self.

This begs an essential question: **is "refugeehood" necessarily traumatic?** By definition, refugees are people who have faced severe threats in their countries of origin, and many experience violence during their flight or in refugee camps. Disruption of social networks and separation from or loss of family members are common consequences of forced migration and are associated with an increased risk for subsequent mental health problems (Kirmayer et al., 2011). For many refugees who have arguably been exposed to a plethora of potentially traumatic events both before, during and after migration—what is potentially lost is the ability to draw on meaningful socio-cultural symbolic resources to make sense of these events as well as the ear of a listening Other to whom and with whom the process of sense-making of potentially traumatic experiences may be addressed.

Yet, I would argue that the experience of refugeehood, like any experience of migration, and indeed any general human experience, is complex. As much as the book has highlighted suffering, my hope is that aspects of growth and development in the face of this suffering have equally been highlighted. In short, the state of "refugeehood" is not necessarily traumatic in and of itself. I would instead return to the above definition of trauma, and argue that experiences of refugeehood may be considered traumatic **when there is no possibility of these experiences being elaborated through semiotic means.** Sadly, this is too often the case. Facing potentially traumatic events, as well as significant ruptures from a sociocultural context in which these events may be made sense of, a vast number of refugees are traumatized by their experiences of migration. We need to bear in mind that it is not only the period before and during migration, but also upon arrival in host communities: a period typically characterized by a social and political marginalization leading to isolation, withdrawal, distrust, non-recognition and rejection, as well as being torn from one's communal and social fabric.

In this sense, a sociocultural understanding of **"refugeehood"** itself would consider it as a social phenomenon, beyond the "traumatized" isolated figures of individual asylum seekers. Rather, it considers "violent displacements as embedded in geo-political systems mediated by human language" (Daiute et al. 2020, p. 15). Refugeehood, in other words, is an embededness in refugee systems. The recent unfolding of the refugee "reception crisis" in Europe is inextricably linked to the development of society as a whole. Responses and reactions to the crisis are indicators of the maturity of society. Instead of focusing on individual refugees, a sociocultural approach would consider the dynamic interrelatedness of individuals and broader "refugee systems."

Implications for Mental Health Clinicians

As summarized by Drožđek and colleagues (2020),

> core aims of all psychotherapeutic interventions for survivors of war and violence are to help them to regain control over their lives, restore self-efficacy and a sense of agency, reattach with humanity, give meaning to traumatic experiences and suffering, and regain hope for the future. These therapy aims go beyond the goals of simply reducing symptoms of PTSD, depression, and other comorbid conditions, although reduction of symptoms and associated suffering are important. (p. 9).

How may mental health clinicians obtain these aims? What might a sociocultural approach teach us about experiences of potentially traumatic events among refugee populations? I now explore the implications of such a sociocultural understanding of "trauma" for mental health clinicians working with refugee populations.

The Role of Narrative Activity

Throughout this book, I have defend the view that we are narrative beings, constructing and reconstructing our Selves through stories, locating our biographies and life projects in discursive webs of shared meaning. One consequence of this sociocultural perspective is that understanding the human capacity to produce, think in, and transact with narrative must play a central role in clinical practice. Narrative capacities, skills, practices, and specific content can contribute to the causes, course, and outcomes of psychopathology as well as to processes of coping, resilience, healing, and recovery. Narrating our lives mediates our lives. For refugees, the activity of narrating is a critical part of their "making sense of what is going on in their environment, trying, and sometimes succeeding against great odds to re-create meaningful sustainable life for themselves, for their children, their communities, and natural environments" (Daiute & Gómez, 2014, p. 157).

We do not just speak through language but *use* language to express meaning in context. People use narrating to interact in the world, to figure out what is going on in their environments, how they fit, and sometimes, how to change things (Daiute et al., 2015). The bridging role of language, therefore, should be central to refine the way that clinicians think about how local illness terms, expressions, and explanations relate to the kinds of problems they diagnose and treat. For example, cultural representations of potentially traumatic events and their sequelae held within language may also serve to articulate modes of experience and adaptation that contribute to resilience and well-being in the face of adversity (Lewis-Fernández & Kirmayer, 2019).

Clinicians, through the mediating impact of language as a cultural tool, may play a key role in facilitating narrative activity: assisting the memories of potentially traumatic events to be elaborated upon, made sense of, and placed within a meaningful temporal framework. It is this narrative activity which allows individuals to reconfigure a sense of themselves and their experiences—both of the past, the present, and the future—in order not to remain stuck within the wordless nothing. Through a process of semiotic mediation, we find the words to confront the wordless nothing. It is not only PTSD which may be used as a cultural tool by mental health clinicians and their refugee clients or patients alike. A sociocultural approach has allowed us to examine the ways in which language *itself* acts as a cultural tool with which to mediate potentially traumatic experiences—for example, in the narrative activity of the psychotherapy session. For many, the therapeutic context itself may function as another cultural tool—the rituals inherent to the therapeutic process unfolding within the session, and developed within the context of a human relationship, serving to facilitate a process of healing and recovery. Here, I return to Daiute's (2014) definition of a cultural tool as "symbolic process developed in human relations for interacting purposefully in the world" (p. 23). Narrative activity within the psychotherapeutic process exemplifies such purposeful interaction.

The Collective Cultural Frame

At the core of this book is the idea that the experiencing of potentially traumatic events has a social and cultural dimension: "the manner in which people understand their afflictions is undoubtedly connected to beliefs about the origins of such afflictions. Such beliefs are central in devising appropriate therapeutic strategies for the alleviation and elimination of the afflications" (Honwana, 2006, p. 229). This book has explored "culture" in all of its dynamic unfolding over time. "Culture" is not static. It changes with experiences of forced migration, and over time, so clinicians should bear in mind the ever-changing local cultural communities and current issues and concerns. They should also be aware of their own personal and professional cultural assumptions (Kirmayer et al., 2011).

Some key implications for mental health clinicians, arising from a sociocultural exploration of experiences of potentially traumatic events among refugees, is the significant influence of collective histories of colonialism, racism, violence, and exploitation which may influence the development of a working alliance built on trust. People from refugee communities come with their own collective histories, living conditions, and social, moral, and political concerns that form the backdrop of their personal experience of potentially traumatic events. For survivors of torture in particular, the clinical situation may remind them of these potentially traumatic events—the interview leading to a sense of being interrogated, as was the case for some research participants. It is essential that clinicians be aware of the sociocultural issues framing experiences of potentially traumatic events. Such experiences may not be framed by refugee patients or clients as an "illness" as such, but rather seen in terms of the events' social, moral, and political meanings. It is this **cultural framing** which substantially determines processes of healing and recovery, responses to therapy and the risk of psychopathology developing. Ignoring these different cultural framings may lead to a patient or client feeling discriminated against, misunderstood, or simply not believed—interfering with trust and disclosure.

Temporality

A sociocultural approach allows us to.

> grasp the dynamics of interactions between resilience, psychological damage, context and time. These interactions are nonlinear, and contingently result in development of psychopathological phenomena when reaching a threshold during a process of accumulating potentially traumatic experiences over a survivors' lifetime (Drožđek et al., 2020, p. 1).

What is highlighted in the approach is the **nonlinear** nature of the unfolding of experience. A sociocultural approach allows us to view the **dynamic and bi-directional** relationship between the sociocultural context and the individual's internal, subjective experience of potentially traumatic events. As noted in the above quote, Drožđek argues that "in order to understand the complexity of this relationship, one should be guided by a string of causation principles and grasp the logic of fluctuation of psychopathology over survivor's life trajectory" (p. 2–3). His model (p. 5) highlights this ever-changing dynamic over time, notably the influence of risk and protective factors within the sociocultural environment having an impact on the trajectory of an individual's mental health. It highlights the roles of potential risk factors as well as potential protective resources, across time and across different scales (for example, the level of the individual, the level of close friends and family, to the macro level of the socio-political environment). In other words, at each stage/age of the individual, there are various risk and protective factors at play at different levels:

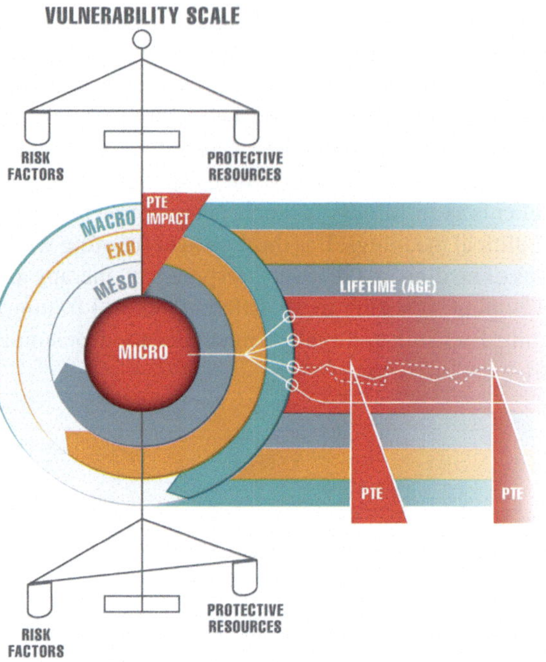

	VULNERA-BILITY	ONGOING STRES	COPING	RESOURCES
1) RESILIENT	LOW	-	ADAPTIVE	+
2) RECOVERING	LOW	-	ADAPTIVE	+
3) DELAYED	MEDIUM	+	MALADAPTIVE	-
4) CHRONIC/ COMPLEX	HIGH	+	MALADAPTIVE	-

In exploring the individual trajectories of refugees impacted by potentially traumatic events, the results of the work similarly highlight the changing impact of the sociocultural environment (including risk and protective factors) in dynamic interaction with individual mental health, as represented in the above model. This calls into question assumptions of a linear trajectory from the experiencing of potentially traumatic events, to the experiencing of post-traumatic symptoms, to healing and recovery:

> Assumptions about trajectories of actions toward presumed progress also implicate temporality, as in the term 'resilience in war' implying that 'war' is a temporary interruption and people can/must recover from such interruptions. When people narrate specific times, they interact with historical time, thereby using time to create meaningful connections of contemporary plights and dreams with events over a broader span of time, place, and consequence. (Daiute & Gómez, 2014, p. 159).

Mental health clinicians need to pay attention to these aspects related to **temporality.** The implications are twofold: firstly, in terms of the nonlinear fluctuation in subjective experiences of potentially traumatic events as noted above, but secondly in understanding the importance of reconstructing a subjectively meaningful temporality within the therapeutic process. For many refugees participating in this research, a significant part of their process of healing and recovery involved the re-establishing of a meaningful "linearity." In line with the above quote, they indeed "create[d] meaningful connections of contemporary plights and dreams with events over a broader span of time, place, and consequence."

Part of mediating potentially traumatic events is, through processes of linguistic elaboration, allowing memories of potentially traumatic events to be placed within a meaningful temporal order; in other words, placed alongside other memories of the past so as not to haunt the present, or the (imagined) future. As Daiute and Gomez (2014) have demonstrated among two of their Colombian research participants, Don Paz and Feniks,

> Don Paz's orientation to the past and Feniks's orientation to the future interact with the physical and symbolic temporalities limiting their lives and holding possible alternatives. While there's no perfect past for Don Paz nor an open future for Feniks, using time to imagine options is an important step. (p. 172).

The authors note that "when people narrate specific times, they interact with historical time, thereby using time to create meaning in relation to contemporary plights and dreams" (p. 163). They show "how people use the cultural tool of imagined time to analyse their circumstances critically and eventually manage those circumstances" (p. 168). Drawing on the work of Ricoeur (1984), they point to how memories, including those of potentially traumatic events, are never set. Rather, the memory of any specific event can differ or appear different depending on the circumstances of recall and sharing. When refugees narrate their experiences of potentially traumatic events, there's inevitably a "present of past things" (Ricoeur, 1984, p. 9). There is similarly a "present of present things" (Ricoeur, 1984, p. 9), the anchoring perspective of narrating time which expresses the narrative purpose and which is intricately related to the unfolding relationship between refugee and mental health clinician, as well as a "present of future things" (Ricoeur, 1984, p. 9). This projection into the future, they note, is imagined and fluid:

> Considering the diverse meaning of explicit and implicit temporality in terms of the context raises implicit questions to guide investigations about how diverse narrators use time to make sense of situations, considering collective goals, and creating narratives of action (p. 167).

In the case studies explored in **chapter seven,** this imagination of possible futures was connected to hope. For many refugees, points of recovery and subsequent growth were inextricably linked to being able to imagine new possible futures. They were also connected to an individual's ability to "question the inevitability of a certain future narrative" (Daiute & Gómez, 2014, p. 166). These possibilities of imagining and creating new futures formed part and parcel of their power to act—integral to processes of healing and recovery from the experience of potentially traumatic events. In the act of imagining the future, in other words through constructing narratives within hypothetical time, individuals "build on [their] own story to create a turning point expressing the awful realities of a suspended life, very possibly with no future" (Daiute & Gómez, 2014, p. 171).

Here, I again return to the point noted above: the experiences of potentially traumatic events are **nonlinear.** While the reconstruction of a meaningful temporality, through semiotic mediation, is integral to processes of healing and recovery from such events, clinicians need to be aware that this is a complex and dynamic process. In analysing Jules' trajectory in **chapter seven,** article five presents a "loop model" of his possibility to imagine. Imagination in this article is conceptualised as a process which creates "loops" out of the present, here-and-now of experiences connected to the material reality of the current environment. The process is seen as being triggered by some disrupting event, which generates a disjunction from the person's unfolding experience of the "real" world, and as unfolding as a loop, which eventually comes back to the current, actual experience (Zittoun & Cerchia, 2013). In concluding this book, and reflecting upon the implications for mental health clinicians, I would like to revisit this conceptualisation. The loop model presented a linear concept of Jules' trajectory. It may not go far enough in capturing nonlinearity. It risks "retain[ing] a monocultural vision of linear time, in contrast to less formal unofficial perspectives occurring in everyday life of communities, and emerging movements" (Daiute & Gómez, 2014, p. 172). The reality is far messier than the model could suggest. Experiencing potentially traumatic events may disrupt a coherent sense of linearity. It may break any subjectively meaningful sense of temporality. Clinicians need to be prepared to meet this "temporal chaos."

One way in which clinicians may pay attention to, and work with, such aspects related to **temporality** is to track nonlinearity within the narrative activity of their refugee clients or patients. Pay attention to the words of the individual in the consulting room:

> The varied use of tense markers [...] and the use of subjunctive in particular provide rich analyses of narrative time. Diverse verbal time markings interact with expected truth and imagination. All narrative time is symbolic, but past and present time markings imply actual experience, while the range of future, conditional, and possible time markings are more clearly imagined times. Narrated past events appear fixed and true because they are reported as having happened. Future, conditional, and hypothetical events have not occurred, so they are imagined, although often overlooked as such. Present tenses appear fixed in another way, often expressing the position of the narrator. The result of this interplay of time settings is the highlighting of meaning in the narrator's imagined time (Daiute & Gómez, 2014, p. 170).

Considering aspects of temporality in narrative activity, and the relationship to the experiencing of potentially traumatic events, is particularly relevant for those refugees still waiting on a decision from the asylum tribunal. Many of the individuals who participated in the research waited months, if not years, for a response from the asylum tribunal. They remained held captive by the potentially traumatic events they had experienced in the past. They reported feeling stuck in time. If the experience of potentially traumatic events is understood as a radical disconnect from a meaningful past, present, and future; lengthy asylum delays function as an external mirror to this internal experience. I refer to the moving account of refugeehood provided by Clementine Wamariya (2018) upon arrival in her host country,

> Time, once again, refused to move in an orderly fashion; the pages of the book lay scattered, unbound. This still happens to me. My life does not feel logical, sequential, or inevitable. There's no sense of action, reaction; no consequence, repercussion; no **plot** (p. 33)

Using language as a cultural tool, the role of the mental health clinician is therefore to assist individuals in constructing and reconstructing meaningful **plots** to their lives. A sociocultural exploration has allowed us to explore how this narrative activity serves to re-establish a meaningful linearity between the experience of potentially traumatic experiences of the past, the present, and hopes for the future.

The Permeable Self

In exploring the impact of the cultural framework on experiences of potentially traumatic events among refugee clients or patients, one key element for consideration is the various ways in which the cultural framework determines the border or boundary of "self" and "Other." As Tang (2007) notes: "cultures differ regarding their dominant ideas about the ontology of self as well as relationship between self and others, between self and the universe, and between life and death" (p. 129). In **chapter eight,** the case of Mr B is given as an example of a research participant who doesn't experience himself so much as an individual but more as having a "family self" based on relational models. The analysis highlights how he frames his experiences of potentially traumatic events within the intersubjective realm of his family network—similar to the South Sudanese research participants presented by Tankink and Richers (2007). Here, it is worth considering that refugee patients or clients from cultural contexts which are more collectivist in orientation may have different degrees of permeability of ego boundaries—in other words, the boundaries between "self" and "Other" may be conceptualised as being more extensive, flexible, or permeable. In clinical practice, this perspective can guide us to a deeper understanding of resilience, healing, and recovery based not only on internal psychology or biological processes but also equally on social-interactional processes. The implications would be to integrate the knowledge of the individual's life-world, their family, and community as the site of both challenges and resources with which to cope, adapt, heal, and recover.

Universality of Experience

Exploring mental health clinicians' work with diverse refugee populations raises questions surrounding the universality of experiences of potentially traumatic events. What is culturally determined and what is universal? It must further be noted that clinicians working with refugee communities face very concrete linguistic barriers. Not only may they be working with translators among populations who don't speak their language—they may be working with individuals for whom there simply are no words for "trauma" or "stress" in their language at all. What are the implications for mediating the experiences of potentially traumatic events in such an instance?

In exploring the exchange between mental health clinicians and refugee victims of torture—as in the case of Brigitte seen in **chapter five**—what strikes me is the way in which symptoms align with those appearing in the definition of PTSD found in the D.S.M. V (APA, 2013). However, despite the universal symptoms (in this particular example, experiencing nightmares), the way in which she understands these symptoms are culturally informed. Language plays a key role in mediating this sense making process—in connecting Brigitte's cultural environment (in this case, African traditional spirituality—a worldview wherein ancestors who have passed away may still cast spells on the living) to the way in which she makes sense of and experiences these symptoms. It also fundamentally frames her process of recovery and post-traumatic growth. Believing the nightmares to indicate her ancestor's continual displeasure with her actions, she continues to feel guilty—a feeling that impedes her own sense of Self, and her plans for the future.

The results of this research may lead us to consider that, while many of the experiences of potentially traumatic events remain universal, including symptoms indicated in the definition of PTSD, the way in which they are framed is culturally determined. It is this cultural framing which mental health clinicians need to pay attention to, as they accompany their refugee clients or patients in their narrative activity. As noted by Kirmayer (2019),

> Beyond engaging with local contexts, attention to culture can advance social psychiatry by revealing both commonalities and variations in the experience and expression of mental disorders. In addition to improving the validity of clinical assessment and the appropriateness of interventions, cross-cultural comparative methods can identify new strategies for adaptation and recovery rooted in local traditions but potentially translatable and transportable to new contexts. (p. 31).

Here, Kirmayer refers to the need to "improve the validity" of clinical assessment—not to stop the activity altogether. Despite cultural variations in experiences of potentially traumatic events, he notes that we need to pay attention to "both **commonalities** and variations in the experience and expression of mental disorders" (my emphasis). Elsewhere, he and colleagues have noted that "understanding suffering in context may also challenge common assumptions about what we assume to be culturally different, but **emerges as similar** across contexts" (Bemme & Kirmayer, 2020, p. 12) (my emphasis). We are all human beings, and much of our experience as human beings is universal. It is therefore worth reflecting on many of the benefits of a PTSD diagnosis for refugee patients or clients. For many, there may be a sense of relief in having one's experience understood. In other words, PTSD as a cultural tool may provide individuals with a framework in which their experiences may be made sense of. I remember discussing symptoms of PTSD with a South Sudanese woman who exclaimed with incredulity "but how can you, as a white woman, know that this is what is happening to me?!" It's possible that at that moment that she had felt seen and understood, that she had been provided with words to explain the "wordless nothing." Such a framing of her experiences meant that she was neither alone, nor crazy. What she had been experiencing was a "normal" reaction to potentially traumatic events.

The construct of PTSD may have some universal applicability, but the focus should be widened to recognize the multiple biosocial, cultural, and political processes that are essential aspects of experiencing potentially traumatic events—as well as resilience and recovery. The experience of these events and related suffering is both personally and socially value-laden:

> The dilemma with the current emphasis on PTSD therefore, is that although the diagnosis may capture a universal pattern of fear conditioning, anxiety, and avoidance behavior, this pattern is only a limited aspect of the range of clinical problems that can be directly related to trauma exposure. Other dimensions of trauma experience have social and cultural meanings and dynamics requiring comparable clinical attention. (Kirmayer et al., 2011, p. 5).

We need to see "beyond the PTSD paradigm" (Drožđek et al., 2020, p. 2), but not disregard it altogether. A key message to be borne in mind is adequately summarized by experts in the *Lancet* commission for global mental health:

> Mental health problems exist along a continuum from mild, time-limited distress to chronic, progressive, and severely disabling conditions. The binary approach to diagnosing mental disorders, although useful for clinical practice, does not accurately reflect the diversity and complexity of mental health needs of individuals or populations. (Patel et al., 2018, p. 1).

As disease models broaden and care practices become collaboratively stepped, shifted and shared among self, family and friends, community leaders, and medical providers—new conceptual and relational issues arise (Patel et al., 2018). A sociocultural framework allows us to understand the importance not only of a specific Other (for example, a psychotherapist) in this process of recovery and post-traumatic growth, but indeed the role of the entire sociocultural context as influencing the development of the individual. Narrative use integrates the individual with society (Daiute et al., 2015). In the following section, I therefore explore some implications for mental health and psychosocial (MHPSS) interventions within humanitarian contexts more generally.

Implications for Mental Health and Psychosocial (MHPSS) Interventions in Humanitarian Settings

Increasing awareness of the substantially elevated mental health and psychosocial needs of refugee populations has led to focused interventions for mental health and psychosocial support (MHPSS) for these groups. However, despite growing attention to MHPSS for emergency-displaced populations, there are still major gaps in programming and support. To foster social integration and improve post-traumatic recovery, it is crucial to better understand and address the specific needs of this highly vulnerable population (Schick et al., 2016). In light of the high prevalence of PTSD symptomatology and given the low uptake of mental care among resettled refugees noted in the literature (Schouler-Ocak et al., 2016; Slewa-Younan et al., 2017), interventions need to consider the myriad of complex and inter-related factors influencing refugee experiences of potentially traumatic events. Such a framework would "connect the risk and protective factors in the material and social conditions of refugees' post-migration lives to broader social, economic, and political factors" (Hynie, 2018, p. 297). Furthermore, to ensure that psychosocial and mental health needs are met, MHPSS should be integrated as part of a continuum of care that is multi-layered. MHPSS is not the domain of one sector. It needs to be realised through coordinated and complementary actions of a multitude of actors within legal and medical activity systems (Faregh et al., 2019).

I base the following recommendations on a review of the literature, current trends in MHPSS interventions within humanitarian settings, and on the implications of the empirical results of this research:

A Community-Based Response

Trauma is a social as well as an individual phenomenon (Daiute, 2016). The sociocultural context in which we live and the quality of relationships we have are central to our mental wellbeing and contribute to risks of developing mental health problems. This is also true in terms of the social context within humanitarian crises. Furthermore, the contexts, roles, values, and demands produced by cultural communities may be a source of disadvantage, structural violence, and suffering as well as providing opportunities for adaptation, healing, and recovery (Kirmayer, 2018). Sociocultural dynamics are therefore integral to trauma trajectories as both a potential source of trauma as well as a source of healing and recovery. Here, I once more refer to results of the research which highlight the important sociocultural resources which participants drew upon to make sense of potentially traumatic events, to recover from these experiences, and, ultimately, to thrive. In the case of Jules explored in **chapter seven,** for example, it was the fact of remembering his father's wisdom pertaining to times of hardship, making friends at church, falling in love, and creating plans for the future with family members in France, that facilitated healing.

The focus on the individual in the modern mental health field tends to underemphasise the importance of social and structural drivers of wellbeing and illness. This calls for strengths and resilience-based approaches to interventions and supports that not only respond to problems, deficits, and prevalence of mental health conditions, but also build on existing strengths and resources within affected communities. We especially need to recognise the role that non-specialists and community members can play. In summary, we need an approach that recognises the sociocultural context of mental health—a perspective that goes beyond a purely individualistic view of treatment and recovery. Rather, as noted by Daiute (2016), focusing on social relations in humanitarian contexts involves building in individual capacities, interactions in communities, and the human right to continue developing these capacities:

> By extending beyond the individual to the individual-in-collective, we [can address] the tensions not only in terms of individual [...] voices, but also in terms of interacting shared narratives, diverse goals and opportunities within and across each context (p. 132).

This social justice approach, Daiute notes, emphasizes what needs to be done, whereas a trauma approach focuses what has been done. At the levels of public health and policy, a sociocultural perspective on trauma necessitates that we consider the powerful effects of structural violence, migration policies, and social inequality as determinants of health. This involves a recognition that social systems have their own dynamics which can amplify experiences of potentially traumatic events or conversely provide sources of collective resilience (Kirmayer, 2019). Any such community-based response should further heed the mediating influence on language in individual and communal experiences of potentially traumatic events and subsequent recovery. This includes, for example, focussing on and facilitating **collective narrative practices** organizing group activities, a dynamic and potentially transforming process allowing members to create solidarity, to reflect critically, and to imagine life in their own way:

> just as narrative has been created by humans to interact, to solve problems, and to change culture over many civilizations, people across circumstances, including those in the least privileged and powerless situations, use narrating to interpret, to debate, to act, and sometimes to transform extremely challenging and tragic life circumstances (Daiute & Gómez, 2014, p. 157).

A Culturally Relevant Response

We need to situate experiences of potentially traumatic events in sociocultural context. Lack of attention to cultural context on the part of providers and decision-makers can lead to mistrust of mental health information and services and reduce motivation to engage with mental healthcare or adhere to treatment (Faregh et al., 2019). Exploring the influence of culture on experiences of potentially traumatic events among refugee populations—both related to their original and current sociocultural context—should be a fundamental consideration in the clinical assessment of this population, as well as the design and delivery of mental health interventions (Hassan et al., 2015; Kirmayer et al., 2018).

Such attention to culture and context in MHPSS interventions could include, for example, attempts to refine diagnostic criteria (finding the right level of generality and specification to work across cultures), the identification of new diagnostic variants, and the inclusion of more contextual assessments (Kirmayer, 2018). Much headway has been made in this regard over recent years. In the most recent version of the D.S.M. (APA, 2013) the term "cultural concepts of distress" has replaced the outdated terminology of culture-bound syndromes—a change intended to signal a broader, more inclusive understanding of culturally specific distress as something that changes over time and does not represent place-specific "exotica" (Kaiser & Jo Weaver, 2019). It should be noted that integrating culture in mental health services and systems is not just an issue for groups that face specific inequities related to their identity and social position but is central to person-centred healthcare for all. Indeed, the sociocultural perspective adopted throughout this book rejects any static or reified notion of "the cultural other ... but with recognition of the developmental, social and political facts of our cultural being" (Kirmayer & Jarvis, 2019, p. 18).

A Longitudinal, Contextually Situated Response

Exposure to ongoing stress in an instable environment, together with individual vulnerabilities, coping styles, and limited availability of protective resources, seems responsible for the maintenance of post-traumatic symptoms over the life trajectory, combined with the decline of resilience by increased intensity or continued exposure to potentially traumatic events (Drožđek et al., 2020). Mental health and psychosocial support (MHPSS) needs do not remain static over time. They shift and change in response to both the external environment and an individual's inner resources. This requires a wide range of supports to be offered in the response, based on individual or community needs, and at different stages of a crisis. Long-term, flexible approaches are needed that take into consideration that the mental health needs of refugees may change over time and that trauma trajectories are inextricably intertwined with the changing sociocultural, political, legal, and economic environment. Briefly put, we need not only to focus on "trauma" from an individual, clinical perspective. We need to understand the ways in which it is inherently connected to the macro level of immigration policies affecting migration trajectories over time: delayed asylum trials, unemployment, constantly changing accommodation arrangements, prolonged detention… these factors do not simply "add to" existing experiences of potentially traumatic events, they multiply and compound it through the constantly reinforcing effect of feedback loops—as shown in the case of Dilraj in **chapter two** (Womersley & Kloetzer, 2018b). What is needed is a "processual reconceptualization of wellbeing and distress" (Kidron et al., 2019, p. 28).

A Depathologizing Response

Diagnosing someone with PTSD does something in the world. A sociocultural approach to understanding experiences of potentially traumatic events among refugees, as adopted in this book, includes considering the concrete legal, political, and social implications of the use of cultural tools, such as medical diagnoses, on the individual. As succinctly summarized by Kirmayer (2018):

> epistemic practices, including medical diagnosis and treatment, serve to bring particular configurations of distress into being by shaping individuals' experience and expressions of distress in ways that then receive confirmation through medical attention and intervention. This social response then stabilizes the disease or disorder as a discrete entity and can increase its prevalence (p. 3).

He notes that calling something a "mental disorder" depends on a series of distinctions: a normative distinction between illness and affliction versus health and wellness; an ontological distinction between afflictions that are bodily, spiritual, or sociomoral and those that.

are specifically mental; and a pragmatic distinction that ascribes the problem to the domain of psychiatry as a discipline, profession, and social institution. A detailed understanding of the cultural construction and consequences of mental disorders, he continues, therefore requires consideration of the institutional apparatus and circuits of power and knowledge that co-constitute forms of suffering and their treatment. He and colleagues have therefore called for "culture-specific etiology, symptomatology, treatment approaches, and outcomes which diverge from biomedical taxonomies and illness constructs" (Kidron et al., 2019, p. 1).

This is not to say that the diagnosis of PTSD should be gotten rid of entirely. To the contrary, the diagnosis does have concrete ramifications for the daily life of the individual which may be to their benefit: not only for their personal psychological rehabilitation in terms of making sense of potentially traumatic events, symptoms and post-traumatic recovery, but also in terms of the political, legal, and social impact of the diagnosis. For many participants, the diagnosis was a validation of their suffering. It offered an important means of social recognition. Research by Kidron and colleagues (2019) among Holocaust descendants, for example, reveals how the "emotive scar" left by exposure to potentially traumatic events was seen by respondents as a culturally valorised form of commemorative remembering and worn as an empowering badge of honour. It is, however, necessary to stress the importance of considering PTSD as a particular cultural tool, within a particular sociocultural environment, understood and used differently by various actors. A sociocultural perspective insists upon the ethical responsibility to consider this concrete impact. This includes paying attention to how and why we diagnose PTSD.

These recommendations are in line with the recent Lancet commission on global mental health and sustainable development (Patel et al., 2018). The commission stresses the fact that psychiatric diagnoses can lead to unhelpful labelling that often oversimplifies and undervalues the complexities of personal circumstances. Moreover, labels can be stigmatizing, and the impact of stigma is often even more burdensome than the symptoms that have led to the diagnosis themselves. Importantly, the commission highlights the need for MHPSS interventions to be based on socioculturally informed narratives of trauma. As an alternative to the categorical diagnostic model, the Lancet commission proposed a staging model, which recognizes opportunities for intervention at all stages of the pathway from well-being to different stages of disorder. In other words, it recommends a rejection of the mental illness-health dichotomy in favour of conceptualising mental health as existing along a continuum and dynamically changing over time. In other words, it rejects the "deficit" narrative inherent to a pathologising framing of experiences of potentially traumatic events, in favour of a concept considering both "wounds and wellness."

A Resiliency-Based, Forward-Looking Response

Given the potentially traumatic impact of forced displacement, as made evident in the research results, the possibility of healing and growth may seem small in comparison. However, the results also attest to the fact that human beings may be quite capable of restoring their identities and (re)finding their place in the world when given the chance to do so. The results highlight the multiple ways in which refugees may show resilience in the face of exposure to potentially traumatic events. They point to ways that resilience and vulnerability may interact, qualifying one another in the process of meaning making. In other words, they reveal the ways that refugee experiences of potentially traumatic events are embedded in complex networks of personal and collective meaning that may give rise to both resilience and vulnerability. Here, the notion of "resilience" is not a reified psychological state, that can be captured by yet another global measure of health and illness but rather "a hermeneutic process of meaning making that shapes the way that selves and communities experience and respond to distress in order to restore or enhance culturally valorized forms of well-being" (Kidron et al., 2019, p. 30). **Resilience** is thus understand from a sociocultural perspective as the capacity of a system to adapt successfully to the challenges that threaten system function, survival, or development. From this perspective, resilience is dynamic. It changes as the capacity for adaptation is distributed across systems. It further depends on the resilience of other systems (Masten, 2014a, b).

This concurrent experience of resilience and vulnerability challenges some key assumptions of "traumatised refugee" narrative. Contrary to the inhuman Narrative of a psychiatric diagnosis, human narratives are "dynamic, subjective, and imaginative of survival, justice, and thriving." (Daiute & Gómez, 2014, p. 157). Refugees are active agents engaging in the new world in which they find themselves. They are not only patients, victims, seekers of asylum. They are dreamers, planners and doers, family members and friends, with hope for the future. They "interpret their circumstances, interlocutors, and options for making lives in this shifting world order" (Daiute et al., 2020, p. 2). This response involves helping refugees make meaning of their experience, focusing on their strengths, as well as fostering an environment where they are able to meet their basic needs. In a very powerful TED Talk, Luma Mufleh (2017), the founder of a refugee youth program and herself an asylum seeker from the Middle East stated, "Don't feel sorry for them, believe in them." So too must we consider experiences of forced migration from a trauma-informed lens, recognizing the unimaginable difficulties refugees have suffered as well as their strengths, resiliency, and capacity for hope (Ringler-Jayanthan *et. al.,* 2020, p. 82). It is as important to consider resilience and wellbeing within local worlds as it is to consider distress (Kaiser & Jo Weaver, 2019), to recognize the strong sense of connection to places left behind while at the same time recognizing the possibilities of a constructive (re)building of connections to people and place (Sampson & Gifford, 2010).

Returning for a brief moment to the theoretical framework of sociocultural psychology informing this work, Dafermos (2015) notes that Vygotsky himself developed a theory that opens up new perspectives for the rethinking and overcoming of a crisis. In contrast to dominant psychological theories that describe the actual developmental level and presents forms of human being, the approach illuminates prospective human development. In other words, rather than seeing someone as "traumatised" (static, present), we need to respect and value their potential for growth and development (dynamic, future orientated). Challenging the concept of adaptation, Dafermos notes how Vygotsky proposed the idea of creative, future oriented activity, that "…makes the human being a creature oriented toward the future, creating the future and thus altering his own present" (Dafermos, 2015, p. 21). Elsewhere, Dafermos (2018) similarly reflects on the link between "crisis" and "creativity" within a sociocultural perspective. Here, he demonstrates how Vygotsky's theory was developed as an attempt at the conceptualization of crucial issues associated with human development that emerged within the process of societal change: "the future focus, the orientation to what might happen rather than what has already happened constitutes a significant dimension of the human creative agency" (p. 233). Striving to overcome crises, Dafarmos argues, people can develop an active, creative, socially oriented activity. While drawing on the idea that individuals' narrative activity always occurs in social relations, a sociocultural perspective allows us to shift from the assumption that powerful actors impose values on less powerful actors (in this case, refugee victims of torture) to an acknowledgment that people in vulnerable positions can act strategically (Daiute et al., 2020).

A resiliency-based intervention from a sociocultural perspective, therefore, should aim to:

- Foster prosocial bonds at every level
- Integrate systems of care
- Provide opportunities for development
- Support culturally based ceremonies fostering resilience
- Support community engagement and collective action.

As we "move away from a categorical biomedical model toward dimensional and transdiagnostic approaches" (Bemme & Kirmayer, 2020, p. 3), we should similarly aim to develop more viable, clinically relevant tools for refugee populations, as well as contribute to a more critical, decentered literature on mental health and illness (Kaiser & Jo Weaver, 2019). This includes a focus on the broader structures or forces that are being contested, whether implicitly or explicitly, through the often-conflicting ways in which "trauma" among refugees is understood. In the ways in which we understand and (re)present narratives of refugee trauma, we must be careful to avoid presenting distress as reflecting solely individual psychopathology or equitably distributed distress. This is essential to avoid victim-blaming through a myopic exploration of only immediate causes of distress (Kaiser & Jo Weaver, 2019). Nowhere is this more relevant than in the context of the current humanitarian crisis of forced displacement.

We need to beware of "priorities and practices [which] amount to a neo-colonial imposition of Western knowledge that threatens traditional and indigenous forms of care and healing" (Bemme & Kirmayer, 2020) p. 4). Furthermore, as argued by Daiute (2017), "defining the problem in individual bodies of those labelled 'refugees' averts the analytic gaze from the broader problem, while a focus on 'refuge' shifts our gaze to the politics of displacement." (p. 12). In other words:

> Issues such as poverty, war, oppression, racism, violence, poor education, unemployment, lack of housing, or other forms of structural violence, critics have argued, may be at risk of being further obscured when distress is reconfigured into a psychiatric condition and only addressed downstream (Bemme & Kirmayer, 2020, p. 11).

Attention to the social and the structural are key means of avoiding these pitfalls. This necessitates a "move away from models dominated by implicit colonial hierarchies, racialized identities, and reified notions of culture as homeostatic or steady-state systems, toward "postcolonial" models of cultures as open, dynamic, heterogeneous, and hybrid social systems that offer individuals resources for self-fashioning and positioning." (Kirmayer, 2018, p. 9). Furthermore, future work should continue to clarify the mechanisms by which societal tensions and dilemmas are transmuted into individual experiences of potentially traumatic experiences as well as resilience, including the extent to which individuals' or families' engagement with narratives of trauma and resilience helps them manage their social predicaments (Lewis-Fernández & Kirmayer, 2019).

My final hope is that this book has gone some small way in providing.

> a rightful encouragement for clinicians and practitioners to consider the ways in which the implicit and explicit models from which we operate impact our understanding of refugees and limit the ways their stories are told, but also [a] springboard through which we learn to truly hear the stories of refugees as those of hope and resilience. That is to say, the way that we hear stories, the level at which we allow ourselves to be truly moved by them and the way that we choose to respond to them moreover, and the things on which we choose to focus are ultimately directly correlated with healing and restoration in those refugees whom we serve. (Neace 2020, p. 16).

References

American Psychiatric Association. (2013). *Diagnostic and statistical manual of mental disorders* (5th ed.). Arlington, VA: American Psychiatric Association.

Aroche, J., & Coello, M. J. (2004). Ethnocultural considerations in the treatment of refugees and asylum seekers. In J. Wilson & B. Drožđek (Eds.), *Broken spirits: The treatment of traumatized asylum seekers, refugees, war and torture victims* (pp. 53–80). New York, NY: Brunner-Routledge.

Bakhtin, M. (1978). *Esthétique et théorie du roman [traduit du russe par Daria Olivier, préface de Michel Aucouturier].* Paris, France: Gallimard.

Bakhtin, M. (1981). *The dialogic imagination (translated by Caryl Emerson and Michael Holquist).* Austin, TX: University of Texas Press.

Bakhtin, M. (1986). The Bildungsroman and its significance in the history of realism. In C. Emerson & M. Holquist (Eds.), *Speech genres and other late essays* (p. 21). Austin, TX: University of Texas Press.

Bélanger-Dumontier, G., & Vachon, M. Review of Refuge and resilience: Promoting resilience and mental health among resettled refugees and forced migrants. *Transcultural Psychiatry, 52,* 274-275.

Bemme, D., & Kirmayer, L. J. (2020). Global Mental Health: Interdisciplinary challenges for a field in motion. *Transcultural Psychiatry, 57*(1), 3–18.

Bennett, J. (2000). The politics of writing. *Agenda, 16*(46), 3–12.

Clot, Y. (2011). 1. Théorie en clinique de l'activité. In B. Maggi (Ed.), *Interpréter l'agir: un défi théorique* (pp. 17–39). France Presses Universitaires de France.

Clot, Y., & Béguin, P. (2004). L'action située dans le développement de l'activité. *Activités, 1*(1–2).

Clot, Y., & Litim, M. (2008). Activité, santé et collectif de travail. *Pratiques Psychologiques, 14*(1), 101–114.

Dafermos, M. (2015). Reflection on the relationship between cultural-historical theory and dialectics. *J Психологическая Наука И Образование, 20*(3), 16–24.
Dafermos, M. (2018). Developing creativity in science: The case of Vygotsky. In M. Dafermos (Ed.), *Rethinking cultural-historical theory* (pp. 215–242). Singapore: Springer.
Dafermos, M., Triliva, S., & Varvantakis, C. (2017). Youth tubing the Greek crisis: A cultural-historical perspective. In M. Kontopodis, C. Varvantakis, & C. Wulf (Eds.), *Global youth in digital trajectories* (pp. 69–96). London: Routledge.
Daiute, C. (2014). *Narrative inquiry: A dynamic approach.* Los Angeles: Sage Publications.
Daiute, C. (2016). A relational approach to human development research and practice in 21st century violence and displacement. *Journal of Human Development, 59*(2–3), 128–151.
Daiute, C. (2017). Narrating refuge. *Europe's Journal of Psychology, 13*(1), 1–15.
Daiute, C., & Gómez, P. B. (2014). Narrating change in and against time in Colombia. *Representations of war, migration, and refugeehood* (pp. 154–176). New York: Routledge.
Daiute, C., & Lightfoot, C. (2004). *Narrative analysis: Studying the development of individuals in society.* London: Sage.
Daiute, C., & Lucić, L. (2010). Situated cultural development among youth separated by war. *International Journal of Intercultural Relations, 34*(6), 615–628.
Daiute, C., Beykont, Z. F., Higson-Smith, C., & Nucci, L. (2006). *International perspectives on youth conflict and development.* Oxford, U.K.: Oxford University Press.
Daiute, C., Todorova, R. S., & Kovács-Cerović, T. (2015). Narrating participation and power relations in a social inclusion program. *Language Communication, 45,* 46–58.
Daiute, C., Cerovic, T. K., Micic, K., Sullu, B., & Vracar, S. (2020). Dynamic Values Negotiating Geo-Political Narratives Across a Migration System. *Qualitative Psychology,* (In Press).
Dauite, C. (In Press). Imagining in Community Engagement. In T. a. G. Zittoun, Vladimir (Ed.), *Handbook of Imagination and Culture.* Oxford University Press.
Dromer, C., & Grandmaison, C. (2007). Le certificat médical, pièce jointe à la demande d'asile en France. *Mémoire de Master,* University d'Evry, Val d'Essonne, France.
Drožđek, B., Rodenburg, J., & Moyene-Jansen, A. (2020). "Hidden" and diverse long-term impacts of exposure to war and violence. *Frontiers in Psychiatry, 10*(975), 1–12.
Faregh, N., Lencucha, R., Ventevogel, P., Dubale, B. W., & Kirmayer, L. J. (2019). Considering culture, context and community in mhGAP implementation and training: Challenges and recommendations from the field. *International Journal of Mental Health Systems, 13*(1), 1–13.
Fox, M. (2002). Finding a way through: From mindlessness to minding. In R. K. Papadopoulos (Ed.), *Therapeutic care for refugees: No place like home* (pp. 103–120). London: Karnac Books.
Garland, C. (2002). *Understanding trauma: A psychoanalytical approach.* Karnac Books.
IASC. (2014). *Inter-Agency Standing Committee (IASC) reference group for mental health and psychosocial support in emergency settings: Recommendations for conducting ethical mental health and psychosocial research in emergency settings.* Geneva: Inter-Agency Standing Committee.
Gilbert, P. (1997). The evolution of social attractiveness and its role in shame, humiliation, guilt and therapy. *British Journal of Medical Psychology, 70*(2), 113–147.
Gilbert, P., & Andrews, B. (1998). *Shame: Interpersonal behavior, psychopathology, and culture.* London: Oxford University Press.
Gilbert, P., & Miles, J. (2014). *Body shame: Conceptualisation, research and treatment.* London: Routledge.
Glăveanu, V. P., Karwowski, M., Jankowska, D. M., & de Saint Laurent, C. (2018). Creative imagination. In T. Zittoun & V. P. Glăveanu (Eds.), *Handbook of imagination and culture* (pp. 1–39). New York, NY: Oxford University Press.
Harré, R. (1986). *The social construction of emotions.* Oxford: Basil Blackwell.
Hassan, G., Kirmayer, L. J., Mekki-Berrada, A., Quosh, C., El Chammay, R., Deville-Stoetzel, J., & Coutts, A. (2015). *Culture, context and the mental health and psychosocial wellbeing of Syrians: a review for mental health and psychosocial support staff working with Syrians affected by armed conflict* (pp. 14–15). Geneva: UNHCR.

Honwana, A. (2006). Child soldiers: Community Healing and rituals in Mozambique and Angola. In C. Daiute, Z. Beykont, C. Higson-Smith, & L. Nucci (Eds.), *International perspectives on youth conflict and development* (pp. 225–244). Oxford, U.K.: Oxford University Press.

Horney, K. (1991). *Neurosis and human growth: The struggle toward self-realization*. New York, NY: WW Norton & Company.

Hviid, P. (2008). "Next year we are small, right?" Different times in children's development. *European Journal of Psychology of Education, 23*(2), 183.

Hynie, M. (2018). The social determinants of refugee mental health in the post-migration context: A critical review. *The Canadian Journal of Psychiatry, 63*(5), 297–303.

Kadianaki, I., & Zittoun, T. (2014). Catalysts and regulators of psychological change in the context of immigration ruptures. In K. R. Cabell & J. Valsiner (Eds.), *The Catalyzing Mind* (pp. 191–207). New York, NY: Springer.

Kaiser, B. N., & Jo Weaver, L. (2019). Culture-bound syndromes, idioms of distress, and cultural concepts of distress: New directions for an old concept in psychological anthropology. *Transcultural Psychiatry, 56*(4), 589–598.

Kidron, C. A., Kotliar, D. M., & Kirmayer, L. J. (2019). Transmitted trauma as badge of honor: Phenomenological accounts of Holocaust descendant resilient vulnerability. *Social Science and Medicine, 239,* 112524.

Kirmayer, L. J. (1996). Landscapes of memory: Trauma, narrative and dissociation. In P. Antze & M. Lambek (Eds.), *Tense past: Cultural essays on memory and trauma* (pp. 173–198). London: Routledge.

Kirmayer, L. J. (2018). Ethno-and Cultural Psychiatry. In H. Callan (Ed.), *The international encyclopedia of anthropology* (pp. 1–11). Hoboken, NJ: Wiley.

Kirmayer, L. J. (2019). Toward an ecosocial psychiatry. *World Social Psychiatry, 1*(1), 30.

Kirmayer, L. J., & Jarvis, G. J. H. (2019). Culturally responsive services as a path to equity in mental healthcare. *Healthcare Papers, 18*(2), 11–23.

Kirmayer, L. J., Rousseau, C., & Measham, T. (2011). Sociocultural Considerations. In D. M. Benedek & G. H. Wynn (Eds.), *Clinical Manual for the Management of PTSD* (pp. 415–444). Washington, DC: American Psychiatric Press.

Kirmayer, L. J., Ban, L., & Jaranson, J. (2018). Cultural logics of emotion: Implications for understanding torture and its sequelae. *Torture Journal, 28*(1), 84–100.

Kloetzer, L., Clot, Y., & Quillerou-Grivot, E. (2015). Stimulating dialogue at work: The activity clinic approach to learning and development. In L. Filliettaz & S. Billett (Eds.), *Francophone perspectives of learning through work* (pp. 49–70). Springer.

Kvale, S. (1996). *Interviews: An introduction to qualitive research interviewing*. London: Sage.

Laban, C. J. (2015). Resilience-oriented treatment of traumatised asylum seekers and refugees. In M. Schouler-Ocak (Ed.), *Trauma and migration* (pp. 191–208). Cham: Springer.

Larrabee, M. J., Weine, S., & Woolcott, P. (2003). "The wordless nothing": Narratives of trauma and extremity. *Human Studies, 26*(3), 353–382.

Lemma, A., & Levy, S. (2004). *The impact of trauma on the psyche: Internal and external processes*. London: Whurr Publishers.

Lester, R. (2013). Back from the edge of existence: A critical anthropology of trauma. *Transcultural Psychiatry, 50*(5), 753–762.

Lewis-Fernández, R., & Kirmayer, L. J. (2019). Cultural concepts of distress and psychiatric disorders: Understanding symptom experience and expression in context. *Transcultural Psychiatry, 56*(4), 786–803.

Linell, P., & Marková, I. (2013). *Dialogical approaches to trust in communication*. Charlotte, NC: IAP.

Marková, I. (2016). *The dialogical mind: Common sense and ethics*. Cambridge: Cambridge University Press.

Masten, A. S. (2014). Global perspectives on resilience in children and youth. *Child Development, 85*(1), 6–20.

Masten, A. S. (2014). Invited commentary: Resilience and positive youth development frameworks in developmental science. *Youth Adolescence, 43,* 1018–1024.

Meili, I., Heim, E., & Maercker, A. (2018). Culturally shared metaphors expand contemporary concepts of resilience and post-traumatic growth: Contrasting an indigenous Brazilian community and a Swiss rural community. *Medical Humanities, 45*(4), 335–345.

Miller, S. (2013). *The Shame Experience.* London: Routledge.

Morgan, G., Melluish, S., & Welham, A. (2017). Exploring the relationship between postmigratory stressors and mental health for asylum seekers and refused asylum seekers in the UK. *Transcultural Psychiatry, 54*(5–6), 653–674.

Morina, N., Akhtar, A., Barth, J., & Schnyder, U. (2018). Psychiatric disorders in refugees and internally displaced persons after forced displacement: A systematic review. *Frontiers in Psychiatry, 9,* 433.

Murray Yang, M. (2011). Still burning: Self-immolation as photographic protest. *Quarterly Journal of Speech, 97*(1), 1–25.

Neace, R. T., Thaier, C., & Nasir, S. (2020). Understanding Refugees: A Complex Discussion. In J. Kottler, S. Banu, & S. Jani (Eds.), *Handbook of refugee experience: Trauma, resilience, and recovery* (pp. 9–20). California Cognella Academic Publishing: San Diego.

Patel, V., Saxena, S., Lund, C., Thornicroft, G., Baingana, F., Bolton, P., et al. (2018). The Lancet Commission on global mental health and sustainable development. *The Lancet, 392*(10157), 1553–1598.

Posel, D. (2005). The scandal of manhood:'Baby rape'and the politicization of sexual violence in post-apartheid South Africa. *Culture, Health, Sexuality, 7*(3), 239–252.

Ricoeur, P. (1984). *Time and narrative* (Vol. 1). Chicago: University of Chicago Press.

Ringler-Jayanthan, E., Neibich-Gianni, M., Brubaker, D., & Naranjo, F. (2020). Integrating trauma-informed care in providing services for refugees and asylum seekers. In J. Kottler, S. Banu, & S. Jani (Eds.), *Handbook of refugee experience: Trauma, resilience, and recovery* (pp. 82–91). San Diego, California: Cognella.

Salgado, J. (2013). Searching for trust in psychotherapy. In T. P. Linell & I. Markova (Eds.), *Dialogical approaches to trust in communication* (pp. 101–119). Charlotte: IAP.

Sampson, R., & Gifford, S. (2010). Place-making, settlement and well-being: The therapeutic landscapes of recently arrived youth with refugee backgrounds. *Journal of Health and Place, 16*(1), 116–131.

Schick, M., Zumwald, A., Knöpfli, B., Nickerson, A., Bryant, R. A., Schnyder, U., et al. (2016). Challenging future, challenging past: The relationship of social integration and psychological impairment in traumatised refugees. *European Journal of Psychotraumatology, 7*(1), 28057.

Schouler-Ocak, M., Wintrob, R., Moussaoui, D., Villasenor Bayardo, S. J., Zhao, X.-D., & Kastrup, M. C. (2016). Background paper on the needs of migrant, refugee and asylum seeker patients around the globe. *International Journal of Culture and Mental Health, 9*(3), 216–232.

Schouler-Ocak, M., Laban, C. J., Bäärnhielm, S., Kastrup, M. C., Dein, S., & Wintrob, R. (2019). Transcultural psychiatry: Refugee, asylum seeker and immigrant patients over the globe. In A. Javad & K. Fountoulakis (Eds.), *Advances in Psychiatry* (pp. 637–655). Cham: Springer.

Shala, M., Morina, N., Gross, C. S., Maercker, A., & Heim, E. (2020). A point in the Heart: Concepts of emotional distress among Albanian-speaking immigrants in Switzerland. *Culture, Medicine, Psychiatry, 44,* 1–34.

Simich, L., & Andermann, E. (2014). *Refuge and resilience: Promoting resilience and mental health among resettled refugees and forced migrants.* Dordrecht: Springer.

Slewa-Younan, S., Yaser, A., Guajardo, M. G. U., Mannan, H., Smith, C. A., & Mond, J. M. (2017). The mental health and help-seeking behaviour of resettled Afghan refugees in Australia. *International Journal of Mental Health Systems, 11*(1), 49.

Steyn, E., & Steyn, J. (2008). Revictimisation of rape victims by the South African Police Service. *Journal of Acta Criminologica: African Journal of Criminology Victimology, 2008*(Special Edition 1), 41–60.

Stone, J., Carson, A., & Sharpe, M. (2005). Functional symptoms and signs in neurology: Assessment and diagnosis. *Neurosurgery, and Psychiatry, 76*(suppl 1), i2–i12.

Sturm, G., Baubet, T., & Moro, M. R. (2007). Mobilising social and symbolic resources in transcultural therapies with refugees and asylum seekers: The story of Mister Diallo. In B. Drožđek & J. Wilson (Eds.), *Voices of trauma: Treating psychological trauma across cultures* (pp. 211–231). New York: Springer.

Sturm, G., Baubet, T., & Moro, M. R. (2010). Culture, trauma, and subjectivity: The French ethnopsychoanalytic approach. *Traumatology, 16*(4), 27–38.

Sucharov, M. S., Buirski, P., & Kottler, A. (2007). Kafka's window and Kohut's mirror: A dialogic journey to the center of traumatic worlds. In P. Buirski & A. Kottler (Eds.), *New Developments in self psychology practice* (pp. 193–206). Lanham: Jason Aranson.

Tang, C.S.-K. (2007). Culturally relevant meanings and their implications on therapy for traumatic grief: Lessons learned from a Chinese female client and her fortune-teller. In B. Drožđek & J. P. Wilson (Eds.), *Voices of trauma: Treating psychological trauma across cultures* (pp. 127–150). New York: Springer.

Tankink, M., & Richters, A. (2007). Silence as a coping strategy: The case of refugee women in the Netherlands from South-Sudan who experienced sexual violence in the context of war. In B. Drožđek & J. Wilson (Eds.), *Voices of trauma: Treating psychological trauma across cultures* (pp. 191–210). New York: Springer.

Van Der Kolk, B. (2015). *The body keeps the score: Brain, mind, and body in the healing of trauma.* Penguin Books.

Wamariya, C., & Weil, E. (2018). *The girl who smiled beads: a story of war and what comes after.* London, UK: Windmill Books.

Womersley, G., & Kloetzer, L. (2018). This is not paranoia, this is real life": Psychosocial interventions for refugee victims of torture in Athens. *Intervention, 16*(2), 95.

Womersley, G., & Kloetzer, L. (2018). Using cultural-historical theory to explore trauma among refugee populations in Europe. *Cultural-Historical Psychology, 14*(1), 87–97.

Womersley, G., & Kloetzer, L. (2018). Being through Doing: The self-immolation of an asylum seeker in Switzerland. *Frontiers in Psychiatry, 9,* 110.

Womersley, G., Kloetzer, L., Van den Bergh, R., Venables, E., Severy, N., Gkionakis, N., et al. (2018). "My mind is not like before": Psychosocial rehabilitation of victims of torture and other forms of ill-treatment in Athens. *Torture Journal, 28*(2), 72–84.

Yassin, N., Taha, A. A., Ghantous, Z., Atoui, M. M., & Forgione, F. (2018). Evaluating a mental health program for Palestinian refugees in Lebanon. *Journal of Immigrant And Minority Health, 20*(2), 388–398.

Zipfel, S., Pfaltz, M. C., & Schnyder, U. (2019). Refugee mental health concerns all of us! *Frontiers in Psychiatry, 10,* 72.

Zittoun, T. (2014). Three dimensions of dialogical movement. *New Ideas in Psychology, 32,* 99–106.

Zittoun, T., & Cerchia, F. (2013). Imagination as expansion of experience. *Integrative Psychological and Behavioral Science, 47*(3), 305–324.

Correction to: Trauma and Resilience Among Displaced Populations

Correction to:
G. Theisen-Womersley, *Trauma and Resilience Among Displaced Populations*,
https://doi.org/10.1007/978-3-030-67712-1

The original version of this book was inadvertently published without open-access funder information. This has been updated in the book.

The updated version of the book can be found at
https://doi.org/10.1007/978-3-030-67712-1

G. Theisen-Womersley, *Trauma and Resilience Among Displaced Populations*,
https://doi.org/10.1007/978-3-030-67712-1_13

The manufacturer's authorised representative in the EU is Springer
Nature Customer Service Centre GmbH, Europaplatz 3, 69115 Heidelberg,
Germany. If you have any concerns regarding our products, please
contact ProductSafety@springernature.com

Printed and bound by CPI Group (UK) Ltd, Croydon, CR0 4YY
07/10/2026
02229460-0001